SMART NANOTECHNOLOGY WITH APPLICATIONS

SMART NANOTECHNOLOGY WITH APPLICATIONS

Edited by Dr. Cherry Bhargava, Dr. Amit Sachdeva, and
Dr. Pardeep Kumar Sharma

CRC Press
Taylor & Francis Group
Boca Raton London New York

CRC Press is an imprint of the
Taylor & Francis Group, an **informa** business

First edition published 2021
by CRC Press
6000 Broken Sound Parkway NW, Suite 300, Boca Raton, FL 33487-2742

and by CRC Press
2 Park Square, Milton Park, Abingdon, Oxon, OX14 4RN

CRC Press is an imprint of Taylor & Francis Group, LLC

Library of Congress Cataloging-in-Publication Data

ISBN: 978-0-367-56316-5 (hbk)
ISBN: 978-1-003-09753-2 (ebk)

Typeset in Times New Roman
by MPS Limited, Dehradun

Contents

Preface

Nanotechnology is a field of research and innovation concerned with building 'things' – generally, materials and devices – on the scale of atoms and molecules. Nanotechnology is rapidly entering the world of smart materials and taking them to the next level. Smart materials are defined as materials with properties engineered to change in a controlled manner under the influence of external stimuli. Some of the external stimuli are temperature, force, moisture, electric charge, and magnetic fields. The proposed book targets the future of nanotechnology in various next level smart industry and disciplines. Nanoparticles can be designed as smart biosensors for plant disease diagnostics and as delivery vehicles for genetic material, probes, and agrichemicals. In the past decade, reports of nanotechnology in phytopathology have grown exponentially. Smart nanomaterials have been integrated into disease management strategies and diagnostics and as molecular tools.

This book covers the basics of nanotechnology and provides a solid understanding of the subject. Starting from a brush-up of the basic quantum mechanics, MEMS/NEMS, and materials science, the book helps to gradually build up an understanding of the various effects of quantum dots, application of nanotechnology in air space and defense systems, and major smart nanomaterials. From mechanical to medicine, nanotechnology has emerged as a multidisciplinary branch that deals with making things of the size of atoms and molecules. The interest of nanotechnology is increasing, especially in the medical field. It has also triggered the emergence of a new field known as nanomedicine.

The book, *Smart Nanotechnology and Its Applications*, offers an introduction of the increasingly developing and growing smart *nanotechnology* field by highlighting the key fundamentals and the application of smart nanotechnology in real life. The book covers the various physical, chemical, and hybrid methods of nanomaterial synthesis and nanofabrication. This book will act as a superb introduction to nanotechnology and nanoscience for students and those intrigued by the nanoworld and its applications.

Editor Biographies

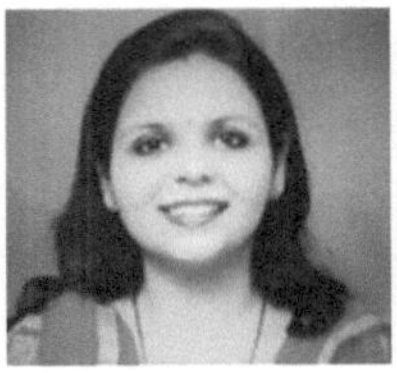

Dr. Cherry Bhargava is working as an Associate Professor and Head, VLSI domain, School of Electrical and Electronics Engineering at Lovely Professional University, Punjab, India. She has more than 15 years of teaching and research experience. She earned her PhD (ECE) from IKG Punjab Technical University, State Govt. University, Punjab, M.Tech (VLSI Design & CAD) from Thapar University, and B. Tech (EIE) from Kurukshetra University. She is GATE qualified with an All India Rank of 428. She has authored about 50 technical research papers in SCI and Scopus indexed quality journals and attended various national/international conferences. She has 16 books to her credit. She has registered two copyrights and filed 21 patents. She is a recipient of various national and international awards for being an outstanding faculty in engineering and an excellent researcher. She is an active reviewer and editorial member of numerous prominent SCI and Scopus indexed journals. Her research area is Nanotechnology and Artificial Intelligence.

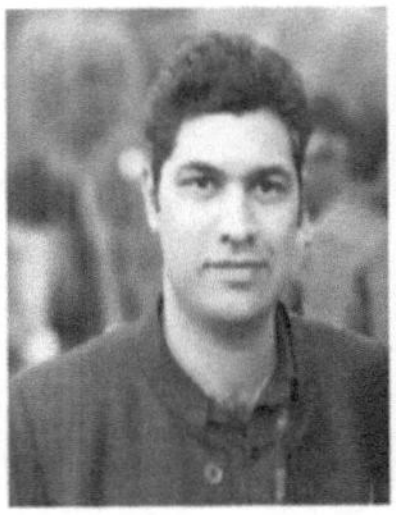

Dr. Pardeep Kumar Sharma is working as an Associate Professor at Lovely Professional University, Punjab, India. He has more than 13 years of teaching experience in the field of Applied Chemistry, Experimental Analysis, Design of Experiments, and Reliability Prediction. He earned his PhD from Lovely Professional University, and has completed his M.Sc. (Applied Chemistry) from Guru Nanak Dev University, Amritsar. He has authored about 20 research papers in SCI and Scopus indexed quality journals and attended various national/ international conferences. He has six books to his credit in the field of nanotechnology and artificial intelligence. He has filed eighteen patents and two copyrights. He is a recipient of various national and international awards. He is an active reviewer of various indexed journals.

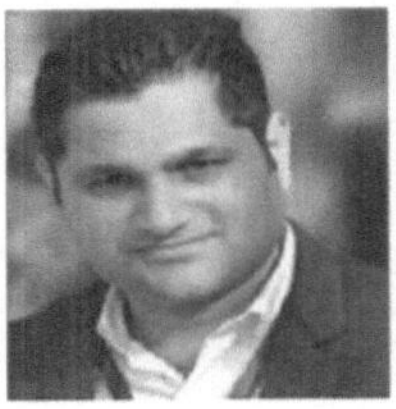

Dr. Amit Sachdeva is working as an Associate Professor at Lovely Professional University, Jalandhar. Punjab, India. He has a teaching experience of more than seven years and his field of specialisation is Material Technology. Dr. Sachdeva has authored around 20 technical research papers in SCI and Scopus indexed quality journals and attended various national/ international conferences. Dr. Sachdeva is also an editorial member of various scientific indexed journals and is a lifetime member of IAENG and IFERP. Dr. Sachdeva has received the Young Scientist Award from University of Malaya, at ICFPAM 2019 organized at Penang Island, Malaysia. He also chaired a session and was also selected as a judge for evaluating poster sessions. He has participated in around 15 international conferences and have also been part of the organising committee in 6 international conferences. Dr. Sachdeva also coordinates all the FDPs along with academia–industry interface incharge of Lovely Professional University.

Contributors

Shivani Arora Abrol
School of Electronics and Electrical Engineering, Lovely Professional University, Punjab, India

Sirajuddin Ahmed
Civil Engineering Department, Jamia Millia Islamia, New Delhi, India

Nitika Anand
Department of Ayurvedic Pharmacy, School of Pharmaceutical Sciences, Lovely Professional University, Punjab, India

Dileep Singh Baghel
Department of Ayurvedic Pharmacy, School of Pharmaceutical Sciences, Lovely Professional University, Punjab, India

Cherry Bhargava
School of Electronics and Electrical Engineering, Lovely Professional University, Punjab, India

Roshan Rajesh Bhatkar
Department of Aerospace Engineering, Amity University, Dubai, UAE

Fazlollah Changani
Department of Environmental Health Engineering, School of Public Health, Tehran University of Medical Sciences, Tehran, Iran

Rekha Chaudhary
School of Electronics and Electrical Engineering, Lovely Professional University, Jalandhar, India

Sachin Chavan
Department of Mechanical Engineering, Bharati Vidyapeeth Deemed to be University College of Engineering, Pune, India

Sudhakar CK
School of Pharmaceutical Sciences, LIT-Pharmacy, Lovely Professional University, Jalandhar, India

Izharul Haq Farooqi
Civil Engineering Department, Aligarh Muslim University, Aligarh, India

Parul Gaur
UIET, Department of Electrical and Electronics Engineering, Punjab University, Chandigarh, India

Ali Asgher Ali Hasan
Department of Aerospace Engineering, Amity University, Dubai, UAE

Chandan Bhogendra Jha
Division of Cyclotron and Radiopharmaceutical Sciences, Institute of Nuclear Medicine and Allied Science, DRDO, New Delhi, India

Iqbaljit Kaur
Department of Ayurvedic Pharmacy, School of Pharmaceutical Sciences, Lovely Professional University, Punjab, India

Simranjeet Kaur
Department of Ayurvedic Pharmacy, School of Pharmaceutical Sciences, Lovely Professional University, Punjab, India

Nadeem A. Khan
Civil Engineering Department, Jamia Millia Islamia, New Delhi, India

Afzal Husain Khan
Civil Engineering Department, Jazan University, Jazan, Saudi Arabia

Vibhu Khanna
Department of Ayurvedic Pharmacy, School of Pharmaceutical Sciences, Lovely Professional University, Punjab, India

Mangesh Pradeep Kulkarni
School of Pharmaceutical Sciences, Lovely Professional University, Punjab, India

Arun Kumar
Department of Ayurvedic Pharmacy, School of Pharmaceutical Sciences, Lovely Professional University, Punjab

Pawan Kumar
Department of Materials Science and Nanotechnology, Deenbandhu Chhotu Ram University of Science and Technology, Haryana, India

Rajesh Kumar
School of Pharmaceutical Sciences, Lovely Professional University, Punjab, India

Rajiv Kumar
University Institute of Pharmaceutical Sciences, Punjab University, Chandigarh, India

Rajnish Kumar
Department of Mechanical Engineering, Deenbandhu Chhotu Ram University of Science and Technology, Haryana, India

Ravinder Kumar
School of Mechanical Engineering, Lovely Professional University, Punjab, India

Vinod Kumar
Department of Bio and Nanotechnology, Guru Jambheshwar University of Science and Technology, Haryana, India

Rashi Mathur
School of Pharmaceutical Sciences, Lovely Professional University, Punjab, India

Amrinder Mehta
School of Mechanical Engineering, Lovely Professional University

Prasantha R. Mudimela
School of Electronics and Electrical Engineering, Lovely Professional University, Jalandhar, India

Gaurav Prashar
School of Mechanical Engineering, Lovely professional university, Punjab, India

Parteek Prasher
Department of Chemistry, University of Petroleum & Energy Studies, Energy Acres, Dehradun, India

Dipen Kumar Rajak
Department of Mechanical Engineering, Sandip Institute of Technology and Research Centre, Nashik, MH-India

Rameela Davanagere Ramesh
Department of Aerospace Engineering, Amity University, Dubai, UAE

Sakshi Sabharwal
Department of Ayurvedic Pharmacy, School of Pharmaceutical Sciences, Lovely Professional University, Punjab, India

Anusha Santhosh
Department of Aerospace Engineering, Amity University, Dubai, UAE

Garima Shandilya
Department of Nanotechnology, Bharati Vidyapeeth Deemed to be University College of Engineering, Pune, India

Pardeep Kumar Sharma
School of Pharmaceutical Sciences, Lovely Professional University, Punjab, India

Ankit Sharma
School of Pharmaceutical Sciences, Lovely Professional University, Phagwara, Punjab, India

Deepika Sharma
School of Pharmaceutical Sciences, Lovely Professional University, Phagwara, Punjab, India

Mousmee Sharma
Department of Chemistry, Uttaranchal University, Arcadia Grant, Dehradun, India

Rajeev Sharma
Department of Electrical Engineering, Guru Nanak Dev Engineering College, Ludhiana

Gagandeep Singh
University Institute of Pharmaceutical Sciences, Punjab University, Chandigarh, India

Gurpal Singh
University Institute of Pharmaceutical Sciences, Punjab University, Chandigarh, India

Gurvinder Singh
School of Pharmaceutical Sciences, Lovely Professional University, Punjab, India

Jaswinder Singh
Department of Mechanical Engineering, DAV University Sarmastpur, Jalandhar, India

Sachin Kumar Singh
School of Pharmaceutical Sciences, Lovely Professional University, Punjab, India

Saurabh Singh
Department of Ayurvedic Pharmacy, School of Pharmaceutical Sciences, Lovely Professional University, Punjab, India

Sharanjit Singh
Department of Mechanical Engineering, DAV University Sarmastpur, Jalandhar, India

Ashish Suttee
School of Pharmaceutical Sciences, Lovely Professional University, Punjab, India

Sarath Raj Nadarajan Assari Syamala
Department of Aerospace Engineering, Amity University, Dubai, UAE

Kirtan Tarwadi
Department of Nanotechnology, Bharati Vidyapeeth Deemed to be University College of Engineering, Pune, India

Divya Thakur
Department of Pharmaceutical Sciences and Drug Research, Punjabi University, Punjab, India

Bakul Tikoo
University Institute of Pharmaceutical Sciences, Punjab University, Chandigarh, India

Sergij Vambol
Life Safety and Law Department, Kharkiv Petro Vasylenko National Technical University of Agriculture, Ukraine

Viola Vambol
Educational and Scientific Department of Occupational Safety and Health, Public Agency, National Scientific and Research Institute of Industrial Safety and Occupational Safety and Health, Ukraine

Mohit Vij
School of Pharmaceutical Sciences, Lovely Professional University, Punjab, India

Rohit Vij
Mittal School of Business, Lovely Professional University, Punjab, India

Hitesh Vasudev
School of Mechanical Engineering, Lovely Professional University, Phagwara, India

Dr. Pankaj Wadhwa
School of Pharmaceutical Sciences, Lovely Professional University, Punjab, India

Sheetu Wadhwa
School of Pharmaceutical Sciences, Lovely Professional University, Punjab, India

Ashok Kumar Yadav
University Institute of Pharmaceutical Sciences, Punjab University, Chandigarh, India

1 The Journey of Nanotechnology in Product Development

From Bench to Bedside

Divya Thakur, Sheetu Wadhwa, Sachin Kumar Singh, Rajesh Kumar, and Rohit Vij

1.1 INTRODUCTION

Nanotechnology is a revolution in the recent times for all disciplines of life and especially in the field of medical research – it has brought a new outlook. The application of nanotechnology (in the range of 1–100 nm) in the field of medicine is generally termed as nanomedicine. Various nanotechnology-based systems in pharmaceutical sciences are explored which includes polymeric nanoparticles, dendrimers, metallic nanoparticles, liposomes, nanocapsules, magnetic nanoparticles, nanogels, and so on. These systems overcome the challenges and non-compliance of existing therapies and exhibit potential advantages, i.e. site-specific drug delivery, improvement in patient compliance, dose frequency reduction, and lesser drug side effects.

Although some nanotechnology-based products are able to overcome these major hiccups, still there are challenges in the pilot plant scale-up, regulation concerns, toxicity issues, impact on the environment, and in their commercialization too [1]). With recent advancements, this technology has demonstrated its propensity towards tissue engineering, nanorobots, bio-sensors, diagnosis, and even drug discovery [2].

Several nanomedicines have achieved the regulatory approval, successfully commercialized, and are available for patients. But more efforts are required to achieve the site-specific target approach with improved pharmacokinetics and effective benefit to ratio risk [3]. This can only be possible when industry collaborators join hands with academic researchers for better understanding of the challenges at the molecular level and to come up with solutions to overcome regulatory issues [4,5].

This chapter focuses on different existing and emerging nanotechnology-based delivery systems, systems being explored at pilot scale for enhanced drug delivery along with the success story of popular nanotechnology-based product 'Ambisome' from bench to bedside.

1.2 EXISTING AND EMERGING NANOTECHNOLOGY-DRIVEN CARRIERS

With the advent of nanotechnology, various nanocarriers are developed. These have great advantages and are classified according to their composition. Few existing and emerging nanocarriers are shown in Figure 1.1 and discussed briefly below [6].

Few other nanotechnology-based pharmaceutical and cosmetics products which reached the market are discussed in Tables 2 and 3. Briefly, liposomes are also called "magic bullets", prepared from both natural and synthetic materials, able to entrap both lipophilic and hydrophilic drugs within the lipid bilayer and aqueous core, respectively, biocompatible, and non-toxic too. But there are few limitations, too, such as instability when stored for longer periods, uptake by reticuloendothelial system (RES) system which leads to low-circulation half-life, selection of apt sterilization method, drug leakage on storage, and other regulatory issues [7]). Another delivery system is

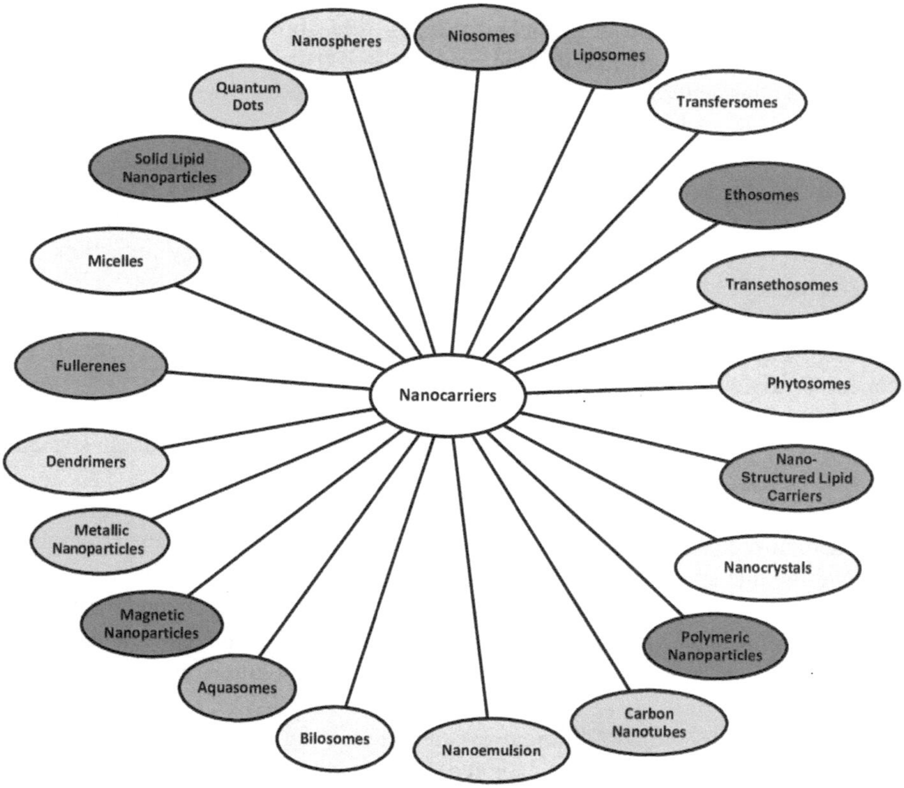

FIGURE 1.1 Nanotechnology-Driven Systems.

niosomes and these are similar in structure to liposomes. Niosomes are composed of non-ionic surfactants. The surfactant molecules tend to orient themselves in such a way that the hydrophilic ends of the non-ionic surfactant point outward, while the hydrophobic ends face each other to form the bilayer [8]. Transfersomes have an inner aqueous core which is surrounded by flexible lipid bilayers made up of edge activators or flexible surfactants [9]. Ethosomal systems are small nano-range vesicles composed of high quantity of alcohol along with water and phospholipid component [10,11]. Another system transethosomes are a combination of both ethosomes and transfersomes having properties and potential of both systems. Phytosomes are plant-based lipid complexes, used widely for the incorporation of phytoconstituents. Bilosomes are composed of bile-salts for the oral delivery of vaccines. Aquasomes are nano-size spherical vesicles enabling the drug and antigen delivery. Emulsomes are nano-size lipid-based particles consisting of lipid assembly and a polar group [12]. Some vesicular systems such as Discomes, Pharmacosomes, Sphingosomes [13], Enzymosomes, Cubosomes [14], Colloidosomes, Micelles, Cryptosomes, Genosomes, Photosome, Erythrosomes, Vesosomes are also explored asnanocarriers [6,15]).

Some non-vesicular carriers such as nanoparticles (polymeric and lipidic) are nano-size range drug delivery systems, widely utilized owing to their advantages over other systems. Solid lipid nanoparticles are another widely used and popular colloidal system which is composed of liquid lipid and solid lipid and has potential to deliver pharmaceuticals, cosmetics, and neutraceuticals. Metallic nanoparticles are developed using gold, silver, platinum, nickel, iron, or their oxides for the delivery of drugs. Carbon nanotubes (CNTs) are made up of carbon in the order of nanometer in size, fabricated as single or multiwalled, and exhibit extensive tensile strength [16]. Quantum dots are another man-made nano-scale structures which have unique optical and electrical properties. Fullerenes are carbon allotropes, composed of carbon atoms which are connected through single and double bond linkage, and form hollow mesh-like structures [17]. Nanoemulsion systems are a mixture of two immiscible liquids, in which one liquid is the dispersed phase which is dispersed into another phase known as the continuous phase [18]. Majority of nanotechnology-based commercialized products such as liposomes, polymeric nanoparticles, micelles, etc. are developed for different types of cancer, incorporating different anti-cancer drugs which generally possess toxicity issues and other side effects (shown in Table 1.1), and some nanotechnology-based marketed cosmeceutical products are discussed in Table 1.2 [15,19]).

1.3 APPLICATIONS AND CHALLENGES OF NANOTECHNOLOGY-BASED DELIVERY SYSTEMS

Nanotechnology-based delivery systems are broadly explored by oral, topical, and transdermal delivery routes for drugs, proteins, peptides, genes, and cosmetics. These systems exhibit site-specific drug targeting, controlled drug delivery, better solubility and bioavailability, improved patient compliance, and as theranostics (in the diagnosis of tumours), etc.

Various advantages and challenges of nanotechnology-based delivery systems are shown in Figure 1.2 [4].

TABLE 1.1
Nanotechnology-Based Marketed Pharmaceutical Products

Marketed Product (Registration Year)	Active Pharmaceutical Ingredient (API)	Nano-carrier	Indication	Route of Administration	Company
Abelcet® (2015)	Amphotericin B	Liposomes	• Invasive fungal infections	Intravenous	Leadiant Biosciences, Inc., USA
Ambisome® (2014)	Amphotericin B	Liposomes	• Invasive fungal infections • Aspergillosis	Intravenous	Gilead Sciences, Inc., USA
Amphotec® (2015)	Amphotericin B	Liposomes	• Invasive aspergillosis	Intravenous	Ben Venue Laboratories, Inc., USA
DaunoXome® (2014)	Daunorubicin	Liposomes	• HIV-associated kaposi's sarcoma	Intravenous	Galen US, Inc., USA
Depocyt® (2015)	Cytarabine	Liposomes	• Lymphomatous meningitis	Intravenous	Pacira Pharmaceuticals, Inc., USA
Depodur® (2014)	Morphine sulfate	Liposomes	• Post-surgical pain management	Epidural	Pacira Pharmaceuticals, Inc., USA
Doxil® (2015)	Doxorubicin	Liposomes	• Ovarian cancer • Kaposi's sarcoma	Intravenous	ALZA Pharmaceuticals, USA
Epaxal® (2016)	Inactivated hepatitis A virus (strain RGSB)	Liposomes	• Hepatitis A	Intramuscular	Crucell, Netherlands

Visudyne® (2015)	Verteporfin (photosensitizer)	Liposomes	• Classic subfoveal choroidal neovascularization due to age-related macular degeneration (AMD)	Intravenous followed by activation of Visudyne® with light from a non-thermal diode laser	Novartis AG, Switzerland
Abraxane® (2014)	Paclitaxel	Protein nanoparticles	• Metastatic breast cancer • Lung cancer • Pancreatic cancer	Intravenous	Abraxis BioScience, LA, CA, USA; Astra Zeneca, London, UK
Adagen® (2015)	Pegademase bovine	Polymeric nanoparticles	• Severe combined immunodeficiency disease (SCID) associated with a deficiency of adenosine deaminase	Intramuscular	Leadiant Biosciences, Inc., USA
Macugen® (2016)	Pegaptanib sodium	Polymeric nanoparticle	• Neovascular (wet) age-related macular degeneration (AMD)	Intravitreal	Gilead Sciences, Inc., USA
Pegasys® (2016)	Pegylated interferonalfa-2a	Polymeric nanoparticle	• Hepatitis C	Intramuscular	Genentech, Inc., USA
Neulasta® (2016)	Pegfilgrastim (PEGylated form of the recombinant human granulocyte colony-stimulating factor)	Polymeric nanoparticle	• Neutropenia for patients with cancer receiving myelosuppressive chemotherapy	Subcutaneous	Amgen, Inc., USA
Somavert® (2016)	Pegvisomant	Polymeric nanoparticle	• Acromegaly	Subcutaneous	Pharmacia and Upjohn Company LLC, Sweden
Genexol PM® (2016)	Paclitaxel			Intravenous	

(*Continued*)

TABLE 1.1 (Continued)

Marketed Product (Registration Year)	Active Pharmaceutical Ingredient (API)	Nano-carrier	Indication	Route of Administration	Company
		Polymeric micelle	• Breast cancer • Non-small cell lung cancer		Samyang Pharmaceutical, Daejeon City, Korea
Diprivan® (2016)	Propofol	Polymeric micelle	• Induction and maintenance of anesthesia	Intravenous	Fresenius Kabi, USA
Restasis® (2016)	Cyclosporine	Polymeric micelle	• Ocular inflammation associated with keratoconjunctivitis sicca • Dry eye syndrome	Ophthalmic (topical)	Allergan, Ireland
Rapamune® (2015)	Sirolimus	Nanocrystals	• Immunosuppressant	Oral	Pfizer Ireland Pharmaceuticals, Ireland
Tricor® (2016)	Fenofibrate	Nanocrystals	• Hypercholesterolemia	Oral	AbbVie, Inc., USA

These drug delivery systems offered promising applications and showed great potential in both preclinical and clinical studies. Few pharmaceutical companies, who worked in the anti-cancer and anti-fungal areas, have been engaged in the translation of liposomes from bench to bedside. As these drugs are toxic in their free forms and exhibit serious side effects too, their loading in these delivery systems can not only overcome the existing challenges but also can provide additional protection to the drugs [20].

However, very few systems are commercialized and can translate from bench to bedside; others suffer from challenges such as batch-to-batch variability, not-so-robust preparation techniques and feasibility issues, instability, variation at pilot-plant scale-up, apt technique of sterilization in case of thermolabile components, and the cost of process and analysis, etc. Other barriers are the lack of infrastructure at research laboratories and inadequate technical competent researchers for the translation of these products from bench to bedside [6]. Several other applications of nanotechnology are in the area of tissue engineering, nanorobots, bio-sensors, diagnosis, and even drug discovery.

Figure 1.3 shows the process of translation of research from bench to bedside with the advancement of nanotechnology.

1.4 SUCCESS STORY OF LIPOSOMAL AMPHOTERICIN B (AMBISOME®)

In 1995, there was a victorious entry of liposomes into the market with PEGylated liposomal formulation, Doxil®. Since then, these novel drug delivery systems were consistently explored for a wide array of their applications in cancer, pain management, viral, fungal diseases, etc., and were successfully translated into the clinics, and reached the patient bedside.

Liposomal Amphotericin B, (AmBisome®, LAmB), manufactured by M/s Gilead Sciences, is a distinctive lipid-based formulation for the treatment of opportunistic fungal pathogens which is in clinical use for 20 years.

Amphotericin B is a polyene anti-mycotic agent with activity against yeasts, molds, and even protozoan parasite *Leishmania spp.* It binds to the sterol present in the fungal cell membrane, i.e. ergosterol, which results in the creation of pores followed by ion leakage and finally fungal cell death. In 1950, an initial formulation of this drug, i.e. amphotericin B deoxycholate (DAmB), was developed and used for many decades. However, there were side effects associated with DAmB such as nephrotoxicity and infusion-linked reactions which urged the formulation scientists to devise a new formulation that retains the anti-fungal activity and reduces toxicity. In light of the above facts, a unilamellar liposomal-based structure for parenteral administration comprising three main ingredients, namely, soy phosphatidylcholine, distearoylphosphatidyl glycerol, and cholesterol (molar ratio – 2:0.8:1), was designed. Soy phosphatidylcholine, a lipid with a unique property of gel to liquid-crystal phase transition point, prevented the hydrolyses of the lipid component on exposure to human body temperature. Distearoylphosphatidyl glycerol was chosen because of the presence of the slight negative charge and fatty acid chain length similar to the hydrophobic part of amphotericin B. Amphotericin B was retained

TABLE 1.2
Nano-Cosmeceutical-based Marketed Products

Marketed Product (Registration Year)	API	Nano-carrier	Application Area	Properties	Manufacturer
Color Ombres dip-dye look (2019)	Silicon dioxide	Nanoparticles	Hair	• Hair dying and nourishment	L'Oreal, France
Eye Tender (2016)	Shea butter, tocopheryl acetate	Liposomes	Eye	• Rapid elimination of lines and wrinkles • Stimulation of fibroblasts and collagen production • Reduction of inflammation	KaraVita, Inc., USA
Nano Nails Líquido 10 ml Frasco com pincel (2018)	Melaleuca (tea tree oil), clove oil	Liposomes	Nails	• Nail fortification • Cutical moisturization • Nail strengthening	Doce Erva Ltda, Brazil
Nanoserum Classic (2015)	Silver, gold, and silicon	Nanoparticles	Skin, vagina	• Skin rejuvenation and soothening • Revitalizant	NanoBeauty, Poland
ReSpimask® VK - Virus Killer (2020)	Copper(II) oxide	Nanoparticles	Face	• Virus and bacteria protection	Respilon Groups. R.O, Czech Republic
Sensitive shaving gel (2015)	Vitamin C and E	Liposomes	Face	• Softening of beard for close and comfortable shave • Protection against micro cuts and irritation	Beiersdorf AG, Germany
Desensin® repair toothpaste (2019)	Hydroxyapatite	Nanoparticles	Teeth	• Reduction of dental hypersensitivity	DENTAID GmbH, Germany

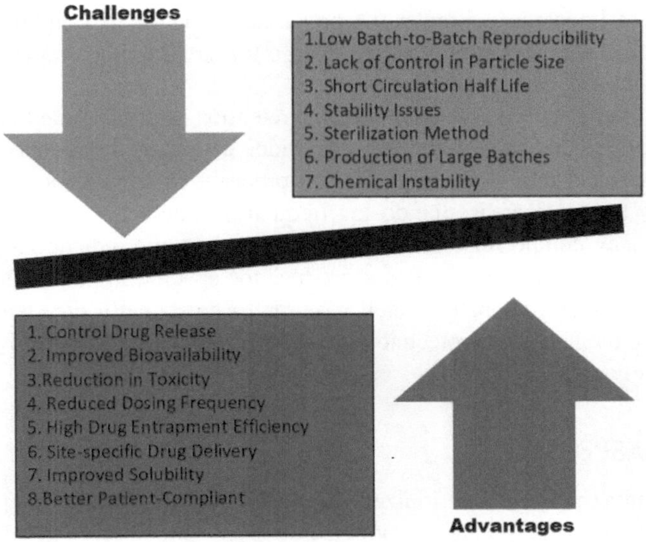

FIGURE 1.2 Advantages and Challenges of Nanotechnology-Based Drug Delivery.

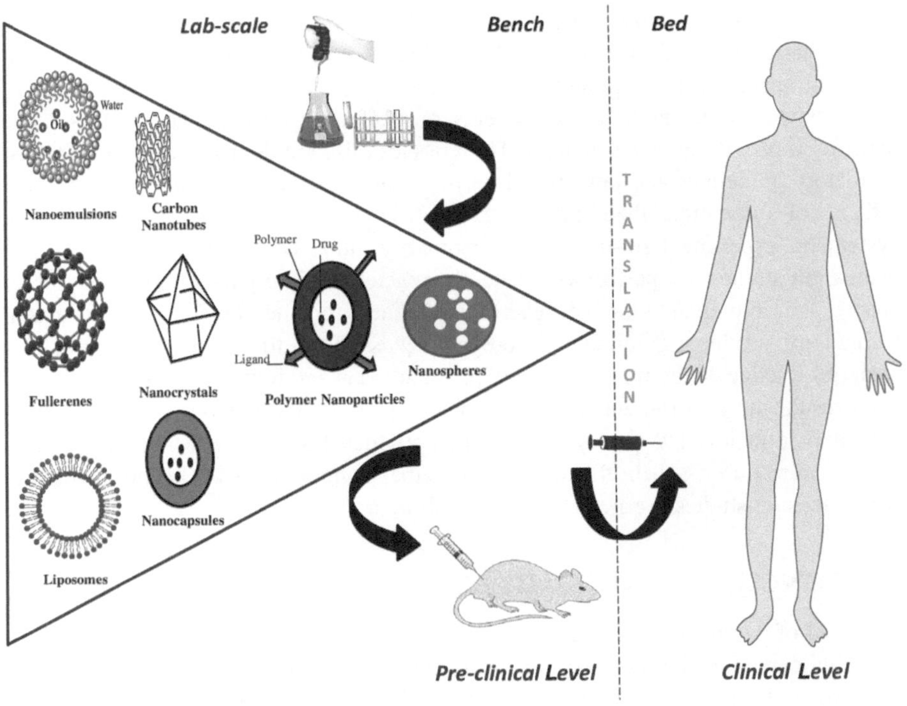

FIGURE 1.3 Translation of Research from Bench to Bedside.

inside the lipid bilayer of liposomes as under the preparatory conditions (slightly acidic), the amino group of the drug with positive charge forms an ionic complex with distearoylphosphatidyl glycerol.

Finally, the addition of cholesterol also facilitated the retention of drug inside the liposome bilayer. Therefore, the final formulation provides a sustained residence time of drug in tissues. According to the experts, this property of Ambisome® is underexploited and may further decrease the dosing frequency, reduce cost as well as toxic effects without any compromise on product efficacy in some indications. Further, there is inadequate clinical data of this product for specific populations such as pregnant women, obese, neonates which requires to be urgently directed [21,22]. This is how with the help of nanotechnology an anti-fungal drug reaches to bedside from bench side.

1.5 REGULATORY ASPECTS

Nanotechnology has amazingly revolutionized both the pharmaceutical and biomedical research by offering plenty of opportunities for the treatment of several dreaded diseases. These technologies offer their support in the development of not only diagnostics and theranostics but also in the development of vaccines and novel delivery strategies as well. Moreover, the gene therapy and immunotherapy have led to open new horizons in the area of personalized medicine system [23].

However, the toxicity issues and undesirable health risks linked with these nanotechnology-based products create challenges and act as barriers in successful clinical translation and regulatory approval as well [20].

Moreover, some nanoparticle systems pose toxicity concerns as well as some harmful impact on the environment. These issues raise the demand for a well-framed regulatory guidelines and laws based on professional ethics to ensure the safety and efficacy of a commercialized product [24,25]. This can be achieved by carrying out systematic experiment set-ups as per regulatory guidance so that possible toxicity evaluation studies are performed. Federal agencies need to play a proactive role to ensure the implementation of federal guidelines for the development of nanotechnology products. Moreover, more awareness need to be created among the societies to educate them regarding the pros and cons and impact of nanotechnology. As a result, the government will get a societal support and feedback in maintaining the safety, efficacy, and quality of developed products [26]. However, in the past, few reports were published on the safety of polymer nanoparticles on healthy cells, but still extensive studies are needed to establish their safety.

1.6 CONCLUSION AND FUTURE PROSPECTS

The field of nanotechnology possesses an immense potential to find its applications in healthcare for the delivery of drugs and cosmetics. The main advantages are targeted approach, controlled drug delivery, improved pharmacokinetics, bioavailability, etc. However, successful commercialization and scale-up of these nanotechnology-based products are still in formative years, and more exhaustive research is required. With the advancement of science and technology, development of innovative polymers, novel systems, and deeper understanding of disease loci at molecular level, it seems that nanotechnology is the future of medicine. Although the success of few nanocarriers is discussed so far, the attention should be focussed toward the development of successful nanotechnology products that can be commercialized and reach beside the bedsides of patients.

REFERENCES

1. Cattaneo, A. G., Gornati, R., Sabbioni, E., Chiriva, M., Cobos, E., Jenkins, M. R. and Bernardini, G. (2010) "Nanotechnology and human health: risks and benefits", *Journal of Applied Toxicology*, 30(8), pp. 730–744.
2. Madaan, T., Pandey, S., and Talegaonkar, S. (2015) "Nanotechnology: A smart drug delivery tool in modern healthcare", *Journal of Chemical and Pharmaceutical Research*, 7(6), pp. 257–264.
3. Havel, H., Finch, G., Strode, P., Wolfgang, M., Zale, S., Bobe, I.,Youssoufian, H., Peterson, M. and Liu, M. (2016) "Nanomedicines: From bench to bedside and beyond", *The AAPS Journal*, 18, pp. 1373–1378. doi: 10.1208/s12248-016-9961-7.
4. Kaur, I. P., Kakkar, V., Deol, P. K., Yadav, M., Singh, S. and Sharma, I. (2014) "Issues and concerns in nanotech product development and its commercialization", *Journal of Controlled Release*, 193, pp. 51–62. doi: 10.1016/j.jconrel.2014.06.005.
5. Prabhakar, U., Maeda, H., Jain, R. K., Sevick-Muraca, E. M., Zamboni, W., Farokhzad, O. C., et al. (2013) "Challenges and key considerations of the enhanced permeability and retention effect for nanomedicine drug delivery in oncology", *Cancer Research*, 73, pp. 2412–2417.
6. Wadhwa, S., Garg, V., Gulati, M., Kapoor, B., Singh, S. K. and Mittal, N. (2019) "Nanovesicles for nanomedicine", *Theory and Practices*, 2000, pp. 1–17.
7. Torchilin, V. P. (2005) "Recent advances with liposomes as pharmaceutical carriers", *Nature Reviews Drug Discovery*, 4, pp. 145–160.
8. Uchegbu, I. F. and Vyas, S. P. (1998) "Non-ionic surfactant based vesicles (niosomes) in drug delivery", *International Journal of Pharmaceutics*, 172, pp. 33–70.
9. Cevc, G. and Blume, G. (2004) "Hydrocortisone and dexamethasone in very deformable drug carriers have increased biological potency, prolonged effect, and reduced therapeutic dosage", *Biochimica et Biophysica Acta*, 1663, pp. 61–73.
10. Patil, R., Patil, S., Patil, S., et al. (2014) "Ethosome: A versatile tool for novel drug delivery system". *Journal of Current Pharma Research* 4, pp. 1172.
11. Touitou, E., Dayan, N., Bergelson, L., et al. (2000) "Ethosomes—novel vesicular carriers for enhanced delivery: characterization and skin penetration properties". *Journal of Controlled Release,* 65, pp. 403–418.
12. Paliwal, R., Paliwal, S. R., Mishra, N., Mehta, A. and Vyas, S. P. (2009) "Engineered chylomicron mimicking carrier emulsome for lymph targeted oral delivery of methotrexate", *International Journal of Pharmaceutics,* 380, pp. 181–188.
13. Saraf, S., Gupta, D., Kaur, C. D., et al. (2011) "Sphingosomes a novel approach to vesicular drug delivery", *International Journal of Current Science Research,* 1, pp. 63–68.
14. Garg, G., Saraf, S. and Saraf, S. (2007) "Cubosomes: an overview", *Biological and Pharmaceutical Bulletin*, 30, pp. 350–353.
15. Santos, A. C., Rodrigues, D., Sequeira, J. A. D., Pereira, I., Simões, A., Costa, D., Peixoto, D., Costa, G. and Veiga, F. (2019) "Nanotechnological breakthroughs in the development of topical phytocompounds-based formulations", *International Journal of Pharmaceutics*, 572, p. 118787. doi: 10.1016/j.ijpharm.2019.118787.

16. Mehra, N. K., Jain, K. and Jain, N. K. (2015) "Pharmaceutical and biomedical applications of surface engineered carbon nanotubes", *Drug Discovery Today*, 20(6), pp. 750–759.
17. Aoshima, H., Kokubo, K., Shirakawa, S., Ito, M., Yamana, S. and Oshima, T. (2009) "Antimicrobial activity of fullerenes and their hydroxylated derivatives", *Biocontrol Science*, 14, pp. 69–72.
18. Baccarin, T. and Lemos-Senna, E. (2017) "Potential application of nanoemulsions for skin delivery of pomegranate peel polyphenols", *American Association of Pharmaceutical Scientists*, 18, pp. 3307–3314.
19. https://product.statnano.com/ (accessed on 20.04.2020).
20. Jain, K., Mehra, N. K. and Jain, N. K. (2015) "Nanotechnology in drug delivery: Safety and toxicity issues", *Current Pharmaceutical Design*, 21, pp. 4252–4261.
21. Bulbake, U., Doppalapudi, S., Kommineni, N., and Khan, W. (2017). "Liposomal formulations in clinical use: An updated review", *Pharmaceutics*, 9(2), p. 12.
22. Stone, N. R., Bicanic, T., Salim, R., and Hope, W. (2016) "Liposomal amphotericin B (AmBisome®): A review of the pharmacokinetics, pharmacodynamics, clinical experience and future directions", *Drugs*, 76(4), pp. 485–500.
23. Zhang, X. Q., Xu, X., Bertrand, N., Pridgen, E., Swami, A. and Farokhzad, O. C. (2012) "Interactions of nanomaterials and biological systems: Implications to personalized nanomedicine", *Advanced Drug Delivery Reviews*, 64(13), pp. 1363–1384.
24. Bowman, D. M. and Fitzharris, M. (2007) "Too small for concern? Public health and nanotechnology", *Australian and New Zealand Journal of Public Health*, 31(4), pp. 382–384.
25. Resnik, D. B. and Tinkle, S. S. (2007) "Ethics in nanomedicine", *Nanomedicine (London)*, 2(3), pp. 345–350.
26. Clausen, I. and Glott, T. (2014) *Development of clinically relevant implantable pressure sensors: Perspectives and challenges*, Sensors (Basel), 14(9), pp. 17686–17702.

2 Advances and Applications of Nanotechnology

Nadeem A. Khan, Sirajuddin Ahmed, Izharul Haq Farooqi, Afzal Husain Khan, Viola Vambol, Sergij Vambol, and Fazlollah Changani

2.1 INTRODUCTION

Modernization and industrialization have led to a huge issue of water sullying through natural and inorganic contaminations. The primary sources of such contamination are pesticides, soil disintegration, metals, colours and so forth. Pharmaceuticals and colours are the most basic toxins that taint wastewater. Wastewater treatment is a noteworthy challenge in the present times because of its variable nature. The currently used materials for wastewater treatment should be examined for high detachment capacities and being prudent and recyclable. These materials can be utilized in different treatment process like adsorption, redox corruption, layer partition and so forth. In these procedures, adsorption is significant for the ebb and flow wastewater treatment. Adsorbents like nanotubes, initiated carbon, graphene and so on are used in the water-treatment process. These days, nanocomposites are increasingly utilized compared with nanoparticles because of their excellent sanitizing capacities. Present-day pollutants, such as colours, pharmaceuticals and several metals, are expelled for adsorption from nanocomposites because of their affinity to metal particles, size and high zone-to-volume proportion. This chapter talks about different nanocomposite materials and their effectiveness for most contaminants found to date.

2.1.1 Wastewater as a Cause of Environmental Degradation

As a rule, water that has been used at home, in enterprises, business establishments, or for other purposes and, after use, has been directed to centralized flows is called "wastewater". Considering the worldwide water-withdrawal data between 1950 and 2010, it was concluded that the worldwide home water-utilization increased by 3.7 times over this period, while water use inside the business locale enhanced by 2.9% by 2010. The suppers and horticulture venture (FAO) of the United Nations (UN) expected that the entire universal water intake utilizing farming area in 2010 was 2769 km^3, which accounts for 69% of the whole water intake.

Since lack of water is among the important unresolved natural issues that the field faces, the search for new, unexplored ways of efficient (sparing) use of water resources is urgently needed. In nature exists a closed circuit of water. Humanity must follow the example of natural processes. This means that wastewater must be treated and used for suitable purposes. And the most appropriate is its reuse in agriculture. For agriculture, treated wastewater is the main water source. This approach is especially relevant in arid areas where there is a lack of water. Additionally, it should be emphasized that a high treatment level needs to be provided before releasing wastewater into the biological environment. This will provide support for a healthy environment. Wastewater poisons are different in different kinds of water (for example, farming, modern, or residential wastewaters). Typically, concoction, natural, and radiological toxins might be found in a steady progression or together in wastewater. Compound toxins might be classified into natural (together with chlorophenols) and inorganic contaminants. The U.S. natural wellbeing association (USEPA) and the part wellbeing organization (WHO) distributed exhaustive pointers for reuse of wastewater, where special attention is directed to the capture of chemical synthetic mixtures from wastewater that must be reused for horticulture, fish farming, animal husbandry and other uses (U.S. Ecological assurance association 2012; worldwide wellbeing manager 2006a, b, c, d). Wastewater from various households contains bacteria and microorganisms, substances of natural origin, and may also contain radioactive particles. Horticultural seepage water includes various composts and pesticides in substantial amounts. Especially, the nature of seepage water is perceived with the measure of its salt content and essential particles (for example Na, Ca, Mg, CO_3, SO_4, Cl), harmful follow factors (for example Disc, Palladium, Mercury, Arsenic), chemical or biological agents for controlling pests and plant diseases (for example paraquat, carbofuran, butachlor, atrazine), notwithstanding the centralizations of plant supplements containing saltpetre and other fertilizers. Then again, wastewater from households and business institutions is regularly exposed to toxin sources, which the concrete compound structures explicitly comprise. New normal squanders can be frequently organically, or by high temperature, corrupted into water and carbon dioxide (CO_2), while inorganic business squanders aren't degradable and must be released after a treatment that could decrease the poor outcomes for the earth and human wellbeing. In any case, the diffusion of toxins from mining ventures pollues water, turning it into wastewater that needs to be dealt with.

Various researchers have found that wastewater that has not been treated pollutes soil, air, and clean water (Chamtouri et al. 2008; Elbana et al. 2013; Karaouzas 2016). Numerous researchers, analysts and tree huggers are continually looking for cheap, sensitive materials that can viably and suitably remove poisons from wastewater. Nanomaterials are considered green substances because of their over-the-top surface spot, receptive synthetic attributes and high capacity for purging up contaminated oceanic answers. Using nanoparticles to improve water quality cure essentially relies on adsorption, oxidation (photocatalysis), and cleansing, just as partition draws near. In this regard, we can reasonably assume that the use of nanoparticles increases the likelihood of removal of toxins from wastewater or decrease in the quantity of these toxic focuses. In particular, the essential objectives of this chapter are: (i) to show the importance and urgent need for nanoparticles, as well as their reactivity study; and (ii) to focus on nanoparticles' usefulness for the removal of inorganic and natural pollutants from wastewater.

2.1.1.1 Nanoparticles' Reactivity

The chemical activity of any substance significantly depends on its surface. Knowing how nanomaterials get their huge surface area will help explain their reactivity. Consider an iron cube with a side size of 0.2 µm, which is segmented into eight equal cubes. We can imagine its subsequent division into eight segments of each of the eight cubes obtained earlier. Thus, the division of each new cube into smaller cubes can be continued again. Let us dwell on 512 cubes (1, eight, sixty-four, 512 cubes for consecutive segmentation, see Figure. 2.1), for which a side length of 200 nm is characteristic, and consequently, the cube surface area is 0.24 μm^2. Therefore, if the cube is segmented sequentially three times, the face period of each smallest cube will be 25 nm, and the total surface area of 512 cubes will be 1.92 μm^2. Obviously, due to this division, the surface area will be increased by eight times, although the cube was segmented only three times. Such a situation will necessarily provide an increase in the threshold energy and chemical activity of nanoparticles. Moreover, thanks to such a figurative explanation, it is seen that nanoparticles have an incredibly large surface location in step with unit mass or quantity "unique floor region". The reactivity of nanomaterials may be ascribed to the floor and the quantum confinement results (Roduner 2006). That is, atoms in the bulk of a substance have more bonding and coordination numbers than atoms on the surface of the nanoparticles. Since state density modification is possible in nanomaterials, they are characterized by means of a discrete energy level set. It should be remembered that the chemical activity of nanomaterials depends on their surface flexure. That is, excess chemical activity is expected to accompany excess flexure (a small radius). The dependence of the nanomaterial reactivity on its surface flexure was emphasized in a study. Also, in this study, it was proved that reactivity is better for a convex surface and worse for a concave surface.

2.1.2 Technologies for Wastewater Treatment using Nanomaterials

Numerous modern researchers demonstrate that nanomaterial-based technologies can effectively reduce contamination and thus have successfully implemented urban wastewater (UWW) treatment. Most extensively studied different nanotechnology applications in wastewater treatment have been developed into the following broad categories:

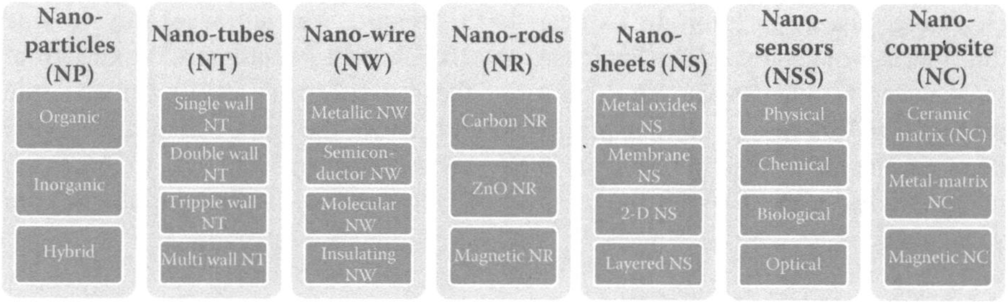

FIGURE 2.1 Nanomaterials (1–100 nm) for Wastewater Clean-Up.

2.1.2.1 Adsorption Processes

Adsorption, a polishing step, is usually adopted with the aim of removal of organic and inorganic pollutants from water and wastewater. Efficient adsorption generally depends on the appropriate surface area, porous structure and active sites. Due to the significant specific surface of nano-adsorbents, more sorption sites are provided, namely, porous mediums and spaces.

2.1.2.2 Carbon-based Nano-adsorbents (CNMs)

Carbon is a pervasive element, and hence it is inexpensive. Also, it is environment-friendly and renewable, and hence, undoubtedly beneficial. Its positive features include a high surface-to-volume ratio, which increases the potential for its use in wastewater treatment. High specific surface and chemical stability, high porosity and low density, ease of regeneration and the possibility of reuse are the qualities of carbon nanomaterials, which have led to a significant scientific interest in them. Due to these qualities, nanoporous carbon, graphene and its derivatives, carbon nanofibers (CNFs) and nanotubes (CNTs), as well as other carbon nanomaterials (CNMs), have been widely used as adsorbents [1].

2.1.2.3 Nano-adsorbents on a Metal Substrate

Particularly effective for wastewater treatment are particles of metal oxides of magnesium, zinc, iron, titanium and alumina (MgO, ZnO, FeO, TiO). Because they are inexpensive, such adsorbents have found widespread use. Iron oxide $(FeO)^-$ based nanomaterials can successfully remove dye, heavy metal and pharmaceutical contamination from wastewater because of their salient features such as small pore size, higher surface area and magnetic characteristics. It was found that the removal efficiency of Cr^{6+} using nanoscale zero-valent iron is higher than using iron powder for the same purpose. In this case, the extraction of Cr^{6+} from the adsorbent was observed to be 4.8 times more than that under the same conditions using iron powder [2]. Similarly, magnetically separable nanoadsorbents, such as FeO nanoparticles, which have a large surface area, have attracted much attention from scientists, since these nanoadsorbents are highly effective for the adsorption of As^{3+} and As^{5+} through electrostatic attraction. Also, other heavy metals (e.g. cobalt, lead, chromium, etc.) can be effectively removed from contaminated water by FeO nanoparticles.

2.1.2.4 Membrane Processes

Membrane-based technologies have found widespread use in water- and wastewater-treatment processes. The membrane-separation process is widely used for water filtration, such as the desalination process for salt separation. This membrane process is also very effective in controlling microbial growth [3]. In recent years, to separate micropollutants and particulate matter, scientists have developed membranes with increased efficiency [4]. Moreover, such membranes effectively remove from contaminated water, organic substances that affect the qualitative characteristics of water (taste, smell, etc.) and various harmful microorganisms.

2.1.2.5 Photocatalysis

Nowadays, photocatalysis is reasonably considered an inexpensive, sustainable and environment-friendly water-treatment technology. This technology has great potential for chemically hazardous enterprises with a large production of contaminated water, such as dye production or textile enterprises [5]. From a study, it was found that about 17–20% or more global industrial waters are water that has been contaminated by the processes of pigmentation and textile processing. Every year on the planet, 7×10^5 tons of different dyestuff types are produced. The synthesis and dyeing processes are accompanied by release into the environment of more than 10–15% harmful chemicals.

2.2 NANOMATERIALS FOR WASTEWATER CLEANUP

The advancement of nano-substances as nano-adsorbents has been found to be effective to get rid of various poisons, for example, natural, inorganic and organic contaminations from water or wastewater. A substantially wide assortment of nano-adsorbents utilized for wastewater treatment rely on different critical factors including pH, temperature, reaction time of working circumstances, size and state of NPs, and technique for test, for example, clump tests or a section. The most critical area of contaminated water treatment is their filtration through nanolayers, nanopowders and nanoparticles to reuse treated water. Various efforts to remediate contaminated waters and improve their quality have been made to create the best water models. Purification should be possible through diminishing pollutants considering the positive allowable cutoff, renovating a harmful concoction to safe conjunction, and additionally to discard organic dangers and pathogens. There is a wide range of nanomaterials that can provide such purification by adsorption of synthetic substances and destruction/inactivation of pathogens, since they have been tested for the treatment of wastewater from the production of paper, water-containing inorganic pollutants, pesticides, dyes, etc. So, the use of nanoscale zero-valent iron as an adsorbent is suitable for capturing toxic or non-biodegradable substances in a unique oxidation system. The explanation for this is the strong dependence of hydroxyl radicals assembling from nanoscale zero-valent iron. The author also examined that nanocomposites progressed by utilizing CNMs including graphene show considerable capacity as receptive adsorbents for removing inorganic and regular contamination from wastewaters. At the same time, further research is still required for large-scope bundles (Gautam and Chattopadhyaya 2016).

Zhang, Guangzhi and Pan [6] surveyed the nanoadsorbents most regularly used for water purification: carbon nanomaterials (CNTs, CNFs, graphene-based nanomaterials and others), nanoparticles of metal and their oxides (nanoscale zero-valent iron, nanoscale iron oxides and others), and precious metal nanoparticles, as gold (Au) and silver (Ag). The inventors of such adsorbents have inferred that they are very promising for the innovative approaches developed in the water-purification field [6]. So, CNTs are very effective for getting rid of contaminants. That is a direct result of their extraordinary adsorption limit and over-the-top pace reaction motor. Carbon nanotubes have been thought of as green impetuses considering their high ability to remove small-scale living beings and infections ([5]). Indeed, a rapid improvement in several projects of nanotechnology for contaminated water-treatment is currently expected (Hasemzadeh et al. 2014). Although nanomaterials create favourable circumstances for contaminated-water treatment, adverse circumstances and hindrances must also be kept in mind. Regarding the use of nanomaterials, some scientists [6–8] touched on such issues as (i) the reliability of the creation of nanomaterials; (ii) the possibility of nanomaterial reuse after their service life (except for nanoparticles); (iii) the unknown destiny of extensive introduction in various fields of science, production, and everyday life. Liu et al. [5] accentuated the designing and similarly modest difficulties for CNTs, which incorporate the same scattering and creation esteem, separately. At the same time, there is a need for comprehensive assessment of the viability and environment-friendliness of the nanomaterials used. An attempt to develop criteria for comprehensive assessment of nanomaterials has also been mentioned in other studies [9]. Additionally, toxicology and assurance challenge for understanding nanomaterials and their utility will finish executions in STP.

2.2.1 Removal of Organic Pollutants using Nano-adsorbents

Common wastewater-contamination-prevention measures include managing and reusing wastewater and releasing it to the environment carefully. Without a doubt, charged nanomaterials can absorb natural anionic toxins. These results demonstrated improved sorption capacity to remove ibuprofen. In an experiment, initiated carbon and typical graphene oxide were found to have the highest sorption capacity. It is well known that organofluorine mixtures have a harmful impact on the environment. Zhang, Guangzhi and Pan [6] utilized nano-ZnO lined cathodes for the debasement of perfluorinated mixtures in the purification of contaminated water and completed execution of electrochemical oxidation framework on 39–66% in 40 minutes. Such disposal productivity is undoubtedly better than using tempered steel plates for the anode and cathode terminals [6]. Unquestionably, natural contaminants represent a genuine threat to ecological sources, principally due to their different classes that need exact cures. In different words, contaminants can be cationic, anionic, insecure, brief or long-chained. Therefore, their disposal from wastewater is a troublesome issue that needs a fused remediation strategy. Thanks to nanomaterials, a ground-breaking choice has been proposed for the purification of contaminated water. The high chemical activity of actualized nanomaterials for the purification of contaminated water can supplement the conventional purification strategies. The probable results of using nanomaterials for the purification of contaminated water include bringing down the predetermined time and power required for the treatment, the types and amounts of the executed concoction mixtures, and improved quality of the managed polluted water.

Figure. 2.2 shows water and wastewater contaminant types classified by their chemical nature. Banerjee et al. (2007) have demonstrated a ground-breaking advancement in the water purification process.

Nanofiltration viability was proved in a pilot-scale test of a layered bioreactor for medical and clinical wastewater treatment. Testing was conducted within 20 days, the results of which were as follows: substance reduction efficiency was 94% for substance oxygen call; 88% for smelling salts; more than 80% for nitrite; 87% for nitrate and 46–68% for phosphorus. At the same time, the contraction of synthetic substances requires high temperature limits, and contamination can limit the nanofiltration product for purging up bad water (Shahmansouri and Bellona 2015).

With regards to the present times, writing assessments and planning wastewater cure principally depend on the utilization of nanomaterials to remember the utility measure, time, treatment estimation as well as the predominant pollutant type. Specific verification steps must be carried out before introducing any nanotechnology:

- Nanomaterials wastewater treatment probability are estimation for decrease the focus to alluring indicator or take out the focused on pollutants.
- Explore the best possible improvement in working conditions and reactor placement.
- Analyze the viability of nanotechnology for immense scope.

Ordinarily, traditional wastewater treatment includes strategies and activities including screening, sedimentation, buoyancy, substance oxidation, layer filtration, sorption, particle change, bright, and others. The effect of blending nanotechnology with conventional treatment for an ideal treatment time is correctly treated polluted

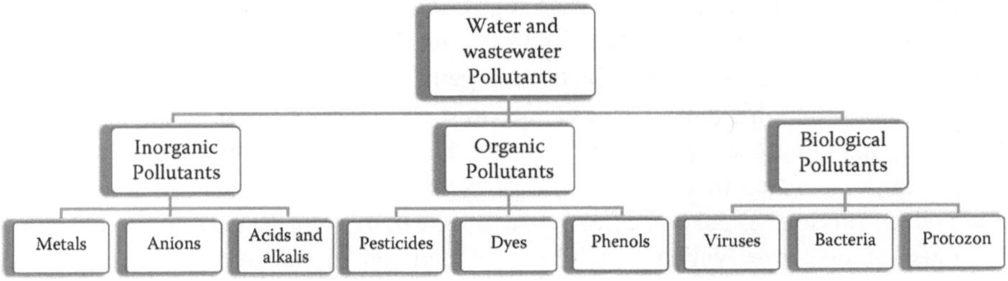

FIGURE 2.2 Water and Wastewater Contaminant Types Classified by Their Chemical Nature.

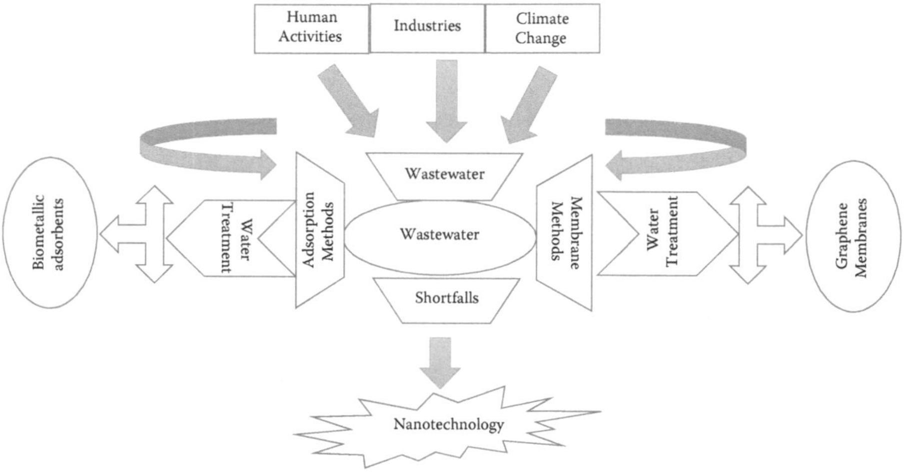

FIGURE 2.3 Water/Wastewater Treatment Techniques.

water. For example, nanoscale zero-valent iron is to a great extent useful in purification of contaminated water. In the primary oxidation method, the outside of 0-valent iron is coated with an iron guide (hydroxides that signal contaminant sorption and decrease responses). Figure 2.2 and Figure 2.3 It is noteworthy to understand that the occurrences as well as utilization of such nanoscale particles for wastewater treatment can cause small to medium level of toxicity and the chemical activity is well described in Figure 2.2 and Figure 2.3.

For instance, CNTs show high efficiency for getting rid of contaminants. That is a direct result of their over-the-top adsorption limit and their unnecessary pace-reaction dynamic. Carbon nanotubes have been contemplated as green impetuses considering their high ability to remove small-scale life forms and infections ([5]; Ren et al. 2011).

2.3 CONCLUSION

In synopsis, water purification using nanoadsorbents is a conceivably encouraging system that has been used lately. Nano-adsorbents are completed for sorption, oxidation, decrease, sanitization and debasement of sewage pollutants. Nanomaterials' adequacy to discard pollution in sewage relies tremendously upon the combination of the nanomaterials', the wastewaters' and the contaminants' qualities. Nanomaterials' reactivity fluctuates depending on its floor, together with floor region, floor repression impact, floor value thickness, quality, and floor ebb and flow, just as the unfaltering quality of nanophase gadget in the sewage. The selection of appropriate nanomaterials for wastewater treatment should consider the nanomaterial's reactivity (the ability for sorption, expulsion effectiveness, and numerous others) notwithstanding the pace of response, which could be a fundamental issue in some cases in the treatment plan. The utilization of the reproduction styles presents a fantastic asset for such purpose. Even though nanoscience is being exponentially developed, the

TABLE 2.1
Nanomaterials for Wastewater Cleanup and Their Removal Efficiencies

Nanoadsorbents	Pollutant species	Adsorption capacity	Reference
Ascorbic acid-stabilized zero	Cd^{2+}	79.58%	[10]
Akaganeite nanocrystals	Cr^{6+}	80 mg/g	[11]
Carbon nanotube supported ceria nanoparticles	Cr^{6+}	30.20 mg/g	[12]
Cobalt ferrite	As^{+3}	24.81 mg/g	[13]
Chitosan-bound Fe_3O_4 nanoparticles	Cu^{2+}	21.5 mg/g	[14]
Gum arabic nanoparticles	Cu^{2+}	38.50	[1]
Hematite	As^{3+}, As^{5+}	2899 ± 71.09 μg/g	[15,16]
Iron NPs modified micro fibrillated cellulose	As^{5+}	2.460 mmol/g	
Manganese ferrite		24.17 mg/g	[13]

absence of guidelines to utilize nanomaterials can be credited to the nonavailability of entire data on nanomaterials. Homegrown-nanomaterials comprising nano-mud are a colossally encouraging methodology in diminishing wastewater pollution.

REFERENCES

1. Banerjee, S. S. and Chen, D. H. (2007). "Fast removal of copper ions by gum arabic modified magnetic nano-adsorbent", *Journal of Hazardous Materials*, 147(3), pp. 792–799. doi: 10.1016/j.jhazmat.2007.01.079.
2. Sharma, Y. C. et al. (2009). "Nano-adsorbents for the removal of metallic pollutants from water and wastewater", *Environmental Technology*, 30(6), pp. 583–609. doi: 10.1080/09593330902838080.
3. Mir-Tutusaus, J. A. et al. (2017). "Pharmaceuticals removal and microbial community assessment in a continuous fungal treatment of non-sterile real hospital wastewater after a coagulation-flocculation pretreatment", *Water Research*, 116, pp. 65–75. doi: 10.1016/j.watres.2017.03.005.
4. Aydin, S. et al. (2019). "Antibiotics in hospital effluents: occurrence, contribution to urban wastewater, removal in a wastewater treatment plant, and environmental risk assessment", *Environmental Science and Pollution Research*, 26(1), pp. 544–558. doi: 10.1007/s11356-018-3563-0.
5. Liu, Z. et al. (2019). "Photocatalytic degradation of dyes over a xylan/PVA/TiO2 composite under visible light irradiation", *Carbohydrate Polymers*, 223(June), pp. 1–10. doi:10.1016/j.carbpol.2019.115081.
6. Zhang, M., Guangzhi, H. and Pan, G. (2009). "Combined DFT and IR evidence on metastable-equilibrium adsorption of arsenate on TiO2 surfaces", *Journal of Colloid and Interface Science*, 338: pp. 284–286.
7. Vambol, S., Vambol, V., Suchikova, Y., Bogdanov, I., and Kondratenko, O. (2018). "Investigation of the porous GaP layers' chemical composition and the quality of the tests carried out", *Journal of Achievements in Materials and Manufacturing Engineering*, 2(86), pp. 49–60. DOI: 10.5604/01.3001.0011.8236.

8. Suhikova, Y. Vambol, S. Vambol, V. Mozaffari, N. and Mozaffari, N. (2019). "Justification of the most rational method for the nanostructure's synthesis on the semiconductors surface", *Journal of Achievements in Materials and Manufacturing Engineering*, 92/1-2, pp. 19–28, DOI: 10.5604/01.3001.0013.3184.
9. Vambol, S. Bogdanov, I. Vambol, V. Suchikova, Y. Lopatina, H. and Tsybuliak, N. (2017). "Research into effect of electrochemical etching conditions on the morphology of porous gallium arsenid", *Eastern-European Journal of Enterprise Technologies*, 6(5/90), pp. 22–31.
10. Savasari, M. et al. (2015). "Optimization of Cd (II) removal from aqueous solution by ascorbic acid-stabilized zero valent iron nanoparticles using response surface methodology", *Journal of Industrial and Engineering Chemistry*. The Korean Society of Industrial and Engineering Chemistry, 21, pp. 1403–1409. doi: 10.1016/j.jiec.2014.06.014.
11. Lazaridis, N. K., Bakoyannakis, D. N. and Deliyanni, E. A. (2005). "Chromium(VI) sorptive removal from aqueous solutions by nanocrystalline akaganèite", *Chemosphere*, 58(1), pp. 65–73. doi: 10.1016/j.chemosphere.2004.09.007.
12. Di, Z. C. et al. (2006). "Chromium adsorption by aligned carbon nanotubes supported ceria nanoparticles", *Chemosphere*, 62(5), pp. 861–865. doi: 10.1016/j.chemosphere.2004.06.044.
13. Martinez-Vargas, S. et al. (2017). "Arsenic adsorption on cobalt and manganese ferrite nanoparticles", *Journal of Materials Science*, 52(11), pp. 6205–6215. doi: 10.1007/s10853-017-0852-9.
14. Chang, Y. C. and Chen, D. H. (2005). "Preparation and adsorption properties of monodisperse chitosan-bound Fe3O4 magnetic nanoparticles for removal of Cu(II) ions", *Journal of Colloid and Interface Science*, 283(2), pp. 446–451. doi: 10.1016/j.jcis.2004.09.010.
15. Dickson, D., Liu, G. and Cai, Y. (2017). "Adsorption kinetics and isotherms of arsenite and arsenate on hematite nanoparticles and aggregates", *Journal of Environmental Management*, 186, pp. 261–267. doi: 10.1016/j.jenvman.2016.07.068.
16. Hokkanen, S. et al. (2015). "Removal of arsenic(V) by magnetic nanoparticle activated microfibrillated cellulose", *Chemical Engineering Journal*, 260, pp. 886–894. doi: 10.1016/j.cej.2014.08.093.
17. Ahmad, R., Kumar, R. and Haseeb, S. (2012). "Adsorption of Cu2+ from aqueous solution onto iron oxide coated eggshell powder: evaluation of equilibrium, isotherms, kinetics, and regeneration capacity", *Arabian Journal of Chemistry*, 5, pp. 353–359.
18. AL-Othman, Z. A. and Inamuddin, Naushad, M. (2011a). "Forward (M2+H+) and reverse (H+M2+) ion exchange kinetics of the heavy metals on polyaniline Ce(IV) molybdate: a simple practical approach for the determination of regeneration and separation capability of ion exchanger", *Chemical Engineering Journal*, 171, pp. 456–463.
19. AL-Othman, Z. A. and Inamuddin, Naushad, M. (2011b). "Adsorption thermodynamics of trichloroacetic acid herbicide on polypyrrole Th(IV) phosphate composite cation-exchanger", *Chemical Engineering Journal*, 169, pp. 38–42.
20. Amin, N. K. (2008). "Removal of reactive dye from aqueous solutions by adsorption onto activated carbons prepared from sugarcane bagasse pith", *Desalination*, 223, pp. 152–161.
21. Andreu, G. and Vidal, T. (2013). "Laccase from pycnoporus cinnabarinus and phenolic compounds: can the efficiency of an enzyme mediator for delignifying kenaf pulp be predicted?", *Bioresource Technology*, 131, pp. 536–540.
22. Andreu, G., Barneto, A. G. and Vidal, T. (2013). "A new biobleaching sequence for kenaf pulp: influence of the chemical nature of the mediator and thermogravimetric analysis of the pulp", *Bioresource Technology*, 130, pp. 431–438.

23. Arfin, T., Jabeen, F. and Kriek, R. J. (2011). "An electrochemical and theoretical comparison of ionic transport through a polystyrene based titanium-vanadium (1:2) phosphate membrane", *Desalination*, 274(1–3), pp. 206–211.
24. Arrad, O. and Sasson, Y. (1989). "Commercial ion exchange resins as catalysts in solid-solid-liquid reactions". *Journal of Organic Chemistry*, 54, pp. 4993–4998.
25. Azelee, N. I. W., Jahim, J. M., Rabu, A., Murad, A. M. A., Bakar, F. D. A. and Illias, R. M. (2014). "Efficient removal of lignin with the maintenance of hemicellulose from kenaf by two-stage pretreatment process", *Carbohydrate Polymers*, 99, pp. 447–453.
26. Barakat, M. A., Ramadan, M. H., Alghamdhi, M. A., Algarny, S. S., Woodcock, H. L. and Kuhn, J. N. (2013). "Remediation of Cu(II), Ni(II) and Cr(III) ions from simulated wastewater by dendrimer titania composites", *Journal of Environmental Management*, 117, pp. 50–57.
27. Barbieri, L., Bonamartini, A. C. and Lancellotti, I. (2000). "Alkaline and alkaline-earth silicate glasses and glass-ceramics from municipal and industrial wastes", *Journal of the European Ceramic Society* 20, pp. 2477–2483.
28. Brzonova, I., Kozliak, E., Kubatova, A., Chebeir, M., and Qin, W., Christopher, L. and Ji, Y. (2014). "Kenaf biomass biodecomposition by basidiomycetes and actinobacteria in submerged fermentation for production of carbohydrates and phenolic compounds", *Bioresource Technology*, 173, pp. 352–360.
29. Bushra, R., Shahadat, M., Nabi, S. A., Raeissi, A. S., Oves, M., Umar, K., Muneer, M. and Ahmad, A. (2014a). "Synthesis, characterization, antimicrobial activity and applications of composite adsorbent for the analysis of organic and inorganic pollutants", *Journal of Hazardous Materials*, 264, pp. 481–489.
30. Bushra, R. and Mohammad, Shahadat M. (2014b). "Synthesis, characterization and applications of nanocomposite materials in diverse fields", *Advances in Environmental Research*, 35, pp. 105–130.
31. Bushra, R., Shahadat, M., Ahmad, A., Nabi, S. A., Raeissi, A. S., Umar, K., Oves, M. and Muneer, M. (2014c). "Synthesis, characterization, antimicrobial activity and applications of composite adsorbent for the analysis of organic and inorganic pollutants", *Journal of Hazardous Material*, 264, pp. 481–489.
32. Bushra, R., Naushad, M., Adnan, R., AL-Othman, Z. A. and Rafatullah, M. (2015). "Polyaniline supported nanocomposite cation exchanger: synthesis, characterization and applications for the efficient removal of Pb2+ ion from aqueous medium", *Journal of Industrial and Engineering Chemistry*, 21, pp. 1112–1118.
33. Bushra, R., Ahmed, A. and Shahadat, Md. (2016). "Mechanism of adsorption on nanomaterials", *Advanced Environmental Analysis*, pp. 90–111.
34. Cabrera, L., Gutierrez, S., Herrasti, P. and Reyman, D. (2010). "Sonoelectrochemical syn- thesis of magnetite", *Physics Procedia*, 3, pp. 89–94.
35. Chen, G. C., He, Z. L., Stoffella, P. J. and Yang, X. E. (2006). "Leaching potential of heavy metals (Cd, Ni, Pb, Cu and Zn) from acidic sandy soil amended with dolomite phosphate rock (DPR) fertilizers", *Journal of Trace Elements in Medicine and Biology*, 20, pp. 127–133.
36. Chena, Y. D., Chena, W. Q., Huang, B. and Huang, M. J. (2013). "Process optimization of K2C2O4-activated carbon from kenaf core using box–Behnken design". *Chemical Engineering Research & Design*, 91, pp. 1783–1789.
37. Cuerda-Correa, E. M., Antonio Macías-Garcia, A., Diez, M. A. D. and Ortiz, A. L. (2008). "Textural and morphological study of activated carbon fibers prepared from kenaf", *Microporous and Mesoporous Materials*, 111, pp. 523–529.
38. Dizge, N., Aydiner, C., Demirbas, E., Kobya, M. and Kara, S. (2008). "Adsorption of reactive dyes from aqueous solutions by fly ash: kinetic and equilibrium studies", *Journal of Hazardous Materials*, 150, pp. 737–746.
39. Duval, C. (1963). *Inorganic Thermogravimetric Analysis*. Elsevier, Amsterdam, p. 315.

40. El-Naggar I. M., Zakaria E. S., Ali I. M., Khalil M. and El-Shahat M. F. (2012). "Chemical studies on polyaniline titanotungstate and its uses to reduction cesium from solutions and polluted milk", *Journal of Environmental Radioactivity*, 112, pp. 108–117.
41. Engstrom, K., Broberg, K., Concha, G., Nermell, B., Warholm, M. and Vahter, M. (2007). "Genetic polymorphisms influencing arsenic metabolism: evidence from Argentina", *Environmental Health Perspectives*, 115(4), pp. 599–605.
42. Engstrom, K., Nermell, B., Concha, G., Stromberg, U., Vahter, M. and Broberg, K. (2009). "Arsenic metabolism is influenced by polymorphisms in genes involved in one-carbon metabolism and reduction reactions", *Mutation Research*, 667(1–2), pp. 4–14.
43. Engstrom, K. S., Vahter, M., Lindh, C., Teichert, F., Singh, R. and Concha, G. (2010). "Low 8-oxo-7, 8-dihydro-20-deoxyguanosine levels and influence of genetic background in an Andean population exposed to high levels of arsenic", *Mutation Research*, 683, pp. 98–105.
44. Gan, S., Zakaria, S., Chia, C. H., Padzil, F. N. M. and Ng, P. (2015). "Effect of hydrothermal pretreatment on solubility and formation of kenaf cellulose membrane and hydrogel", *Carbohydrate Polymers*, 115, pp. 62–68.
45. Hao, A., Zhao, H. and Chen, J. Y. (2013). "Kenaf/polypropylene nonwoven composites: the influence of manufacturing conditions on mechanical, thermal, and acoustical performance", *Composites Part B*, 54, pp. 44–51.
46. Hasfalina, C. M., Maryam, R. Z., Luqman, C. A. and Rashid, M. (2012). "Adsorption of copper (II) from aqueous medium in fixed-bed column by kenaf fibres", *APCBEE Procedia*, 3, pp. 255–263.
47. Inagaki, M., Nishikawa, T., Sakuratani, K., Katakura, T., Konno, H. and Morozumi, E. (2004). "Carbonization of kenaf to prepare highly-microporous carbons". *Lett Ed/ Carbon*, 42, pp. 885–901.
48. Institute of Medicine, Food and Nutrition Board (2001). *Dietary Reference Intakes for Vitamin A, Vitamin K, Arsenic, Boron, Chromium, Copper, Iodine, Iron, Manganese, Molybdenum, Nickel, Silicon, Vanadium, and Zinc.* National Academy Press, Washington, DC.
49. Ip, A. W. M., Barford, J. P. and McKay, G. (2010). "Acomparative study onthe kinetics andmechanisms of removal of reactive black 5 by adsorption onto activated carbons and bone char", *Chemical Engineering Journal*, 157, pp. 434–442.
50. Irmak, S. and Ozturk, I. (2010). "Hydrogen rich gas production by thermocatalytic decomposition of kenaf biomass", *International Journal of Hydrogen Energy*, 35, pp. 5312–5317.
51. Ishrat, U. and Rafiuddin, (2012). "Synthesis, characterization and electrical properties of titanium molybdate composite membrane". *Desalination*, 286, pp. 8–15.
52. Jeun, J., Min, B. L., Young, J. L., Hyun, K. P. and Park, J. K. (2015). "An irradiation-alkaline pretreatment of kenaf core for improving the sugar yield", *Renewable Energy*, 79, pp. 51–55.
53. John, M. J., Bellmann, C. and Anandjiwala, R. D. (2010). "Kenaf–polypropylene composites: effect of amphiphilic coupling agent on surface properties of fibres and composites", *Carbohydrate Polymers*, 82, pp. 549– 554.
54. Khalil, Hpsa, Yusra, Afi, Bhat, A. H. and Jawaid, M. (2010). "Cell wall ultrastructure, anatomy, lignin distribution, and chemical comp osition of Malaysian cultivated kenaf fiber", *Industrial Crops and Products*, 31, pp. 113–121.
55. Khan, A. A. and Akhtar, T. (2008). "Preparation, physico-chemical characterization and electrical conductivity measurement studies of an organic–inorganic nanocomposite cation-exchanger: poly-otoluidine Zr(IV) phosphate", *Electrochim Acta*, 53, pp. 5540–5548.
56. Khan, A. A. and Alam, M. M. (2003). "Synthesis, characterization and analytical applications of a new and novel 'organic–inorganic' compositematerial as a cation exchanger and Cd(II) ion-selective membrane electrode: polyaniline Sn(IV) tungstoarsenate", *Reactive and Functional Polymers*, 55, pp. 277–290.

57. Khan, A. A. and Baig, U. (2012). "Electrically conductive membrane of polyaniline–titanium (IV)phosphate cation exchange nanocomposite: applicable for detection of Pb(II) using its ion-selective electrode", *Journal of Industrial Engineering and Chemistry*, 18(6), pp. 1937–1944.
58. Khan, A. A. and Baig, U. (2013). "Electrical conductivity and ammonia sensing studies on in situ polymerized poly(3-methythiophene)-titanium(IV)molybdophosphate cation exchange nanocomposite", *Sensors and Actuators: B* 177, pp. 1089–1097.
59. Khan, A. A. and Inamuddin, A. M. M. (2005). "Determination and separation of Pb2+ from aqueous solutions using a fibrous type organic–inorganic hybrid cation-exchange material: Polypyrrole thorium (IV) phosphate", *Reactive and Functional Polymers*, 63, pp. 119–133.
60. Khan, A. A. and Innamuddin, (2006). "Application of Hg(II) sensitive polyaniline Sn(IV) phosphate composite cation exchange material in determination of Hg2+ from aqueous solutions and in making ion selective membrane electrode", *Sensors and Actuators B*, 120, pp. 10–18.
61. Khan, A. A. and Paquiza, L. (2011a). "Characterization and ion-exchange behavior of thermally stable nanocomposite polyaniline zirconium titanium phosphate: its analytical application in separation of toxic metals", *Desalination*, 265(1–3), pp. 242–254.
62. Khan, A. A. and Paquiza, L. (2011b). "Analysis of mercury ions in effluents using potentiometric sensor based on nanocomposite cation exchanger polyaniline–zirconium titanium phosphate", *Desalination* 272(1–3), pp. 278–285.
63. Khan, A. A. and Shaheen, S. (2012). "Thermal stability and electrical properties of conducting polymer based 'polymeric–inorganic' composites: poly-o-anisidine and poly-o-toluidine Sn(IV) tungstate", *Materials Research Bulletin* 47, pp. 4414–4441.
64. Khan, A. A. and Shaheen, S. (2014). "Chronopotentiometric and electroanalytical studies of Ni(II) selective polyaniline Zr(IV) molybdophosphate ion exchange membrane electrode", *Journal of Electroanalytical Chemistry*, 714–715, pp. 38–44.
65. Khan, A. A. and Shaheen, S. (2015). "Preparation, characterization and kinetics of ion exchange studies of Ni2+ selective polyaniline–Zr(IV)molybdophosphate nanocomposite cation exchanger", *Journal of Industrial Engineering and Chemistry*, 26, pp. 157–166.
66. Khan, S., Cao, Q., Zheng, Y. M., Huang, Y. Z. and Zlm, Y. G. (2008). "Health risks of heavy metals in contaminated soils and food crops irrigated with wastewater in Beijing, China", *Environmental Pollution*, 152, pp. 686–692.
67. Khan, A. A., Baig, U. and Khalid, M. (2011). "Ammonia vapor sensing properties of polyaniline–titanium (IV)phosphate cation exchange nanocomposite", *Journal of Hazardous Materials*, 186(2–3), pp. 2037–2042.
68. Khan, A. A., Baig, U. and Khalid, M. (2013). "Electrically conductive polyaniline-titanium (IV) molybdophosphate cation exchange nanocomposite: synthesis, characterization and alcohol vapour sensing properties", *Journal of Industrial and Engineering Chemistry*, 19, pp. 1226–1233.
69. Khan, M. D. A., Akhtar, A., Nabi, S. A. and Khan, M. A. (2014). "Synthesis, characterization, and photocatalytic activity of polyaniline-Sn(IV)iodophosphate nanocomposite: its application in wastewater detoxification", *Industrial & Engineering Chemistry Research*, 53, pp. 15253–15260.
70. Khan, A. A., Rao, R. A. K., Alam, N. and Shaheen, S. (2015). "Formaldehyde sensing properties and electrical conductivity of newly synthesized Polypyrrole-zirconium(IV) selenoiodate cation exchange nanocomposite", *Sensors and Actuators B*, 211, pp. 419–427.
71. Rao, C. N. R. (1963b) *Chemical Applications of Infrared Spectroscopy*. Academic, New York, p. 338.
72. Rawat, M., Ramanathan, A. L. and Subramanian, V. (2009). "Quantification and distribution of heavy metals from small-scale industrial areas of Kanpur City, India", *Journal of Hazardous Materials*, 172, pp. 1145–1149.

73. Shahadat, M. and Bushra, R. (2015). "Synthesis, characterization and significant applications of PANI-Zr (IV)sulphosalicylate nanocomposite". *Advances in Nanotechnology*, 13, pp. 81–206.
74. Shahadat, M., Nabi, S. A., Bushra, R., Raeissi, A. S., Umar, K. and Ansari, M. O. (2012). "Synthesis, characterization, photolytic degradation, electrical conductivity and applications of nanocomposite adsorbent for the treatment of pollutants". *RSC Advances*, 2, pp. 7207–7220.
75. Shahadat, M., Teng, T. T., Rafatullah, M. and Arshad, M. (2015). "Titanium-based nanocomposite materials: review of recent advances and perspectives". *Colloids and Surfaces B: Biointerfaces*, 126, pp. 121–137.
76. Sharif, J., Mohamad, S. F., Othman, N. A. F., Bakaruddin, N. A., Osman, H. N. and Güven, O. (2013). "Graft copolymerization of glycidyl methacrylate onto delignified kenaf fibers through pre-irradiation technique". *Radiation Physics and Chemistry*, 91, pp. 125–131.
77. Sharma, G., Pathania, D., Naushad, M. and Kothiyal, N. C. (2014). "Fabrication, characterization and antimicrobial activity of polyaniline Th(IV) tungstomolybdophosphate nanocomposite material: efficient removal of toxic metal ions from water". *Chemical Engineering Journal*, 251, pp. 413–421.
78. Silverstein, R. M., Bassler, G. C. and Morrill, T. C. (1981). Chapter 3: *Spectrometric Identification of Organic Compounds*, 4th ed. Wiley, New York, p. 111.
79. Sud, D., Mahajan, G., Kaur, M. P. (2008). Agricultural waste material as potential adsorbent for sequestering heavy metal ions from aqueous solutions – a review. *Bioresource Technology*, 99, pp. 6017–6027.
80. Sun, D., Zhang, W. Y. and Liu, X. (2010). "Adsorption of anionic dyes fromaqueous solution on fly ash". *Journal of Hazardous Materials*, 181, pp. 335–342.
81. Tennakone K. and Wijayantha K. G. U. (1998). "Heavy-metal extraction from aqueous medium with immobilized TiO2 photocatalyst and a solid sacrificial agent". *Journal of Photochemistry and Photobiology A: Chemistry*, 113(1), pp. 89–92.
82. Topp N. E. and Pepper K. W. (1949). "Properties of ion-exchange resins in relation to their structure. Part I. Titration curves". *Journal of the Chemical Society*, 1949, pp. 3299–3303.
83. Vatutsina O. M., Soldatov V. S., Sokolova V. I., Johann J., Bissen M. and Weissenbacher A. (2007). "A new hybrid (polymer/inorganic) fibrous sorbent for arsenic removal from drinking water". *Reactive and Functional Polymers*, 67, pp. 184–201.
84. Xie L., Jiang R., Zhu F., Liu H. and Ouyang G. (2014). "Application of functionalized magnetic nanoparticles in sample preparation". *Analytical and Bioanalytical Chemistry*, 406, pp. 377–399.
85. Yang Y. and Wang P. (2006). "Preparation and characterizations of a new PS/TiO2 hybrid membrane by sol-gel process". *Polymer*, 47(8), pp. 2683–2688.

3 Significance and Administration of Nanotechnology in the Armed Forces and Defense Sector

Ali Asgher Ali Hasan, Roshan Rajesh Bhatkar, and Sarath Raj Nadarajan Assari Syamala

3.1 INTRODUCTION

Great endeavors are made in current engineering industries to reduce the weight of merchandise and the overall size of products. Engineering at the nano-scale provides us with plenty of opportunities to learn the behavior of materials at the scale of one billionth of a meter. Challenges are met with time and time again to invent merchandise that is lighter, smaller, tougher, smarter and cheaper. Nano-science and its applications are concerned with the ongoing progress of diverse fields of scientific research and engineering applications. This may include (but is not limited to) disciplines or departments of field research such as: biotechnology, advanced electronics, genetic engineering, materials sciences (which can have further diversified applications in civil, mechanical and aerospace engineering domains), applied chemistry, information technology and data analysis and so forth [1]. The advancement of studies such as nano-science and its applications got its inspiration when the renowned physicist Richard Feynman emphasized engineering precision at the atomic scales in one of his discussions "There's Plenty of Room at the Bottom" in around 1959 [2]. Challenges in the aerospace industries encompass obstacles such as over-increasing obligation to manufacture and use eco-friendly technology, which is well relevant to the aerospace sphere where tons of harmful greenhouse gases are exhausted into the open atmosphere during the manufacturing and operation of both aircraft and spacecraft alike. Deliberating about aerial pollution, further complication arises when defense and ordnance manufacturing and application is taken into consideration. Considering challenges in the engineering sphere, obstacles arise within the sector such as manufacturing lightweight craft, utilization of materials for greater strength of the craft, specific stress bearing capacity, specific fracture toughness, corrosion resistance, high-temperature resistance, etc. Further challenges become apparent when contemplating the task of maintenance of operating cruise or launch vehicles. The primary impediment in military aerospace is predominantly based on researches in stealth-based technology that can allow friendly craft to infiltrate enemy territories, all undetected throughout the mission including the weapon drop and precision strike phase of the mission. This chapter is meant to try resolving all the existing challenges in the civil and military aerospace by incorporating the grand researches conducted in the novel nanotechnology discipline throughout past decades.

Employment of nanotechnology in the sphere of defense-fortification and warfare was well established before the foundations of modern nano-science technology and engineering were even laid in the mid-20th century. Gunpowder, for instance, was discovered in the early eleventh century, which was the earliest form of nanotechnology deployed in the armed forces. Subsequently in the eighteenth, nineteenth and twentieth centuries, State-organized military and local militia developed a vast range of ordnance and armaments in their armed forces. These precursory advancements in explosive and ballistic weaponry consequently led to precision engineering of sophisticated explosive and propellant based nano-particles compounds that have lead us to compact rifles and hypersonic cruise guided missiles. However, contemporary warfare's armaments comprise a scope of engineering research much greater than just explosives and propellants. In this chapter, we shall discourse purposefully about nanotechnology applications deployed in contemporary military and defense hardware such as (i) Stealth and camouflage; (ii) Nanoparticle based propellants; (iii) Administration of nano-science in military (high-impact resistant) armor and; (iv) Further research scopes and futuristic prospects in nano-technology in contemporary and futuristic warfare.

3.2 ENHANCED PROPELLANTS

Propellants are energy rich substances that are used as fuels in aircraft that propel them into the air from the ground using non air-breathing engines. The primary example of such an engine is a rocket engine. Rocket engines are primarily used in varieties of high-velocity aircrafts and inter-atmospheric or orbital launch vehicles. The former are simply known as a 'rockets' in popular culture. Rockets, however, are just engines that can propel the aircraft without the necessity to suck in air like air-breathing engines, such as jets. The mechanics of such an engine and its capability to propel the aircraft entirely depends on the mixture of fuel and oxidizer stored in huge quantities within the aircraft. This is evident if one looks at the average amount of fuel in a launch vehicle in terms of percentage with respect to the entire launch vehicle's mass. On average, a staggering 85% of the overall mass at launch of an orbital vehicle is nothing but fuel (propellant). However, the use of propellants in military rockets vary according to the need of the armament used in the field and the former again depends on the mission type and sensitivity. Furthermore, those used in military fortifications are of lower explosive power to have a controlled rate of combustion, which is enough to propel the ordnance. They are used in a variety of armaments in the armed forces' inventory that can comprise (but is not is limited to) a vast range of hand-held projectile weapons such as, artillery, mortars and tank shells. They are the ultimate driving forces of different kinds of Air to Air (AAM), Air to Ground (AAG), Surface to Air (SAM), Anti-ship, Anti-Submarine, Anti-Tanks and Anti-Aircraft (AA) missiles. All the preceding types of missiles are powered using rocket engines for ease of maintenance and fast deployment. Inter-continental cruise missiles are an exception here as they operate at supersonic and hypersonic velocities with the help of air-breathing ramjet or scramjet engines. Inter-continental cruise missiles do not utilize rocket engines because these are advanced missiles developed to target faraway hostile co-ordinates. Air-breathing engines mentioned previously are desired due to their relative simplicity and lower frontal area. Generally, all common, short-range missiles use solid propellants as fuel, but ballistic missiles, which are very large and generally have a long-range of warhead delivery, use liquid propellants as their primary fuel. The majority of long-range missiles comprise of multiple stages of engine operations. They are constructed this way to improve the missiles' operative performance. For instance, a submarine launched Surface to Air Missile (SAM) may initially use solid propellant based rocket boosters, but can transition to a liquid propellant based gas-turbine jet engine propulsion system.

In the upcoming section, we will discuss further upon the different types of propellants used in the armed forces to launch propulsive ordinances directed towards enemy/hostile locations. Further, we may examine the effects of metallic nanoparticles on enhancing the combustion properties of ammonium perchlorate oxidizer in solid rocket propellants.

3.2.1 Solid Propellants

Solid propellants are energy rich particulate compounds that, by their chemical virtues, exhibit solid-state crystalline structure. Gunpowder is commonly used as a propellant in military applications in ballistic projectile weapon. Another example of high-energy substance is an explosive. It is identical to a propellant, but differs only when the rate of combustion factor is considered. This is to say that the rate of combustion of propellants is slightly lower than that of high impact explosives. Furthermore, propellants burn gradually and in a controlled manner, whereas explosives' combustion process is spontaneous and mostly uncontrolled.

Synthesis of solid propellants consists of adding oxidizer, which is of the powdered form, to a liquid fuel to form a semi-solid state substance. This jelly like semi-solid substance matter is molded to form the substance into the desired shape. Further, the mold is then left to cure at well-defined temperature and pressure [3].

Nitrocellulose is of the utmost importance in manufacturing solid-state propellants for use in military armaments. Due to nitrocellulose's property of excellent oxygen balance, perfect explosive and propulsive behavior, it is used in nearly all short to medium range launched ballistic ordnances like tank shells, mortar, ballistic projectile weapon mercenaries, rocket propelled rockets (RPG) and etc.

Solid propellants, based on their synthesis and different compounds constituted in their synthesis, are explained below based on additives dissolved for synthesis as follows [4,5]:

Single-Based Propellants: These propellants consist primarily of nitrocellulose as their main propulsive agent. Ordnance inventory examples comprising single-based propellant systems mainly consist of short-range ballistic operation such as tank shells, cannons, howitzers, airborne ordnance on helicopter or fixed winged war aircraft and anti-aircraft missiles or anti-aircraft projectile weaponries.

Double-Based Propellants: These propellants consist of nitrocellulose as the first base with a second base of nitroglycerine, along with flame stabilizers. These propellants are used in a larger range of field operation than the single-based propellants. The example of these weapons include sniper rifles, mortar shells, Rocket-Propelled Grenades (RPG) etc.

Triple-Based Propellants: These propellants are nothing but extensions of the previous two categories, with an additional nitro-base. Along with nitrocellulose and nitroglycerine, these propellants consist of another nitro-base, known as nitroquanidine. These propellants are an advance over the first two propellants; however, triple-based propellants have limited military use. In the military, triple-based propellants are utilized in cannons and tanks.

Composite propellants: Composite propellants are generally used in large range missiles such as in Inter-Continental Ballistic Missiles (ICBM). The propellant consists of 90% of the total mass of the missile at the launch. The propellants in these kinds of missiles are made of a hybrid of high calorific fuels (such as kerosene, petrol or pure metallic aluminum) and a combustible binder such as synthetic rubber or HTPB [3,6].

The systematic combination of substances that form the basis of solid rocket propellant synthesis ensures both propulsive and destructive powers of the ordnance and, most importantly, ensures controlled combustion of high energy substances to propel different military armament ordnances such as bullets from firearms, canons, missiles, artillery, mortars and tank shells to the targeted hostile locales.

3.2.1.1 Solid Rocket Propellant Fundamentals

Solid propellant grain configuration: Grain configuration is a distinctive property of the aircraft operating on a rocket based engine. If put easily, grain configuration defines the changing state or shape of the rocket engine during the flight. That is to say that the burning surface of the propellant engine keeps changing due to constant combustion in its mid-air cruise. Furthermore, the overall consumption of propellant mostly depends on the quantity and quality of the burning surface available to the burning flame or the igniter. Moreover, the rate of propellant consumption per unit time is also almost entirely dependent on the internal ballistic variables which the engine and its propellants are subjected to. Any grain configuration is classified as neutral, regressive or progressive depending entirely on the variation of thrust, pressure and temperature. Either it can be constant, decreasing or increasing respectively.

Web fraction: It is the ratio of the web thickness to the superficial radius of the grain and is generally larger than unity for end burners since the length of the propellant is considered the web thickness and for open internal configurations, the web fraction is smaller than unity.

Volumetric fill fraction: It is the ratio of the volume of propellant to the volume of the chamber that is maximized (nearly to unity) for end burners as there is no open space left.

Mass burning rate: It is a very crucial factor or property regarding the operation of rocket engines utilizing solid rocket propellants. It is important for engineers who are involved with fuel efficiency constraints while designing and manufacturing the rocket because the mass burning rate directly co-relates to mass flow rate and overall thrust vector of the rocket. This very much intuitive because if the burn rate of the rocket engine increases, then ultimately the mass flow rate and thrust will increase, but propellant stored within the rocket motor will exhaust rapidly. Therefore, there are certain variables here that engineers can control with innovative designs, both of the structure of the rocket motor as well as with the type of solid propellants they are using. The rate of generation of exhaust (product) gases produced during the burning of solid rocket propellants can be calculated by the following equation:

$$\dot{m} = A_b * r * \rho_b \tag{3.1}$$

Where,

$\dot{m}$ = *Mass Flow Rate*;

A_b = *Burn Area* (m^2);

r = *Burn rate of Solid Propellant* (m/s);

ρ_b = *Density of Solid Rocket Propellant* (kg/m^3);

From the continuity equation, the mass flow rate generated must be equal to the sum of the mass storage per time in the rocket motor container mass and the mass flow rate out of the nozzle. Mathematically,

$$A_b r B_b = \frac{d(\rho_c V_c)}{dt} + \frac{A_t P_c}{C^*} \tag{3.2}$$

Where, the subscript 'c' represents any numeric value and C* is the special expression that represents the characteristic velocity, which is a non-physical physical entity that is used to compare different rocket performances. It is noteworthy to bear in mind that the storage term in the precursory equation is neglected because a small mass of gaseous propellants is mixed with the solid propellants, which is required to fill in the left over volumes by the same. So after neglecting the storage term, the above equation can be re-written as the following equation to obtain the chamber pressure within the rocket motor walls [14].

$$P_c = \frac{A_b r \rho_b C^*}{A_t} \quad (3.3)$$

3.2.2 Liquid Propellants

Liquid propellants are energy rich compounds, which chemically and physically exhibit liquid state characteristics. Fluid based propellants have a limited utility in the armed forces due to all the complications that arise during their storage, handling and field operation. However, they are used in long-range missiles that carry warhead payloads to inter-continental distances or to deliver certain payloads to space (Earth's orbit or a completely different planet). Even in the long-range missiles lineup, we have ballistic missiles and cruise missiles, which have two stages of engine operation. The first stage consists of the initial propulsion thrust provided by rocket boosters that utilize solid propellant. During its cruise phase i.e. the second phase, the missile transitions to air-breathing propulsion systems such as ramjets or scramjets until the warhead is delivered. Liquid propellants are generally divided into two types: (i) Hypergolic propellants in which the fuel starts oxidizing (or burning) the moment when it is exposed to the oxidizer. The former happens without the help of any external stimulus such as spark ignition setup. (ii) Non-Hypergolic propellants where the fuel and oxidizer meet but do not self-ignite. Non-Hypergolic propellants require an external agent to cause the mixture of fuel and oxidizer to commence the combustion process. All orbital launch vehicles use non-hypergolic propellants as their initial boost to lift off the launch pad by the help of booster rockets. Liquid propellants can consist entirely of either oxidizers (such as liquid oxygen), fuels (such as pure kerosene or petrol) or monopropellants such as hydrogen peroxide or hydrazine. Monopropellants are commonly chosen to be the propellant in most long-range ballistic missiles as they are generally a mixture of both oxidizer and fuel in one single unit. Liquid propellants generally ignite when the fuel encounters the oxidizer.

Similarly to solid propellants, liquid propellants are classified further based on their synthesis in proportions with other similar, high-energy releasing chemical base additives such as the combination of fuels and oxidizers. This categorization of liquid propellant based on monopropellant or bipropellant base combustion behavior is as follows [4,7]:

Single-Based Liquid Propellants: Recognized as monopropellants where there is a singular base propellant ignited using an ignition assembly. The most widely used monopropellant is hydrazine (N_2H_4). The decomposition of hydrazine occurs at two stages of chemical reaction. The first stage of reaction is where two molecules of hydrazine break down to two molecules of ammonia and hydrogen gas. The precursory reaction is exothermic in nature and releases huge amount of heat to initiate the lift off. The second stage is where ammonia decomposes further into individual nitrogen and hydrogen molecules. The second stage of reaction is endothermic in nature and happens at an expense of reduction in thrust by reducing the initial amounts of energy required to perform a successful lift-off. More examples of Single-Base Liquid Propellants are: nitro methane, methyl or dimethyl derivatives of hydrazine such as the symmetrical mono-methyl hydrazine or the unsymmetrical dimethyl hydrazine, hydrogen peroxide (stable at ordinary temperatures but decompose to hot unstable gases at elevated temperatures) and etc. [8,9].

Double-Based Liquid Propellants: As the name suggests, here we have two high-energy releasing compounds, which initiate the combustion process the moment they are added together. In double-based liquid propellant systems, the two high-energy releasing chemicals are: (i) Fuel and; (ii) Oxidizer. Fuel can either be kerosene (RP-01), alcohol, hydrazine, and its derivatives (UDMH or MMH) along with liquid hydrogen. Oxidizers can be nitric acid (HNO3), nitrogen tetroxide, liquid oxygen, and liquid fluorine. Liquid oxygen and liquid fluorine are the optimum fuel oxidizers, but they have to be stored in cryogenic environments that pose a major constraint in the utility of these two strong fuel oxidizing agents [8,9].

In rocket motors, which are designed based on double-based liquid propellant engine technology; both the fuel and the oxidizers are stored in separate storage tanks and mixed together in a completely different tank. The flow of these energy-rich liquids can be facilitated through designing a complex web of pipes, servos, pumps and valves. When these liquids meet, they react such that the oxidizer, being a perfect oxidizing agent, oxidizes the fuel mixture mixed with a small volume of liquid hydrogen. The resulting exothermic reaction releases immense amounts of light and heat energy. This energy is liberated gradually and in a controlled manner (engineers ensure that detonation does not happen) and this high energy is utilized as a mechanical up-lift force for the rocket through precision engineering and designing of nozzles from where the energy rich exhaust exists the rocket motor and the launch vehicle finally lifts off the ground.

Other types of rocket propellants include gas propellants, electric (ion) propellants or electric thrusters and nuclear propellants. Further moving down through this chapter, we shall discuss about the status of contemporary research activities on the application of nanotechnology in developing efficient propellants that can be deployed successfully in the defense sector.

3.2.3 Applications of Nano-Catalysts in the Decomposition of Ammonium Perchlorate (AP) in Solid Rocket Propellants

In this subsection, we will briefly deliberate about the deployment of certain metallic nanoparticles as additives that act as a catalyst during the decomposition reaction of ammonium perchlorate during combustion that can provide us with high propulsive capability and reliability, which is required in the rocket manufacturing industry [10]. Ammonium perchlorate is seen within the aerospace industry as a potent oxidizer of fuels in solid propellant based rocket motors. Ammonium Perchlorate starts to decompose at temperatures above 150 degrees Celsius. There are certain benefits of ammonium perchlorate in using it as an oxidizer of fuel in the solid propellant based rocket motors. (i) It ensures sufficient supply of oxygen during the fuel combustion process; (ii) It may also be deployed as a potent filler in the binder matrix in manufacturing composite rocket propellants to ensure structural coherence and sturdiness of the propellant compound and; (iii) Checks the burning rate of the propellant during the rocket's operation and avoids the release of a sudden burst of energy that can lead to a mid-air detonation. As stated earlier, the combustion process of ammonium perchlorate begins above temperatures of 150 degrees Celsius. The decomposition of ammonium perchlorate itself happens in stages. Many structural and chemical changes occur during the stages, (i) Reaching temperatures equal to 250 degrees Celsius, ammonium perchlorate crystal undergoes a transition from an orthorhombic crystalline structure to a cubic crystalline structure. This change of the crystalline structural geometry requires the compound to absorb energy from its ambient surroundings, hence the reaction is an endothermic reaction; (ii) further increment in temperatures to 350 degrees Celsius, it is observed to show a low rate of decomposition with minimal release of useful energy. Furthermore, at this stage almost 30% of the compound is said to be either decomposed or sublimed; (iii) Above or equal to temperatures of 450 degrees Celsius, the compound under examination is shown to release high amounts of energy during its decomposition. Hence, this stage is the absolute exothermic reaction during the chemical and thermodynamic decomposition of ammonium perchlorate.

Composites of ammonium perchlorate (AP) and certain nanoparticles are prepared by grinding and mixing processes. The process of preparing the AP composite involves a certain number of steps to ensure the effectivity of the reinforcement to strengthen the application of the matrix (AP). Steps involving the AP-nanoparticle involve (but are not limited to): (i) sonication of the nanoparticles is performed (provided that the nanoparticles were dissolved in the either solution first) to agitate the reinforcements to change their normal properties and make them more soluble to the matrix. (ii) The particle slurry is then ground manually until the ether is evaporated; (iii) These particles are then placed in an oven to cure for at least 30 minutes. These nanoparticles cause a drastic change in the chemical and physical properties/characteristics of AP compound ranging from quantum level effects to molecular interface level to physical and characteristic integrity of the compound as a whole:

Thermal properties: AP matrix reinforced with nanoparticles show a characteristic reduction in the melting point of the compound due to the nanoparticle's small atomic size and high specific surface atomic density. Furthermore, due to the previous reasons, the melting and crystallization temperature always turns out to be less.

Magnetic properties: AP reinforced with nanoparticles exhibit amazing and interesting magnetic behavior often portraying high end-to-end molecular coercivity or even super magnetism.

Improved catalytic properties: Since, nanoparticles are so small, it improves their surface atomic contact with other particles and enhances their ability to interact with other particles on nano-scales. This provides us with a superior absorption rate that leads to improved catalytic properties of the compound.

3.2.3.1 Catalytic Effect of Nickel nanoparticles with Ammonium Perchlorate

As demonstrated by various experiments conducted in hopes of understanding the behavior of nanoparticles' catalytic properties in the decomposition reaction of ammonium perchlorate (AP), it was found that nickel nanoparticles when acting as reinforcements in the nano-nickel and AP composite, they tended to enhance the combustion efficiency of ammonium perchlorate and its combustion velocity.

Experiments to compare the micro particle and nanoparticle of nickel particles were performed and the comparison is illustrated in the following figure:

From Figure 3.1, it is evident that the nickel nanoparticles had a significant effect on the catalytic properties of AP in reducing the peak temperatures of the energy released in the decomposition reaction of AP during its combustion. The value of T_H reduces from 477.2 degrees Celsius to 363.7 degrees Celsius.

3.2.3.2 Catalytic Effect of Copper nanoparticles on Ammonium Perchlorate

The effect of copper nanoparticles are discussed in detail in the following manuscripts [11,12]. In the experiments conducted in [10], it was found that the addition of micron or nano sized copper particles had a negligible effect on the catalytic properties of the crystalline shape transformation of the ammonium perchlorate (AP). Furthermore, about 287.6 and 347 degrees Celsius were observed as high and low exothermic temperature peaks respectively for the composite (Cu-AP), which improved catalytic effect of Cu nano-scale particles when compared with micro scale copper particles at minimum and maximum peak temperatures. When these particles were dissolved into the AP matrix, the heat released from decomposition rose to about 1.300 kJ/g from 0.436 kJ/g.

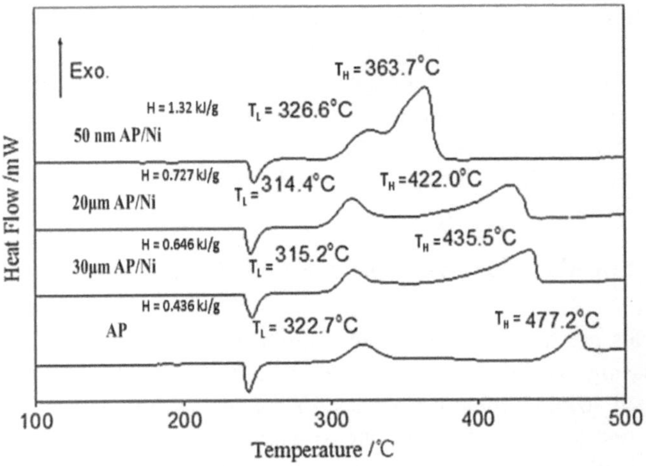

FIGURE 3.1 Graphical Representation of Variation in Heat Flow plotted against Temperature for AP/Ni [10].

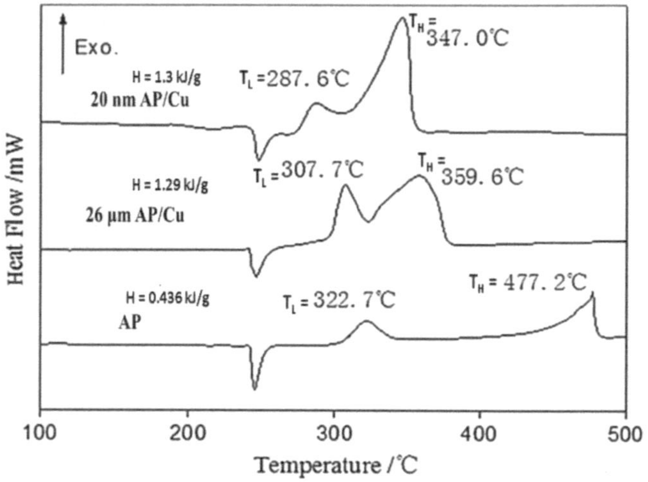

FIGURE 3.2 Graphical Representation of Variation in Heat Flow plotted against Temperature for AP/Cu [10].

From Figure 3.2, it is observed that the decomposition enthalpy of AP is the highest in the 20 nm Cu/AP solid composite propellant, when contrasted with the 26 µm Cu/AP composite propellant and pure ammonium perchlorate. The experimental values of maximum and minimum exothermic temperatures and heat generation illustrated in the graph is based on the nano-Cu content in AP, 26 µm AP/Cu and 20 nm AP/Cu i.e. 0 wt%, 1 wt%, 5 wt% nano-Cu content respectively and for 10 wt%, of nano-Cu content, the maximum and minimum exothermic temperatures and heat generation experimental values are 342.7 and 303.4 degrees Celsius and 1.3 kJ/g respectively. From these experimental values, it is observed that the nano-Cu content gradually incremented. First a decrease in the minimum exothermic temperature and then a sharp increasing temperature level at higher nano-Cu content is witnessed. However, in maximum cases, minimum exothermic peak temperatures of nano-Cu/AP composites were distinctly less in contrast with those of chaste/undoped AP. This phenomenon expresses the obvious influence of nano-Cu on the minimum temperature thermal disintegration of AP. Reversibly, with the nano-Cu increasing, the high exothermic peak temperature decremented step by step. After 10 wt% increment of copper nanoparticles, the T_H decreased by 134.5 to become 342.7 degrees Celsius. Moreover, the decomposition heat was seen clearly increasing up till 5 wt% then remained constant.

Thus, on AP decomposition, 20 nm Cu particles showed a better catalytic behavior in contrast with 26 mm particles.

3.2.3.3 Catalytic Effect of Aluminum nanoparticles with Ammonium Perchlorate

Aluminum micro particles are used to enhance the combustion properties of different high energy releasing compounds due to their high calorific value. Other reasons for choosing small sized aluminum particles for enhancing the combustion process for high energy releasing materials are due to its larger particulate surface area combined with its small size. Aluminum particles' maximum surface area can be utilized to catalyze the combustion reaction and due to their small size, can have maximum mobility within the matrix compound.

As demonstrated by the recorded observations, obtained by performing various experiments using nano/micro Al and AP, the following conclusions can be made. These observations are illustrated in the following figure:

The experimental values of maximum and minimum exothermic temperatures and heat generation illustrated in the graph are based on the nano-Al content in AP, 25 μm AP/Al and 30 nm AP/Al i.e. 0 wt%, 1 wt%, 5 wt% nano-Al content respectively and for 10 wt%, of nano-Al content, the maximum and minimum exothermic temperatures and heat generation experimental values are 420.7 and 329.6 degrees Celsius, 1.436 kJ/g respectively. From the results of the experiment, the decrease in maximum exothermic peak temperature is observed with rise in the content. The least minimum exothermic peak temperature is observed at 1 wt % of nano-Al and heat generated on decomposition increased between 0 and 1 wt % by 0.501 kJ/g, which was lower when compared to 5 wt % and 10 wt% of nano-Al/AP content, as shown by Figure 3.3.

Thus, on AP decomposition, 30 nm Al particles showed a better catalytic behavior in contrast with 25 μm particles, with increase in value of H, and decrease in T_H value.

From the three mentioned metallic nanoparticles in this section, the copper nanoparticles showed the best catalytic behavior at maximum exothermic temperatures followed by nickel nanoparticle and then again followed by aluminum nanoparticles.

3.3 NANOTECHNOLOGY ENHANCED MILITARY UTILITY ARMORS

The materials currently used in military vehicles are stronger in nature but they are also heavier because of the stiffness of the material. Here is where nanotechnology can help. It can provide the same structural properties at a lighter weight. They are also environmentally friendly and flexible in nature. The application of light materials is necessary in tanks, fighter jets, etc. [13].

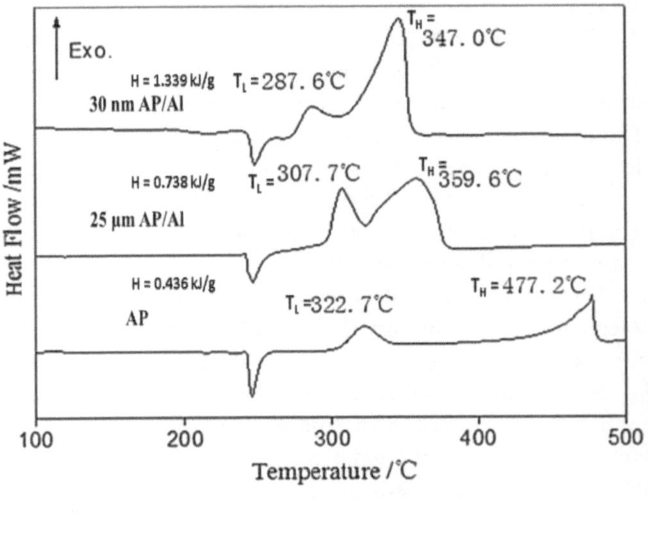

FIGURE 3.3 Graphical Representation of Variation in Heat Flow plotted against Temperature for AP/Al [10].

3.3.1 Polymers

Polymers are a part of our day-to-day lives. Any product that is a plastic or resin is a polymer, for example, many cell phone cases are polymers like Thermoplastic Polyurethane (TPU), which is flexible and durable in nature. The chemical body of a polymer is made up of a continuous chain of molecules. These chains will be in a linear shape i.e. a straight-line string or in a branched form i.e. in a cross-linked shape. To manufacture an armored polymer, it needs to go through a polymerization reaction so that it can modify its chemical properties through physical transformation for the production of the fiber. The structure of the polymer is made into a nano-metric scaled particle by introducing the nanomaterials in the following regions of the manufacturing process:

Nano-reactors: These kinds of reactors have existed in nature in the form of nuclei in cells. They are manufactured from a few kinds of viruses or molecules of polymers. They are the nano-container for chemical reactions to take place. By using a nano-reactor, one can understand the type of reaction and effect of spatial interaction taking place between the free molecules from which the researchers can design new materials [13,14].

Micro-reactors: These reactors are more commonly used for chemical reactions than the nano-reactors. Everything in this reactor is performed at a microscopic level. The physical structure of the reactors consists of three things – Micro-mixer, Micro-heat exchanger, and Micro-separator. It is commonly used because of the ease of design, construct, and usage. In addition, it allows scaling of the newer design of products at a lower cost.

Catalysts: They are the neutral materials that increase the rate of the chemical reaction without practically taking part in the reaction. But for polymeric materials, the physical structure can be affected and can improve the resulting properties. Nanomaterials are introduced to the chemical reaction to obtain small size particles. This can be done by scaling the size of the catalyst molecule to nano-meters.

Molecular Structure Design and Reagents: It is important to consider the chemical structure of the reagents for obtaining nanomaterials. For polymers, two factors are considered, selection of the aromatic rings and size of the molecular mass. The aromatic rings increase the stiffness of the polymeric material and the electric charges from these rings can increase the mechanical strength by increasing the crystallinity of the polymer [15].

Molecular Mass: The mechanical strength of the polymer can be determined by the molecular mass of the polymer, the higher the mass, the higher would be the strength and vice versa. Hence, it is recommended that the polymer must be of high molecular mass for military armor applications. For polymers like polyamides or polyester, there are two ways in which the molecular mass can be increased - Solid State Polymerization (SSP) and Swollen-State-Polymerization (SWSP) reactions. In the case of SSP, the polymer granules are dried in a vacuum chamber and the temperature is gradually increased. With the help of the vacuum, the remaining amount of oligomers are extracted. This process depends upon the type of polymer, the boundary conditions. In SWSP, a solvent is used to swell the polymer initially, and then only the oligomers are extracted from the granules under a vacuumed environment [16].

3.3.2 Carbon Nano-forms

The most common impact resistive material that we know of is steel, but there are other materials that have been discovered which are equivalent to steel or are higher impact resistive than steel. One such discovery is Carbon Nanotubes (CNTs'), discovered by Professor Lijima in the year 1991. Their impact resistive value is approximately 100 times higher than steel. Many other nano forms can result from carbon, which can be used as reinforcements for nanocomposites. CNTs' are of two types, Single-Walled Carbon Nanotubes (SWCNTs') and Multi-Walled Carbon Nanotubes (MWCNTs'). The size of carbon atoms is approximately less than 10 nm [17].

3.3.3 Nanocomposites

It is the combination of two or more than two polymeric materials along with either ceramics or metal. Composite manufacturing helps in introducing the separate properties of the material into a single product for the desired application. For nanocomposites, nano-fillers are introduced at the matrix level of the composite. These fillers are reinforcements. For the application of armored nanocomposites, they are required to be ballistic and flexible in nature [12]. The industrial methodology followed to manufacture a nanocomposite for armor based application is mentioned below:

Melt Processing: The filler and polymer are softened by the application of heat. This is a common practice followed in manufacturing industries but it is not suitable to soften polymers with high molecular weight and also with high stiffness values, which are commonly found in polyaramides having aromatic rings.

Mixing of the Solution: The polymer combined with the filler is dissolved in a solvent, later additional armor fillers are added into it like Carbon Nanotubes (CNTs'), and the solution is mixed thoroughly. Sometimes, CNTs' stick together and are not mixed well in the solution; this is why ultrasound methods are used to separate these CNTs' in the solution. As the mixture is stirred, heat is applied to it. Later the mixture is evaporated and is condensed back again for reusing it and the nanocomposite product is obtained from the mold. Considering the nano-scaled particles, the surface area increases during mixing the solution, thus the bond between the particles becomes stronger. Here is a clear reason why nanotechnology can help the future of manufacturing armored products [18].

On-site Polymerization: In the above-mentioned processes, the CNTs' were added after mixing the solution of the polymer and filler. But in this process, they are added at the very start of the process of polymerization, directly into the reactor along with a few reagents and mixed together. The entire process takes about eight hours to obtain a fine solution with strong bonds between the particles providing improved physical properties to the composite. Later, the solution is extruded in the form of fiber from the reactor using an extruder screw [19].

Alternative Method – Nanocomposite from Latex: There are many other ways to manufacture nanocomposites and one of them is by using latex, which is already a liquid state mixture of nano-scaled polymer particles of many different sizes. In this latex mixture, a nano filler is added into it and stirred thoroughly using a mechanical mixer. The pH levels of the mixture can be altered by adding acidic solvent or additives. After mixing of the solution, the latex starts to harden and the remaining liquid in the mixture is separated to obtain the nanocomposite from the mold.

3.3.4 Armors made of Smart Nanomaterials

A few nanomaterials are versatile in their functional nature. These materials are Smart Nanomaterials, which can perform autonomously to improve armor's lifespan. For military applications, they can provide protection to devices and to military personnel. In military terminology, these materials are reactive materials. They have a set mechanism to react against the impact. The armor includes a sensor, data processing or storage, communication, projection signal, and an actuator. The entire mechanism is situated in the strand of the nanomaterial [20].

3.3.4.1 Memory Materials

Just like human beings, materials like alloys, metals, ceramics, polymers, composites, etc., can exhibit a property called memory. This memory can make the materials return to their programmed shape. This recovery of the original shape is known as shape memory. The deformation of the shape is done by exposing the material to higher temperatures. Ceramics are very constrained when it comes to deformation as they are very fragile and are prone to cracking at a microscopic scale, whereas polymers are not so prone to cracking. Nano-scaled polymers that are cross-linked in nature can vary their shape with the help of variation in pH values of the material. Materials like actuators, possess electric field. For example, piezoelectric material is an electrical actuators. It can give out electrical energy just by the action of external forces. Following the preceding discussion, nanomaterials can be introduced for the protection of the actuator when woven into the clothing, allowing it to provide power to low powered instruments [21].

3.4 STEALTH IN MILITARY AVIATION AND NANOTECHNOLOGY

Nature understands stealth, and consequently evolved countless creatures whose survival depended upon blending with the environment long before "Homo Sapiens" discovered that it even existed. This idea of "not being detected" is crucial in military technology as it is more lethal and cost effective. I In nature a new born fawn in the tall grasses of the African savannah becomes camouflaged and undetectable as prey by hunters. A snake coiled in an area in a rainforest remaining undetected by enemy or prey alike is all because of its lack of the contrast so needed for ordinary detection. I In the military, exercises such as spying, reinforced infiltration, aerial reconnaissance missions/operations require stealth as a primary requirement. Throughout history we are aware of several military raids performed without even being recognized until the end. Many countries maintain confidentiality based on their ever-developing stealth technology [22]. The Spanish conquest of Mexico over Aztec people of South America also represents a fine example of military victory with stealth reinforcement [23].

Nevertheless, modern times have their own problems. Since the First World War (WWI), reconnaissance missions and spying have become a wide spread problem. WW-I. was the first time in history that aircraft and modern weapons were ever used Consequently, nations had to develop technology to bypass this problem of aerial reconnaissance and bombing. Engineers thus developed RADAR to counter the latter problem. In modern times, RADAR poses a high level threat to reconnaissance missions, interception of friendly aircrafts by enemy interceptors, friendly ships intercepted by enemy guided anti-ship bombs and radio-guided missiles, intercontinental ballistic missiles, supersonic cruise missiles and even space satellites equipped with radio jamming equipment. Moreover, radio signature by a friendly aircraft enables enemy aircraft missile's RADAR guided navigational abilities. This applies for surface to air missile ordinance and guided bombs (like the Luftwaffe's Fritz-x during the Second World War) which could be dropped from a bomber aircraft on a friendly navy vessel due to the vessel's radio signature [24].

3.4.1 Significance of Stealth in Military Aviation in post-modern times

It has been well understood that in modern times, the left overs of the radio and infrared footprints have dire consequences as they can be detected by normal monostatic RADARs we use nowadays. Even after these hurdles, air superiority is the first priority for any force operating on a mission. Following the Second World War (WW-II), when we saw the Youm Kippur (1974) war between Israel and the Arabian league, use of RADAR proved catastrophic for both the American and Israeli air forces as they suffered a high casuality of downed aircrafts as they were detected by the Arabs [25]. This could have been the other way around if the aircraft could have controlled their spectrum visibility through conventional monostatic RADARs. This proves that air-superiority is a key element in deciding the victorious course of war in modern times. The United States Department of Defense defines 'strategic air warfare' as "air combat and supporting operations designed to effect through the systematic applications of force to a selected series of vital targets, the progressive distribution and disintegration of the enemy's war-making capacity to a point where the enemy no longer retains the ability or the will to wage war. Vital targets may include key manufacturing systems, sources of raw material, critical material, stockpiles, and power systems [26]." It's also known that keeping an eye on enemy movements during a war is very important. To a small extent, its generally possible by aircraft (interceptors and special reconnaissance aircrafts). Aircraft over a battlefield provide a bird's eye view over an expanded range of enemy land which is crucial to attain air superiority or, air supremacy. Air superiority is defined by the U.S. Chiefs of Staffs as "That degree of dominance in the air battle of one force over another which permits the conduct of operations by the former and its related land, sea and air forces at a given time and place without prohibitive interference by the opposing force" [26]. It can only be achieved through reduction in aircraft's visible, infrared and radio electro-magnetic signatures (or footprints) in the airspace while flying above the enemy domain whilst operating.

3.4.2 RADAR-History and Principle of Operation

Axis and Allied nations developed RADARs in secrecy during 1934 and 1939 [27]. The initial theory behind the whole module was connected to radio waves. Even before RADAR, the microwave part of the radio spectrum was used in many navigational aids. The history of RADARs started in around 1886 with Heinrich Hertz's experiments with radio waves where he found out that these waves were reflected back after striking a metallic object [28]. In 1904, a German engineer, Hulsmeyer, registered a patent on using electro-magnetic waves in obstacle detecting and as a navigational aids in ships [29]. In 1922, Marconi proposed the use of "short radio waves" for radio aids [30]. Then, from this experimental and practical knowledge being in hand, the use and concept of RADAR equipment gradually rose. During this period, however, there was not any absolute use of RADAR technology. It was during WW-II that the importance of the concept was appraised. In that same year, when Marconi proposed his concept of "short waves", Dr. A. Hoyt Taylor and his associates in the U.S Naval Research labs were researching high frequency radio communication from one end to the other. It was during this time they discovered that there was a loss of interception of electro-magnetic wave signals when two ships passed between the transmitter and the receiver. This led them to conclude that their search (using radio waves) could be used to detect enemy ships [31]. Further study by Lawrence Hyland from the U.S Navy Research Laboratories in 1930 showed that it was actually practical and feasible to use RADAR to detect ships and aircraft by using continuous waves. He discovered however that there were fluctuations in his RADAR readings. He found out that this was due to all aircraft on low altitude while taking off or landing transmitting very small amounts out of their total radiated energy. This led to a conclusion by the experts that continuous waves were a failure conducting long-range airspace and coasts surveillance [32]. Continuous waves were however, considerations when the aircraft is high in altitude and only the short-range area was under consideration. This opened gates for researchers to quote pulse-wave RADAR surveillance to be far more effective than the regular continuous waves. During the WW-II, as Britain was under a constant threat of bombing of its settlements by the German Luftwaffe aerial fighters and bombers, it was in the hands of Britain to protect its people. Therefore, Britain realized the importance of the necessity of research in the RDF (Radio and Direction Finding) based early warning system against aerial enemy raiders Robert Wattson further developed RDF and RADAR (Radio Detection and Ranging) was praised for its military applications [33].

3.4.3 Concept of RADAR cross-section

The problem encountered while making an aircraft less isotropic (a theoretical point from which, any electro-magnetic radiation or sound waves propagates in the same intensity in all directions) to incoming long range radio pulses from monostatic or multi-static RADARs is a difficult challenge to engineers. To overcome this, engineers during the cold war came across a method to reduce the RADAR cross-section of the aircraft. The RADAR cross-section of any object is generally a measure of its visibility on the enemy RADAR.

A beam of energy radiates energy in all directions and spreads apart as it travels (though, the radiated energy's intensity remains constant throughout the course of its propagation as the RADAR itself is isotropic in nature). Now, according to the principle of RADAR operation, the emitted radiation hits the target and returns to the receiver, where it is then decoded. However, the amount of energy arriving back at the receiver is inversely proportional to the target's range raised to the fourth power. On calculations, one can find that it takes about 95% reduction in the left behind electro-magnetic spectrum residues by the operating aircraft to reduce the RADAR's detection/recognition capabilities by just 50%. In addition, 99% reduction in electro-magnetic spectrum residues left behind the operating aircraft to reduce the RADAR's detection/recognition capacity by just 67% [34].

The American F117-A is not the only military vehicle/craft to operate on stealth in human history. The German U-boat/submarine U480 may have been the first military aircraft to operate in a quasy-stealth mode. The German U-boat featured an anechoic tile rubber coating, one layer at which contained circular air pockets to suppress sonar.

As we mentioned earlier, for stealth, it is necessary for any aerial vehicle to reduce the amount or (if possible) dampen the amount of radiation reflected back by the craft. This can be done by reducing the RADAR cross-section of the aircraft in operation. The idea to reduce the RADAR cross-section of an aircraft first appeared when after the WW-II, a British bomber aircraft (Avro Vulcan) showed a remarkably small/minor deflection in the way the reflected wave reverted. According to government sources of 1963, the aircraft was occasionally known to fluctuate its position on the RADAR screen or sometimes completely disappear from the screen [35].

RADAR cross-section can be defined as the "hypothetical area that would intercept the incident power at the target, which if scattered isotopically, would produce the same echo power at the RADAR as the actual target" [27]. RADAR cross-section also depends upon a variety of other internal as well as external factors such as; (i) Material used over the skin; (ii) Overall structural design of the craft; (iii) Amount of dependence of electronic circuits and avionics on board the aircraft; (iv) Speed; (v) Exhaust from the engine nozzle; (vi) Distance from the transmitter/receiver; (vii) Terrain of location of the beacon and etc.

The RADAR cross-section can be found out by the following mathematical formula: -

$$\text{RCS} = \lim_{r\to\infty} 4\pi r^2 * \left[\frac{|E_s|^2}{|E_i|^2}\right] \tag{3.4}$$

Where,

'E_s' represents the scattering field;

'E_i' represents the incident field;

'r' represents range or distance between the transmitter and the target aircraft.

The unit of measurement of RADAR cross-section is same as that of area. [S.I units, m^2]. The Scattering of RADAR waves by improving the surface shape and structure of the aircraft is shown in Figure 3.4.

3.4.4 Nanotechnology in Improving Stealth in Military Aviation

To neutralize the effect of RADAR, the RADAR Cross Section (RCS) needs to decrease. As discussed in the earlier subsection, the RCS depends on a variety of factors; therefore, one can easily make changes in the corresponding factors of aircraft design. The primary design parameters where engineers make a difference is either in the surface structure (or shape) of the aircraft or choosing materials which are efficient RADAR absorbents. Other design parameters may include reducing the aircraft's RCS and subsequently reducing the aircraft's radio signatures.

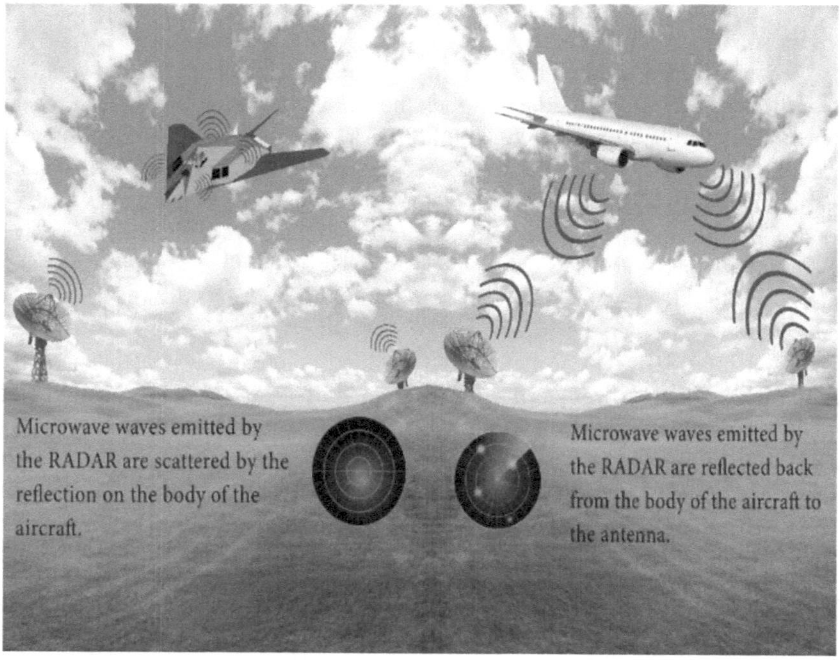

FIGURE 3.4 Scattering of RADAR waves by improving the surface shape and structure of the aircraft.

This can be done by minimizing the electronic utilities such as sensors and various amounts of avionics. However, this compromises the overall efficiency and performance of the aircraft and has a potential to produce unnecessary hindrances in the overall execution of the mission. Moreover, microwave absorbing materials is always in prevailing in the market, besides the military aviation department who use the network range of 1–20 GH like GSM, mobile telecom services, and satellite communications through VHF and UHF frequencies. Since these all services operate on the same network bandwidth, it is necessary to avoid hindrances with other networks within the same range. Therefore, it is always a better idea to shield them with radio wave absorbent materials. The RADAR cross-sections are shown in Figure 3.5.

In material science and engineering, we study the behavior of materials on micro and nano scales and subsequently engineer new materials, which possess physical properties, and material characteristics, which heavily depend on the configuration of particles or substances at these miniscule levels. Therefore, while designing a RADAR absorbent material, we tend to observe the behavior of normal light when it reflects back from a highly reflective surface (such as a mirror). We find that, maximum

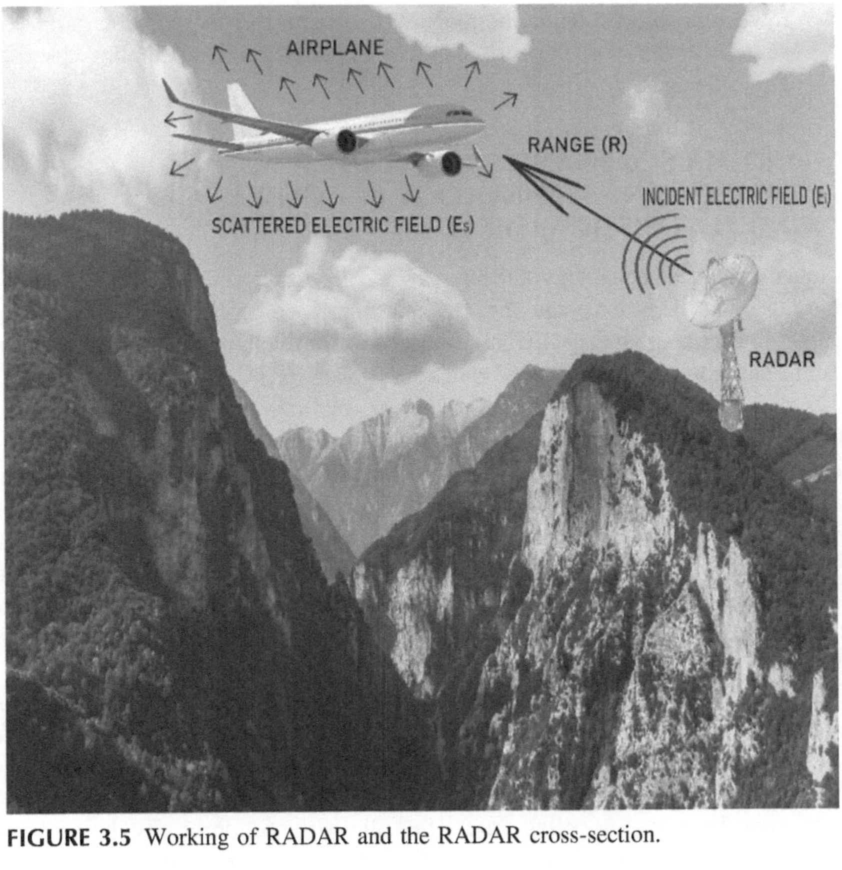

FIGURE 3.5 Working of RADAR and the RADAR cross-section.

reflectivity is obtained when light (being an EM wave) incidents on material at a right angle. The reflectance is found to be minimum when the light hits the material at more than 180 degrees. Similarly, we can arrange nanoparticles in RADAR absorbing materials to reduce the overall reflectance. RADAR generally uses microwaves. Microwaves are electromagnetic radiation, which radiate between 0.3 GH to 300 GH of frequency. The following are the types of RADAR absorbing materials:

Resonant absorber: It is thin and flexible to coat complex surfaces when compared to different absorbers; it is chosen in places where there is absolute no need of bandwidth. It is commonly used in stealth-based aircrafts as it improves the performance of RADAR and antenna patterns.

Broadband absorber: In contrast with resonant absorbers, where high energy is reflected from the back face, broadband absorbers require noticeable loss in network range such that the reflected energy from the back face is able to leave as a low energy reflection from the material. A material of a larger thickness in terms of wavelength can obtain this level of loss in network.

Magnetic absorbers: It can vary the absorption of microwaves. Example of this absorber contain the following micro or nanoparticles: ferrites, iron and cobalt-nickel alloy nano/micro particles. They are termed as effective microwave absorbers, when the magnetic properties of the absorber are strong. Magnetic properties like permeability can be used to calculate the absorption of microwaves.

3.5 FURTHER SCOPE AND PROSPECTS OF APPLIED NANOTECHNOLOGY IN CONTEMPORARY AND FUTURISTIC WARFARE

Attributable to nanotechnology enhanced material's variegated properties by its own virtues that possesses excellent material and substance properties like high tensile strength, impact bearing capacity, large surface area to volume ratio, outstanding heat resisting and conducting properties, and exceptional corrosion resisting properties. It makes nanotechnology deployable for civil and military aerospace in the next 10–20 years [1]. Contemporaneous studies and examinations in the nanotechnology regime of scientific and technological enquiry consist of the following issues: (i) Rudimentary or foundational nanotechnological phenomenon and processes; (ii) Further progress in the understanding of nano-materials (or nano-particles) and their subsequent applications in the aeronautical and astronautical industry; (iii) Advancements in further study of nanoscale electronic devices such as sensors; (iv) Nanotechnology relating to environmental and contemporary issues regarding environmental protection and human health and industrial safety protocols.

The utility of nano technology will provide us with tremendous changes in the contemporary warfare scenario. Advancements in nanotechnology will bring a vast and undeniable change in existing weapon and troop mobilization technologies such as: unmanned combat vehicles, stealth and camouflage, guided ordinance, lighter and efficient firearms, propellants etc. The following section briefly deliberates on some of the futuristic warfare hardware that utilizes nanotechnology to its aid:

Amphibious Rifle: It is a Russian concept of a gas-operated rifle that is supposed to neutralize threats on both water and land.

Counter Defilade Target Engagement (CDTE): It is a grenade launcher with semi-automatic type airburst launch maneuver with laser precision strike technology.

Extreme accuracy tasked projectile ordinance: This weapon is a projectile launch weapon that has homing technology to its launched projectile (bullet) to the hostile target.

Adaptive camouflage: It is observed that chameleons change their color to match the ambient color environment to hide from external threats. Likewise, nanotechnology can be utilized to create such a military uniform. This can be used to conceal firearms, armored armed vehicles etc to infiltrate enemy territories.

Universal human load carrier: This is the first instance of cybernetics used in the military by human soldiers. The concept of a universal human load carrier is to design a mechanical soldier outfit that can aid the soldier to carry war equipment that is heavy and causes a hindrance to troop mobility across battlefields.

Other novel technology adapted in futuristic warfare may include weapons like long range hypersonic missile systems, high power microwave weapons, laser weapons, particle beam weapons and much more [36–43].

REFERENCES

1. Edwards, E., Brantley, C. and Ruffin, P. B., 2017. Overview of nanotechnology in military and aerospace applications. Nanotechnol. *Commer. Manuf. Process. Prod*, pp. 133–176.
2. Richard, P. F., 1959. There's Plenty of Room at the Bottom. In Annual Meeting of the American Physical Society, (1959), December 29.
3. Davenas, A., 2003. Development of modern solid propellants. *Journal of propulsion and power*, 19(6), pp. 1108–1128.
4. Agrawal, J. P., 2010. *High Energy Materials: Propellants, Explosives and Pyrotechnics*. John Wiley & Sons, New Delhi, India.
5. Akhavan, J., 2011. *The Chemistry of Explosives*. Royal Society of Chemistry, Cambridge, UK.
6. Lengellé, G., Duterque, J. and Trubert, J. F., 2002. Combustion of solid propellants (No. RTO-EN-023). *Office National D'etudes Et De Recherches Aerospatiales Chatillon (France) Energetics Dept.*
7. Goebel, D. M. and Katz, I., 2008. *Fundamentals of Electric Propulsion: Ion and Hall Thrusters (Vol. 1)*. John Wiley & Sons, Pasadena, California, USA.
8. Kent, J. A. ed., 1992. *Riegel's Handbook of Industrial Chemistry* Van Nostrand Reinhold, New York City, USA. pp. 368–370.
9. Kumar, N. and Dixit, A., 2019. Nanotechnology-Driven Explosives and Propellants. In *Nanotechnology for Defence Applications* (pp. 81–115). Springer, Cham.
10. Li, F. S., Jiang, W., Liu, J., Wang, Y. J. and Hao, G. Z., 2016. Applications of nanocatalysts in solid rocket propellants. *Energetic Nanomaterials* Elsevier, Amsterdam, Netherlands. pp. 95–120.

11. Fengqi, Z., Pei, C. H. E. N., Dong, Y. A. N. G., Shangwen, L. and Cuimei, Y., 2001. Effects of nanometer metal powders on thermal decomposition characteristics of RDX. *Journal-Nanjing University Of Science and Technology*, 25(4; ISSU 119), pp. 420–423.
12. Gallardo, P. S. and Feynman, R. P., 2019. Nanotechnology-Aided Armor. Nanotechnology in the Defense Industry: *Advances, Innovation, and Practical Applications*, p. 109.
13. Xu, C., Xu, K., Gu, H., Zheng, R., Liu, H., Zhang, X., Guo, Z. and Xu, B., 2004. Dopamine as a robust anchor to immobilize functional molecules on the iron oxide shell of magnetic nanoparticles. *Journal of the American Chemical Society*, 126(32), pp. 9938–9939.
14. Hearle, J. W. ed., 2001. *High-performance fibres*. Elsevier, Boca Raton, Florida, USA.
15. Zhu, J., Ding, Y., Agarwal, S., Greiner, A., Zhang, H. and Hou, H., 2017. Nanofibre preparation of non-processable polymers by solid-state polymerization of molecularly self-assembled monomers. *Nanoscale*, 9(46), pp. 18169–18174.
16. Khan, W., Sharma, R. and Saini, P., 2016. Carbon Nanotube-Based Polymer Composites: Synthesis, Properties and Applications Carbon Nanotubes-Current Progress of their *Polymer Composites*.
17. Hazell, P. J., 2015. *Armour: Materials, Theory, and Design*. CRC Press, Boca Raton, Florida, USA.
18. Sainsbury, T., Erickson, K., Okawa, D., Zonte, C. S., Fréchet, J. M. and Zettl, A., 2010. Kevlar functionalized carbon nanotubes for next-generation composites. *Chemistry of Materials*, 22(6), pp. 2164–2171.
19. Wong, K. K. W., 2010. Transforming the military: the energy imperative.
20. Chang, L. C. and Read, T. A., 1951. Plastic deformation and diffusionless phase changes in metals—The gold-cadmium beta phase. *JOM*, 3(1), pp. 47–52.
21. Liu, L. L., Li, F. S., Yang, Y., Tan, L. H. and Zhang, Q. S., 2005. Effect of nanometer Cu powder on thermal decomposition of ammonium perchlorate. *Chinese Journal of Inorganic Chemistry*, 21(10), pp. 1525–1530.
22. Sharon, M., Silvestre, A. and Lopez Rodriguez, C. S., Nanotechnology in the Defense Industry.
23. Wilson, P. B., 2019. Tactical Missile Performance for Single and Multi-Wire Embedded Propellant Configurations with Discontinuities.
24. the awsemer. 2012. how via uses disguises. [ONLINE] Available at: https://theawesomer.com/how-cia-disguises-work/499424/. [Accessed 21 April 2020].
25. new world encyclopedia. 2013. battle of Tenochtitlan. [ONLINE] Available at: https://www.newworldencyclopedia.org/entry/Battle_of_Tenochtitlan. [Accessed 21 April 2020].
26. USAAF Wright Field Air Technical Service Command, T-2 Intelligence Department (1946). WF 12-105, Captured Film, 'Fritz X' German Radio-Controlled Dive Bomb. The Digital Implosion. Event occurs at 13:45 to 15:00. Archived from the original (YouTube) on April 27, 2012. Retrieved April 22, 2020.
27. Nordeen, Lon (1990). *Fighters Over Israel*. New York: Orion Books. ISBN 0-517-56603-6.
28. Joint Chiefs of Staff. Dictionary of Military and Associated Terms, Department of Defense, Washington DC, January 1986.
29. Virtualmuseum.Ca, C., 1843. *Sworn to Secrecy: Canadians on radar, 1940–1945*, 1st ed. Virtual Museum, Canada.
30. "Heinrich Hertz Produces and Detects Radio Waves in 1888." Science and Its Times: Understanding the Social Significance of Scientific Discovery. Retrieved January 05, 2019 from Encyclopedia.com: https://www.encyclopedia.com/science/encyclopedias-almanacs-transcripts-and-maps/heinrich-hertz-produces-and-detects-radio-waves-1888.
31. Hollmann, M. "Christian Huelsmeyer, the inventor," in RADAR World:http://www.RADARworld.org/huelsmeyer.html.

32. Marconi RADAR History/Franklin and Round. MarconiRADARhistory.pbworks.com. archived from the original on 25 April 2018. Retrieved on 25 April 2018.
33. L. A. Hyland, *RADAR pioneer, 92; Howard Hughe's Top Executive*. New York Times. 26 November 1989.
34. "Making waves: Robert Watson-Watt, the pioneer of RADAR". BBC. 16 February 2017. Archived from the original on 28 February 2017.
35. Bahret, W., 1993. *The beginnings of stealth technology*. 1st ed. United States: IEEE.
36. Sweetman, Bill. "The Bomber that RADAR cannot see." *New Scientist*, 4 March 1982.
37. New Hampshire Section/ IEEE/ AES society // aes.cs.unh.edu.
38. Figure by MIT/ OCW // aess.cs.unh.edu.
39. C. N. Ghosh, Directed Energy Weapons, https://www.idsa-india.org/an-feb-7-01.html
40. Kopp, C., 1996. *The electromagnetic bomb-a weapon of electrical mass destruction*. MONASH UNIV CLAYTON (AUSTRALIA).
41. www.electronicsforum.com. 2014. Directed Energy Weapons: High-Power Microwaves. [ONLINE] Available at: https://www.electronicsforu.com/market-verticals/directed-energy-weapons-high-power-microwaves. [Accessed 20 April 2020].
42. Kochems, A. and Gudgel, A., 2006. The Viability of Directed-Energy Weapons. *The Heritage Foundation Online*, (1931), p. 1.
43. Dunlap Jr, C. J., 2007. Air-minded considerations for joint counterinsurgency doctrine. Air and Space Power *Journal*, 21(4), p. 63.

4 Implementation of Nanotechnology in the Aerospace and Aviation Industry

Rameela Davanagere Ramesh, Anusha Santhosh, and Sarath Raj Nadarajan Assari Syamala

4.1 INTRODUCTION

The aviation and aerospace sector is considered to be one of the most significant heavy commercial enterprises. In such an industry, efficiency is the topmost priority and hence it is imperative to revolutionize the known material science. One of the many proposed ideas that was best suited to this industry is nanotechnology. Nanotechnology deals with matter at the nanoscale where the rules of traditional physics are not applicable. This endows nanomaterials with improved properties. Nanotechnology works with particles of the size 1 nanometer [nm] = $10^{-9}\,nm$ [1]. It has the ability to enhance the functionalities of current products. It is currently a booming industry, creating a wave of impact [2]. The unconventional combination of exceptional properties of thermal, mechanical, and electrical conductivities enables evolution of lighter weight and durable structures that could reform the concept of aircraft and spacecraft [3]. Due to these features, nanotechnology finds many applications in this area. In this chapter, we look into the role of nanotechnology in the field of aerospace and aviation and its further applications. Because of its ease of use, toughness, and prolonged material life, it finds use in sealants, adhesives, and nanocoatings. Nanomaterials, particularly carbon nanotubes (CNTs), are used for load-bearing structures due to their high yield and tensile strength, durability, low weight, and low maintenance requirement. Single-walled carbon nanotubes (SWCNTs), with their high thermal and electrical conductivity, are used to manufacture the components of nanoelectronics. There are many more implementations of nanostructured materials in the aerospace/space industry other than the aviation industry. Radiation shielding, energy storage and generation, heat shields, and self-healing materials are a few of the many applications in this sector.

As the concept of nanotechnology is relatively new, there is still more to explore in the safety realms. We deal with the risks and benefits involved in handling these materials on an everyday basis. Nanosafety training and protection methods have been summarized and discussed in detail. The futuristic scope of nanomaterials for the benefit of space exploration and better performance of the aviation sector has also been reviewed.

4.2 NANOTECHNOLOGY IN AERONAUTICS

Materials used for aircraft part construction should possess the qualities of high tensile and yield strength, corrosion resistance, and low weight, among many others. Focus has been drawn onto nanomaterials for the fact that they are light materials with good properties and are effective in making aircraft components that are in high demand, enabling them to be used for many applications throughout the industry. Ceramic nanoparticles, like barium strontium titanate, are used to make supercapacitors. Data-storage media employ various magnetic nanoparticles (iron oxides). CNTs can also be used to manufacture devices to store hydrogen [2]. The benefits of nanomaterials do not end here. Considering the advantages nanotechnology has got to offer, a perfect material with enhanced properties would be attainable, keeping the cost factor in mind.

4.2.1 Airframe Structures

There are a wide variety of applications of nanomaterials and nanocomposites that can offer excellent mechanical properties required for application in the aviation industry. Aviation requires a high level of perfection and attention to detailing, as it deals with the lives of people, and, therefore, the materials required for design and manufacturing need to be carefully chosen [3]. Materials that are used for the construction of aircraft parts should possess qualities such as high tensile strength, low weight, high yield strength, and corrosion resistance, among many others, which make them ideal for use in airframe structures [1].

Modern aviation demands more requirement of materials with exceptional multifunctional and mechanical properties. Carbon-based nanomaterials, like CNTs, are seen to be highly demanded, compared to other forms of composites available for use. They are used as fillers as they provide high toughness, strength, and stiffness along with appreciable electrical and thermal properties. They can be used to manufacture aircraft brake discs and self-healing composites. CNTs enhance the electrical conductivity of composite panels, thus making the aircraft less susceptible to damages from electric discharge. Self-healing nanocomposite materials could be efficient to construct vehicle parts [4].

Nanostructured metals also exhibit enhanced properties compared to their parent component. These metals consist of nanoscale crystallites; exhibit high yield strength and tensile strength; are intelligence-guided and smart; and have low density [4]. They can act as strengthening agents for load-carrying structures like frames or stringers. Nanocomposites can be combined with nanoadditive integrated ceramic matrix, which can prove to be a key for the radomes of hypersonic planes. Due to their collaborated properties of relatively low cost, barrier properties, and low weight, epoxy nanocomposites have shown to be a reasonable substitute to titanium oxide for use in nacelles of aircraft [5].

Currently, magnesium is the most employed nanocomposite, which exhibits desirable properties. It has also been suggested as a friction-modifying agent to allow easy movement of structures [6]. These include carbides, metals, and other ceramics. Various additives like multiwalled carbon nanotubes (MWCNT), SWCNT, ZnO, and nanoparticles and many others are used as they decrease UV degradation, reduce cracks on the surface of the component, and protect the thickness of the film. Nanomaterials can be used for their electrostatic discharge and electromagnetic (EMI)-shielding properties and provide solutions to structures that are resistant to lightning strikes [7]. The probable enforcement of CNTs in aeronautical fields can be seen in commercial airplanes such as Airbus A380 and Boeing 787 [8]. Passenger aircraft such as Boeing 747 and 767 consist of nanocomposite composition in parts of their control surfaces (ailerons, rudders, and elevators), fairings, doors, etc. [9].

4.2.2 Nanoelectronics

Since the past few years, nanoelectronics has been booming due to its capabilities such as light weight and reduced power consumption. Components used in the aircraft, space shuttles, ground stations, etc. need to be extremely reliable as they should be able to withstand intense temperature and pressure at any given time [2]. To make computers and electronic devices faster and powerful, carbon nanotubes are used, as they have properties similar to silicon and other semiconductors but can work at a molecular level as well, unlike the rest. Few of the properties that make nanotubes a good choice for this industry are their resistance to heat, high tensile strength, relative chemical inactivity, and good ductility. Graphite is an unusual material, as it comes under the semi-metal category. Combining graphite's properties with the quantum rules of energy level and electron waves, we obtain carbon nanotubes, which are excellent conductors. They are used in Boeing EA-18G Growler as well as in most stealth aircraft [10]. SWCNT is a game-changer for the electrical and electronics industry [11].

One of the essential factors in aviation is the comfort and happiness of passengers; hence, entertainment systems need to be improved. For instance, flat screens are manufactured using CNTs, which provide a wider viewing angle, lighter display, and lower energy consumption. For electromagnetic wave shielding and electrostatic dispersion in electronic devices, conductive plastics fabricated with nanotubes can be used. Aircraft weight can be reduced by replacing heavy copper wires with nanotube-improved plastics wires [12].

4.2.3 Sealants and Adhesives

Nanotechnology finds use in adhesives and sealants, predominantly for aircraft. Adhesives are products that act as a glue between various solid materials and help in surface reinforcement. Adhesives and sealants have an edge over other types of joining methods as they prove to be more effective than their counterpart mechanical fasteners by providing the advantages of low weight, labor reduction, ease of use, and many more [13]. These adhesives and sealants involving nanoparticles can easily outperform traditional coatings, due to their uniqueness in the industry. They can soon become an exclusive solution in the aeronautical industry.

Nanocoatings can be taken up as the next alternative in line offering additional properties of long life, hydrophobicity, toughness, durability, and oleophobicity [14]. These can protect the aircraft from different climatic extremities and atmospheres that can hamper the quality of the sealant in addition to providing a barrier from atmospheric contaminants. It protects the surface from harmful exposure to ultraviolet rays, bugs, and many other concerning factors. They also repel dirt, which contributes to reduced cleaning costs for the aircraft and other associated parts. It provides a lasting surface finish to the product and extends the shelf life more than an average sealant would. Its hydrophobicity finds use in deciding applications, which is one of the primary thoughts of line for an aircraft in flight [15]. Their weatherability translates properties of anti-icing to the fluid, which, in turn, proves to be beneficial to be put in practice. Additionally, ceramic adhesives are also delivered to bonds that require resistance to flex and vibration. Nanosealants are used in access doors, on fuel tanks, as well as in cabins of the aircraft as they offer exceptional resistance to unwanted leakage of fluids like oils and water [16]. They are also used as windshield and firewall sealants [17].

That being said, conventional adhesives and sealants also have a few limitations. They do not have an extended shelf life and contain resins that impair when exposed to solvents, heat, light, etc. To get the most out of them, they need to be on extremely clean surfaces [18]. They are highly reactive to ambient atmosphere, which limits their use in any extreme environment and exposes them to bacterial degradation. The only way of examining the component after the adhesive has been applied is by conducting a series of destructive tests. They fail to provide superior strength and can only support loads to a certain extent. This is where we require products that can promote the shelf lives as well as improve the mechanical properties and enhance their applications. A solution to this problem is using a radiant-cured adhesive. They are solvent-free and sustain more degradation than a regular adhesive. They can be used on small- and large-volume operations, equally imparting the same properties throughout. Water-based adhesives are also used, which essentially offer low viscosity to the adhesive to employ water as the transporter medium [19].

4.3 NANOTECHNOLOGY IN AEROSPACE

Nano carbon–carbon composites are used as a base in the aerospace industry, primarily for space vehicles, missiles, and re-entry shuttles. Nanotechnology has had a broad influence on advanced developments of energy-storage devices, self-healing materials, heat shields, radiation shielding, etc. This is due to its unique multifunctional aspects of increased sensitivity, large thrust fuel, low power consumption, excellent fault tolerance, and a lot more [2].

4.3.1 Energy Storage and Generation

Energy generation and storage needs to be dealt with at a microlevel to achieve the necessary results. This area, energy generation and storage, covers a substantial part of the entire vehicular system. A space shuttle has an immense amount of energy and data cables. This signifies the need for a revolutionary technology in energy storage and distribution. Major advancements have been made in storage devices, such as batteries, photovoltaics, energy supply, and many others [20]. The means of storage of energy will be of primary importance in future missions as they are going to be more prolonged and more self-dependent. Therefore, increasing the efficiency of storage and generation is taken as a priority. They are mainly established through minimization of mass and maximization of capacity and reliability. One of the recent methods of doing so is the latest photovoltaic cell that employs quantum dots and rods, which are linked together by CNTs. They are known to exhibit enhanced properties of energy distribution while in smaller proportions. Photovoltaic materials could also be used to gear up power generation [2].

Solar cells are used commonly as energy-saving tools to cut down on additional power requirement. Nanomaterials could provide a boost for this purpose. These can make solar cells work with more durability and efficiency. Proton Exchange Membrane (PEM) is another type of fuel cell that is used to serve as a boost to this energy saving. They provide the assurance of usage of improved materials, reliability, and optimization [21]. Nanotechnology provides systems with higher strength and lower resistance to energy flow, which is said to significantly increase the specific power. CNTs play a major role in flexibility of the photovoltaics used and improvement of the charge transportation to yield a higher amount of solar energy. These technologies are utilized in conformal methodologies and can be unified with outer assemblies of the vehicle or structure to deliver a supplementary source of energy to charge the onboard electricals. For batteries and related structures, nanostructured electrodes prove to be more beneficial in comparison to conventional lithium ion [22]. They can reduce the overall weight and enhance functionality. The main devices for storage of energy would be rechargeable, primary batteries and capacitors. Primary batteries have been found to be used in several planetary probes and capsules, such as Mars Landers (MER), Genesis, Stardust, etc. Orbital missions such as Mars Global Surveyor, TOPEX, and Mars rovers (Opportunity and Spirit) make use of rechargeable batteries as well as advanced capacitors for their missions [23]. The different forms of CNTs are shown in Figure 4.1.

CNTs have been replaced with copper wires to offer lighter weight in use and lower gauge. They are used in the energy-generation systems present in vehicular structures and Extravehicular Activity suits. Moreover, an additional advantage of CNT wires is that they are corrosion resistant and ductile, compared to copper wires. This makes them safer for application and increases durability [24]. Nanomaterials are being tested for their desirable properties. They have a higher surface area and greater reactivity in comparison with their traditional counterparts. This allows larger energy and power distributions. Another take on this technology is the technique of integrating numerous systems, which could offer larger mass

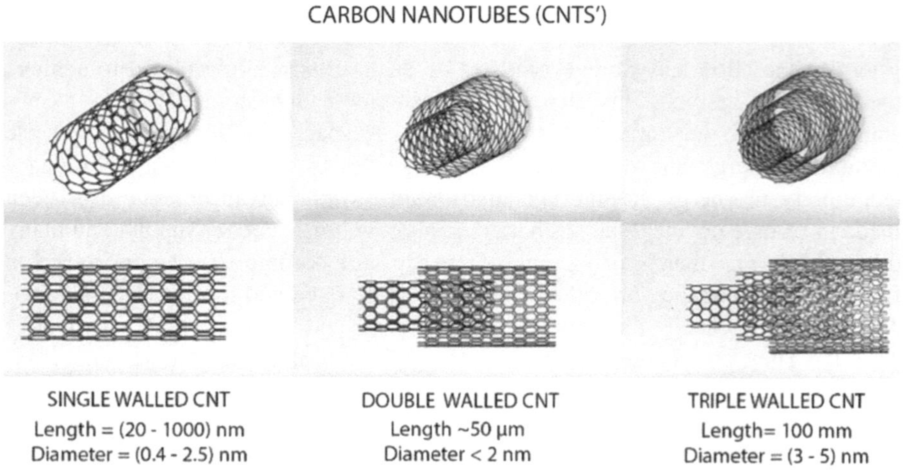

FIGURE 4.1 Diagrams of Different Forms of CNT.

savings compared to an individual system's savings on its own [25]. These could be further developed to make provisions for auxiliary power to the vehicle.

4.3.2 Self-Healing Nanomaterials

Self-healing of a material means the ability of the material to regain its structural integrity and repair its damages automatically [26]. However, in some cases, self-healing is induced by an external factor, such as temperature and pressure. Self-healing is extremely useful when we need to prolong a material's life or when repair or any kind of human intervention is almost impossible or formidable due to harsh conditions (physical or chemical). Due to these factors, self-healing materials are finding use in the space sector [27]. We know that space is uncertain and space debris is a huge challenge that the space industry is facing. One of the most shielded crafts right now is the International Space Station (ISS), and it is crucial that the craft be highly protected due to the billions spent on it as well as the lives of the astronauts involved.

The ISS, older spacecraft, and satellites used a type of shield called the Whipple shield. It consists of three layers, which are separated by a gap known as standoff. The outermost layer is known as the "bumper" and is composed of a narrow lamina of aluminium. The middle layer is a high-strength cloth whereas the last layer is the surface of the spacecraft. If any foreign particle impacts the bumpers, its speed is reduced and the force may even cause the particle to break up. As the number of man-made missions is increasing rapidly, the chances of collision are high; hence, there is a need for better protection [28].

Students from the University of Michigan came up with a solution: a material that can seal anything within seconds. This material is made up of liquid resin called thiol-ene-trialkylborane. It is sandwiched between two polymer panels that create an airtight seal. The resin remains as long as the seal is unbroken. If the seal is broken, the air inside the craft reacts with the resin and forms a solid seal that stops the loss of air from the craft. All this happens within seconds, which makes it extremely efficient to be used in spacecraft, spacesuits, etc. [29].

4.3.3 Heat Shields

Heat shields are designed as brakes of the spacecraft that prevent the overheating of the spacecraft by either absorbing, reflecting, or dissipating heat. This, in turn, prevents the spacecraft from crashing while it is re-entering the earth's atmosphere. Nanomaterials are essential for this process. The Mars Science Laboratory (MSL) spacecraft, which carried Curiosity, went through the most extreme atmospheric entry that ever took place. MSL was protected by a lightweight, thin, carbon-based heat shield material. This material is known as PICA [Phenolic Impregnated Carbon Ablator] and is widely used for heat shields by National Aeronautics and Space Administration (NASA) as well as Space Exploration Technologies Corporation (SPACEX) [30].

Researchers and scientists at the State Florida University have developed a lightweight heat shield using advanced nanomaterials that can endure the impact of hypersonic speeds as well. These shields are composed of a thin, flexible skin that can be applied to the airframe to protect as well as support the structure. These compressed layers are 500 times stronger than steel. Under the flame test, this material can maintain its flexibility and strength, while dispersing heat away from the base layer at temperatures up to 1,900 °C (3450 °F) [31].

4.3.4 Radiation Shielding

The space, as vacuum as it is, contains radiations like Galactic Cosmic Radiation (GCR) and Solar Particle Events (SPE). To top it all, the interaction of SPE and GCR with the superseding matter (space vehicle components like landers or the vehicle itself) produces neutrons, which need to be taken care of. Both GCR and SPE contain supercharged particles with high energy, which upon being struck can cause immense destruction. Neutron particles can emit gamma rays. Nanoparticles made of gadolinium have neutron-shielding capabilities. They have the unique property of having the cross-section of highest absorption of neutrons. For this reason, nanoparticles of boron can also be employed for the same purpose. A certain isotope of boron, boron 10, is used for the same and can even be considered better at neutron shielding than gadolinium. But heavier elements are exempted from use in shielding because they have higher atomicity, which can lead to production of further radiation when exposed to radiation [32].

The shielding from GCR can be considered the most challenging among all due to its capacity to react, even at small levels. This can be taken advantage of to use hydrogen as a shielding element. Hydrogen, in its pure form, cannot be used; hence, materials that contain hydrogen are used. A very common material is hydrogen bound with CNTs or particularly boron nitride nanotubes (BNNT). It is effective at fragmenting the high energy ions that are present in these radiations. But the main drawback would be its insufficient strength to be used for load-carrying structures in aerospace [33].

A lot is being done to improve radiation protection and to make use of the materials in the spacecraft body, which makes it multifunctional in terms of use as the hull and for radiation shielding. These materials need to be light weight and should be stable structurally. Boron nanotubes can be employed in the spacecraft hulls, which are nanosensor-integrated. These can help in quickly alerting the vehicle's electrical systems in cases of any changes in the surrounding [34]. Figure 4.2 shows environmental space hazards.

An area to be focused on in terms of radiation protection is the onboard electricals. The electrical systems are found to tolerate the radiations more effectively once their proportions are altered and decreased [35]. Lighter elements like hydrogen are effective for per unit mass shielding, and elements that are heavier can be used for per unit thickness shielding against Bremsstrahlung radiation and even electrons [36]. Studies have also proved that nanofoams can be an excellent tolerant against radiation due to their ability to divert any electrons that come their way, but they are still under observation and scrutiny [37].

4.4 ENVIRONMENTAL HEALTH AND SAFETY: RISKS AND BENEFITS

Safety is the primary concern with nanotechnology where human exposure is inevitable. The main concern is reducing the exposure of humans to nanoparticles. Nanomaterials can find their way into the body via derma, ingestion, and inhalation

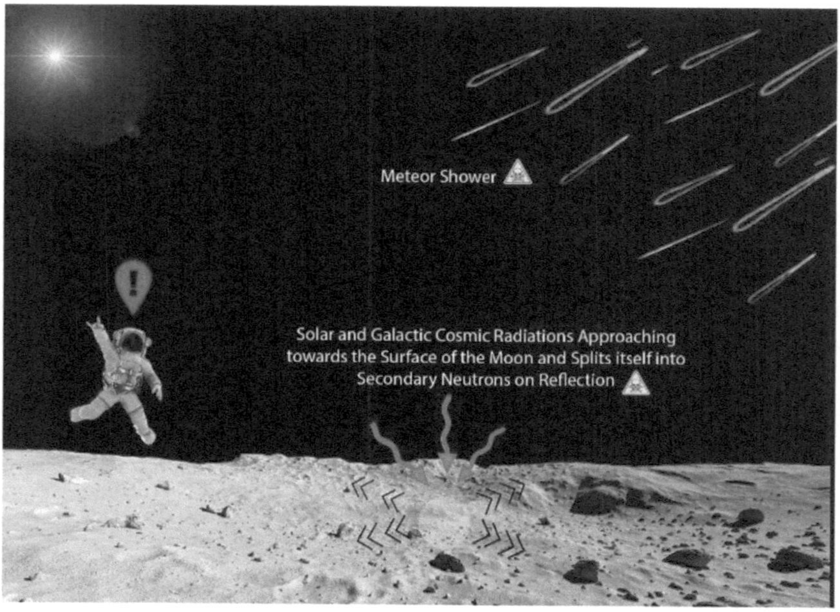

FIGURE 4.2 Environmental Space Hazards.

of particles, which can lead to asthma, cancer of the lung, colon and liver, bronchitis, Alzheimer's disease, heart diseases, etc. Materials such as platinum, gold, and silver, not being toxic at micro- or macroscale, can become fatal at nanoscale. The properties of nanomaterials vary highly compared to their larger counterparts, and hence the existing standards of Environmental Health and Safety (EHS) aspects cannot be applied to these. The working environment of those involved in the manufacturing of the same should be improved for the above reason [38].

4.4.1 Health Risks

People working at companies involved in manufacturing and/or using nanomaterials, as well as the laboratories that work with nanoscience and nanotech materials for research, come into close contact with these particles. It can be assumed with certainty that the current standard safety measures for the exposure of these materials cannot be applied to the exposure of these nanomaterials. It is imperative for these research works to take place as the known applications of nanotechnology are capitalized by industrial and commercial entities [39]. It is theorized that carbon nanoparticles move to the bloodstream from the lungs instead of releasing clotting agents. CNTs are presumably expected to have severe toxic effects on human health, such as lung cancer or asbestosis, as they bear structural resemblance to asbestos, which also causes these diseases [40]. For example, upon burning of waste such as batteries, textiles, etc., nanoparticles can be separated from CNTs. They don't breakdown below the temperature of 850 °C; hence, they can be inhaled or may be introduced into the food chain. One more example that can be thought of is the application and direct contact of nanomaterial clothing, which can penetrate the human body [41]. This is concerning as astronauts need to spend several months in contact with these materials.

The biological toxicity of some materials is given below:

- SWCNT [1.4 nm]: Temporary inflammation and injury to the cells at low exposure rate.
- MWCNT [10–20 nm]: High exposure results in degradation of immune cells in the lung due to alveolar macrophages.
- PEG quantum dots [10 nm]: The quantum dots retain in bone marrow, spleen, and liver.
- Alumina [116 nm]: It leads to the adsorption of protein Bovine Serum Albumin [BSA] with time.
- Quartz [1.5 × 10^{-3} nm]: Leads to high toxicity in the pulmonary region.
- Polytetrafluoroethylene [20 nm]: Results in cell death at mere 15 minutes of continuous exposure [38].

4.4.2 Safety Risks

The safety risk of nanostructured materials can be reduced by limiting the hazardous exposure of the nanoparticle [42]. The most serious and troublesome challenges that can be caused by nanomaterials are fire, explosion, and catalytic reactions. A few nanoparticles such as carbon-based materials, sulfur, hydrocarbons, aluminum, and magnesium, along with forming combustible mixtures and dusts, can also be responsible for the ignition for lethal fires and explosions [38].

4.4.2.1 Fire

Fire can be the outcome of contact of the nanoscale particle surface and dissipation into combustible gas, which is similar to that of explosion. There are different types of combustion reactions that arise from air-borne nanoparticles that depend on the rate of fuel consumption but they all are similar in terms of the duration, power, and speed [43]. In a broad sense, it can be assumed that for a fire to breakout in the workplace, three factors are necessary:

- Oxygen in the atmosphere as well as gases with peroxide and oxygen
- Flammable dust and organic/inorganic materials
- Ignition source to generate heat.

Lack of any one of these can prevent combustion; however, there can be substitutes of these factors, such as an ignition source, which may include chemical strikes and lightning strikes [44].

4.4.2.2 Explosion

When a nanoparticle explodes, it releases enough dust when the atmospheric conditions are just right. When nanoparticles become gasified, they may also lead to an explosion. When exposed to dry air and hot room temperatures, nanoparticles can be easily turned into a combustible mixture because of their exceptionally small size [38]. While warm air currents rise, they mix with the air and the absence of humidity prevents agglomeration. Accidental ignition can take place as the nanoparticles, if dispersed, are suspended in the air as a fuel and can easily react with oxygen, which is already present. This ignition can create a friction heat, flame, electric spark, or chemical reaction, which can cause combustion to take place [45].

Periodically, gas explosion can cause dusts that land on the surface and in turn cause a secondary dust explosion. This chain reaction can escalate pretty fast with increased volume and pressure in the surrounding and may lead to severe damage to property and disastrous injuries. This kind of explosion can be seen in underground mining activity where coal dust and gas interact in the air and explode when the right mixture is reached [46]. By understanding the growth and development of gasification into combustible gas, we can avert unnecessary explosions and accidents.

4.4.2.3 Catalytic Reactions

A few nanomaterials have nanopores that decrease the ignition temperature and increase the reaction speed. Any sort of spill or leakage of nanoparticles is extremely harmful as these incidents can cause a catalytic reaction that causes the manufacturing of these byproducts, which are lethal. Moreover, a few nanoparticles, while they come in direct contact with their surfaces, cause corrosion on aircraft materials, equipment, devices, etc. [47]. This process is known as nanocorrosion. The damage that happens at the molecular level can sometimes escape detection, which makes the structure vulnerable to failure, which is extremely dangerous for an aircraft [48].

4.4.3 Environmental Benefits

Using nanotechnology can benefit the environment in the right way and enhance its productivity. Eco-friendliness can be made most out of this technology, provided that the ill-effects of using it are taken care of. Benefits are, not limited to, reduction in consumption of fuel, thus saving fuel costs, environment-conscious outer coatings, etc. Nanotechnology has the potential to decrease raw material demand, thereby saving energy and water resources and minimizing greenhouse gases [49]. They have surely made a sustainability factor in the environment. Another positive impact on the environment can be the decrement of human footprint as technology evolves over time [50].

Nanomaterials portray a variety of unique features including that of high mechanical properties, prolonged durability, increased life capability, coatings that are water and dirt resistant, and many more, which make them a fascinating product to be dealt with. They are also made into insulation to improve energy competence and into lighter weight materials to curb the loss of energy during transportation [49]. Nanoparticles play a crucial part in water treatment. Nanofiltration is used for dealing with wastewater at various places. They help in controlling air pollution to an extent by using gold and CNT mixtures, which have the ability to absorb sulphur dioxide, carbon dioxide, and likewise, harmful gases. Particular nanosensors can be used to detect the pollutants in the environment, thus enabling us to take actions at the right time [51]. Thus, nanotechnology keeps in mind the customer's needs as well as the thought of a greener environment.

4.4.4 Safety Benefits

The main goal of using nanomaterials and particles is their promise of delivering a safe and sound environment to work with products. They improve the safety of aviation and aerospace vehicles tremendously. All products used on the vehicle are designed to enhance the comfort and safety of the passengers as well as crew on board. From the electrical systems to the nanoparticles used on the structure, they are all thoroughly investigated to ensure maximum performance and security to the assembly [52].

4.4.5 Nano Safety Training

Occupational exposure occurs usually during use, development of the material, laboratory research, and recycling or disposal of waste. Accurate training and education is imperative to all workers dealing with nanotechnology research, development, and manufacturing. They could also be trained to identify risky and unsafe materials so that they would be able to take precautions before opening them [53].

Training should also be provided to employees who are working with composite design as well so that they are able to create parts that don't require much machining and processing, thus reducing the risk involved. Industrial workers can start implementing a new process where the nanomaterials are kept in isolation to avoid contamination. If the nanoparticles are being produced on the site, then the least toxic material can be chosen and the process should be tailored to best suit its toxicity. Another precaution is called functionalization, which is a chemical treatment that can stabilize particles by coating them and making them less toxic [38].

4.4.6 Protection Methods

A necessity while working with nanomaterials would be Personal Protection Equipment (PPE) for all workers during the process of material processing, packing, and transporting. When present in bulk, nanomaterials forms finite powder. When used as a reinforcement or in a resin, they get agitated to become airborne and stay in the air for many days, even for weeks, which can affect the workers' health if inhaled [54]. After being impregnated with the resin, the final composite when machined releases dust along with other particles. Even the paint particles sprayed can pose an issue of inhalation or contact if not properly equipped with goggles, nitrile gloves, safety shields, and disposable suits in case of any process. Employees should also make use of respirators to filter the particles to avoid their infiltration into the body. Another point of focus apart from the respiratory issue is contact of the nanoparticles with the skin, especially when there is a cut or a wound that is open. Shoes that are anti-static can be employed to avoid setting sparks by accident to any nanoscale particles that might have fallen on the shoe [55].

The best way to prevent more contamination is to isolate the room where composite production takes place. One could also take a sample of concentration levels of nanoparticles in the air before and after the procedure to conclude the amount of dust particles the employees are being subjected to and then take necessary actions regarding their health aspects as well as to ensure a completely safe working environment. A High Efficiency Particulate Air [HEPA] type filter is used for nanoparticle filtration present in the atmosphere [56]. The equipment and machinery should be regularly kept clean of any dust that may land on them and can lead to short circuits, if in the vicinity of any electricals. If an Abrasive Water Jet (AWJ) has been used for machining, the water would then contain the composite dust, which could be drained leading to water contamination [38].

Active strategies for containment of the harmful particles produced at each level of production should be implemented for the benefit of the workers. A manufacturer should have a clear idea of the risks that a nanomaterial can impose on an employee and should educate the employee accordingly by mentioning the toxicity amount, degradation methods, and so on. The manufacturer should take a record of the measures undertaken in case a material becomes lethal with time. It is best that the personnel as well as the customers are less exposed to these particles in order to reduce the risk faced. Therefore, workplace assessment to ensure the conditions are fit to carry out nanoparticle manufacture is to be carried out [57].

4.5 FUTURE ASPECTS

The futuristic outlook of nanotechnology is promising for aeronautics and aerospace owing to its distinctive characteristics. Increased job creation and improved economy are the envisioned byproducts of this advancing technology. The forthcoming engineering science is predicted to be predominately established on nanotechnology. In this section, we look more in detail with respect to this regard.

4.5.1 Aviation

The future of aviation has a lot to offer in the field of engineering and with the help of nanotechnology, things have become more reliable and accessible. Materials that have greater strength-to-weight ratio and, at the same time a lower density, can be developed. Research is being done regarding the same. Nanocomposite materials mimic all desirable mechanical properties required in the industry, making it the sole solution to be employed. Nanomaterials would be able to address the essential necessities of flight like consumption of energy (be it fuel or electrical), comfort, and ease of travel. Hence, choosing the right material for the right purpose is of great significance. Ceramic- or polymer-based nanomaterials can upgrade the thermal and structural properties. Nevertheless, there is yet a lot to be explored for a wider range of usage in the nanoscale [58].

The use of nanotechnology can be extended to electronic and photonic devices. They can implement effective use of materials and technology in the most efficient manner making them cheaper, faster, and more reliable than before. The main advantage would be their power consumption being low and the mechanism being operational in stringent conditions. They are also used to manufacture biodegradable polymers with improved functionalities. These can be experimented on further to develop smart panels and converters that have greater structural integrity. Nanosensors can prove to be cost-effective. There will be challenges in changing the basic elements of nanomaterials into highly engineered concepts but the possibilities of nanotechnology in this industry will never end [59].

4.5.2 Space Suits

Space suits have been subjected to consideration under nanotechnology. Space suits should be protected from radiation in outer space. Also, self-repairing nanomaterials can be used to curb the issue of the astronauts denting their suits while traveling or at any time during a mission. These could be placed between the inner and outer surface of the suit that can patch up any puncture that can lead to oxygen escaping. Certain nanomaterials that have high durability and strength can be used to manufacture space suits, provided they are light weight as well. For this purpose, CNT composites could be used. The radiation is applicable to astronauts as well which is why nanosensors could be used to keep track of their health condition [60]. This could be fitted with the suit itself, which can give information about the astronaut's heart rate, blood pressure, and other essentials. This also could be worked out with bio-nanorobots fitted in the suits. They can fix any dents caused along with assisting the astronauts with the

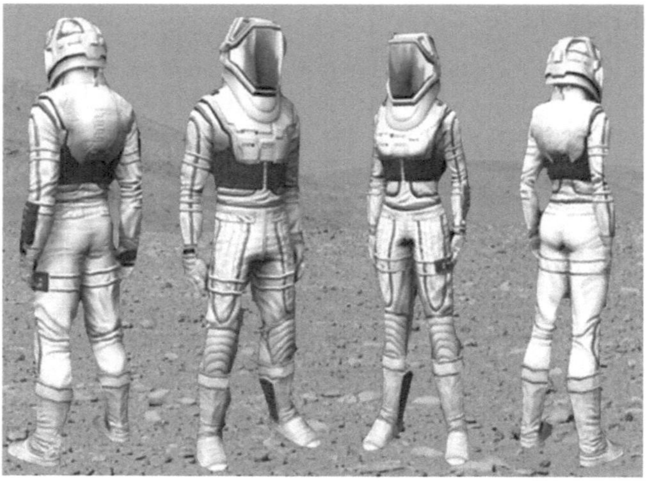

FIGURE 4.3 Conceptual Design.

necessary drugs required in case of any variations in their health condition [61]. The conceptual design is shown in Figure 4.3.

4.5.3 Nanorobotics

Nanorobotics is the study of robotics at the nanometer as well as macrometer scales that are capable of maneuvering items that have nanoscale dimensions [62]. Currently, we already have robots (rovers) on Mars – Curiosity, Spirit, and Opportunity. They are a great success in terms of space exploration, with the only drawback of being slow and the range of their movement being short. There is tremendous research being conducted using these rovers and their missions. But these rovers could come with a swarm of nanobots that once released into the planet would travel with atmospheric wind or across the surface into larger areas and would be able to collect more data in great detail and in a lesser amount of time [60].

Nanorobots can also find use in repairing space suits of astronauts while they are working, which stops them from going back to the station immediately. Using nanotechnology and AI, we would be able to create nanobots that can enable themselves to be self-sufficient and communicative with the ground station. Nanobots will be able to collect chemical or biological samples and communicate them with the spacecraft or the mission control station back on earth for further analysis [63]. For dense atmospheres or stormy gaseous planets where sending a rover is not advisable, nanobots can be deployed from the orbiter that can gather data about the wind current, chemical composition of the planets, and storm patterns and report its findings to the orbiter [60]. This would allow us to prepare for the next rover or man missions for the progress of humanity.

4.5.4 Space Elevators

Another take on nanotechnology in space applications could be in building a space elevator. This device could potentially act as a machine for delivering cargo directly to space. This reduces intermittent costs of fuel or any worries regarding power consumption as they employ solar cells. These could hypothetically travel about 90000 km with freight and back the same distance. They are held with the help of cables which could be made of CNTs which would provide the required strength and toughness along with other properties. This elevator will be connected to an anchor that will be put in the earth's orbital rotation and at the same time, the bottom of the elevator will be linked to a station back on the earth. The elevator supports individual segments (like brackets) powered by the solar cells to travel vertically like a monorail. It is a very cost-efficient project in many perspectives. This is just one of the ideas put forth, and this design consists of several flaws and is currently under detailed consideration [64]. The space elevators are shown in Figure 4.4.

4.5.5 Space Colonization

Space exploration can be tricky and risky and compared to the technology that we currently possess, it is extremely inefficient. Considering the amount of money spent on space missions, and the lives of astronauts and satellites lost, we would say that we need a new and refreshing technology to prevent these disasters from happening again. Nanotechnology keeps proving to be a game changer in every industry possible. Using these nanomaterials for the colonization of Mars or any other planet will be extremely efficient as their properties allows us to take on the next phase of space exploration. Few of the applications where nanotechnology could be used are for life support environments, propulsive fuels, structural materials, etc. [65]. Water is thought to be absent on M ars as it has no water bodies

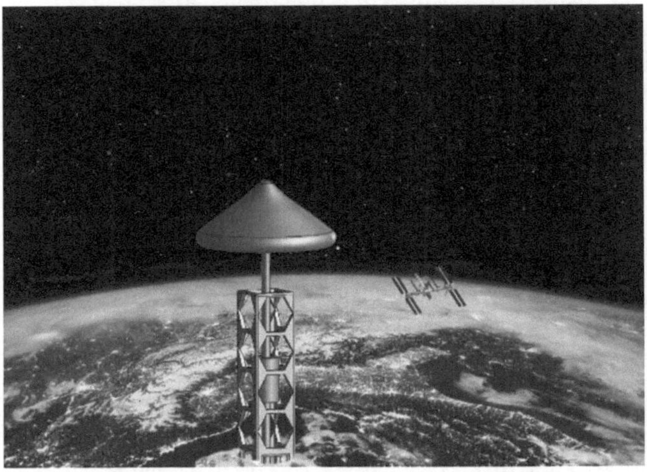

FIGURE 4.4 Space Elevators.

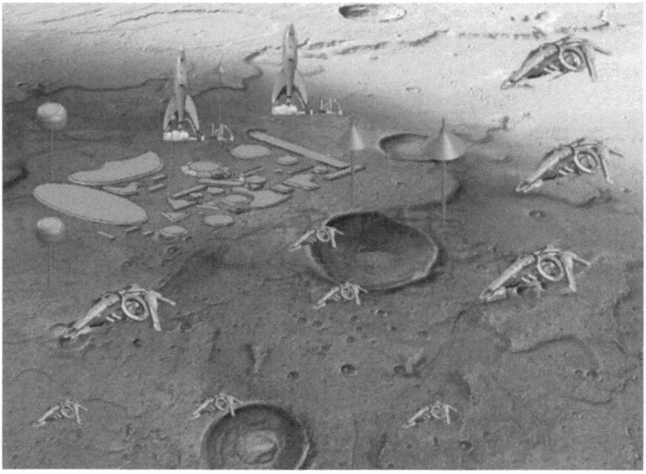

FIGURE 4.5 Space Colonization.

compared to the Earth. But latest research from NASA explores water deposits which could possibly be of aid to human exploration [66]. The space colonization is depicted in Figure 4.5.

4.6 CONCLUSION

Nanoscience is an empowering technology, which affects the aerospace and aviation industry and brings about advancements in composites, electronics, manufacturing, etc. Overall, these sectors are expected to enforce nanostructured materials on a massive scale in the near future. Nanomaterials have properties of corrosion resistivity, reusability, and low maintenance, which makes them more durable, enabling them to find applications in this field of action. There are a number of applications of nanocomposites and materials, taking into consideration the desirable properties they provide. Safety of the workplace should be the primary concern when dealing with a new technology. Complete responsibility must be taken by the employer of the organization to ensure the protection of staff and machinery at all times. Technology is still being looked upon from different perspectives and more is being done to improve its usability. Keeping in mind the limitations it possesses, we can be rest assured that there is still going to be an increment in its utility. It is certain that by the next 20 years, we can see the rise of nanotechnology in various fields of applications and this science will develop into a full-fledged technology.

REFERENCES

1. Meyyappan, M. (2007). "Nanotechnology in aerospace applications (No. RTO-EN-AVT-129BIS)", MM Associates, Moffett Field, CA.
2. Meador, M. A., Files, B., Li, J., Manohara, H., Powell, D. and Siochi, E. J. (2010). *Draft Nanotechnology Roadmap*: National Aeronautics and Space Administration.

3. Khan W., Sharma, R. and Saini, P. (2016). "Carbon nanotube-based polymer composites: Synthesis, properties and applications", *Carbon Nanotubes - Current Progress of their Polymer Composites.*
4. Mathew, J., Joy, J. and George S. C. (2019). "Potential applications of nanotechnology in transportation: A review", *Journal of King Saud University - Science*, 31(4), pp. 586–594.
5. Kumar, I. (2015) "NANOCRAFT- An Aircraft with Nanotechnology", *International Journal for Research in Applied Science & Engineering Technology (IJRASET)*, 3(2), pp. 1–6.
6. Senesky, D. G. and Koehne, J. E. (2016). "Nanotechnology for Aerospace, USA",
7. Reinste Nano Ventures. (2020). Available at: http://www.reinste.com/pdf/Nanomaterials%20for%20Aviation.pdf (Accessed: 18th April 2020).
8. Saito, Y. and Uemura, S. (2000). "Field emission from carbon nanotubes and its application to electron sources", *Carbon*, 38, pp. 169–182.
9. Cheung, K. C. and Gershenfeld, N. (2013). "Reversibly assembled cellular composite materials", *Science*, 341, pp. 1219–1221.
10. Nath, V. and Mandal, J. K. (2018). *Nanoelectronics, Circuits and Communication Systems: Proceeding of NCCS 2017*, Vol. 511, Springer, Singapore.
11. Garber, C. (2020). "Nanotechnology circuit boards", Available at: https://www.nanowerk.com/spotlight/spotid=3316.php (Accessed: 13th April 2020).
12. Thandlawala, A. "NanoTechnology in aerospace", [Online]. Available at: https://www.academia.edu/6781200/NANOTECHNOLOGY_IN_AEROSPACE (Accessed: 10th April 2020).
13. Yadav, T. and Vecoven, A. (2015). "Adhesives and sealants nanotechnology", PPG Industries Ohio Inc. , U.S. Patent 8,932,632.
14. Ultimate Paint Protection (2020). Available at: https://www.ultimatepaintprotection.aero/ (Accessed: 20th April 2020).
15. Nano Drops (2017). "WhaT Is Nano Coating?, Available at: https://nanodrops.co.uk/about-us/what-is-nano-coating.html.
16. Pröbster, Manfred. (2009). "Formulations, properties and applications", *Adhesion: Adhesives & Sealants*, 6(4), pp. 16–20.
17. Klososki, J. M. and Wolf, A. T. (2009). "The history of sealants", *Handbook of Sealant Technology*. Mittal, K. L. and A. Pizzi, (eds.). CRC Press, Boca Raton, FL, p. 4.
18. MASTERBOND (2020). "Advantages of Adhesives Over Mechanical Assembly", Available at: https://www.masterbond.com/techtips/advantages-adhesives-over-mechanical-assembly (Accessed: 17th April 2020).
19. Frost, S. (2020). "Nanocoatings for the Aerospace Industry", Available at: https://www.aerospacemanufacturinganddesign.com/article/aerospace-manufacturing-design-nanotechnologies-frost-sullivan-amd-032811/ (Accessed: 17th April 2020).
20. Kamaruddin, K. (2016). *Graphene and Nanotechnology Applications for Space Technology*, Malaysia.
21. Ginter, S., et al. (1998). "Spacecraft energy storage systems", *IEEE Aerospace and Electronic Systems Magazine*, 13(5), pp. 27–32.
22. Smay, J. W. (18 March 1997). "Spacecraft energy storage, attitude steering and momentum management system", U.S. Patent No. 5,611,505.
23. Surampudi, R. (2017). "Energy Storage Technologies for Future Planetary Science Missions".
24. Robinson, W., et al. (1997). "Spacecraft energy storage systems", Proceedings of the IEEE 1997 National Aerospace and Electronics Conference. NAECON 1997 IEEE Vol. 2.
25. Gandel, M. G. (1978). "Energy storage requirements for spacecraft", *Journal of Power Sources*, 3, pp. 277–289.
26. Zhai, L., Narkar A. and Ahn K. (2019). "Self-healing polymers with nanomaterials and nanostructures", *Nano Today*, 30, p. 100826.
27. Vincenzo, A. and Moreno, M. (2009). "Self-healing at the nanoscale", 1, pp. 74–88.

28. Hofmann, D. C., Hamill, L., Christiansen, E. and Nutt, S. (2015). "Hypervelocity impact testing of a metallic glass-stuffed whipple shield", *Advanced Engineering Materials*, 17(9), pp. 1313–1322.
29. Whitwam, R. (2015). "Self-healing material could patch up damaged spacecraft in under a second", Available at: https://www.extremetech.com/extreme/213063-self-healing-material-could-patch-up-damaged-spacecraft-in-under-a-second.
30. Roberts, G. Jr. (2017). "The heat is on", Available at: https://newscenter.lbl.gov/2017/02/22/building-heat-shield-mars-mission/.
31. David, S. (2020). "Carbon nanotubes key to next-gen heat shields for hypersonic aircraft", Available at: https://newatlas.com/good-thinking/carbon-nanotubes-buckypaper-heat-shield-hypersonic-fsu/.
32. Thibeault, S. A., Kang, J. H., Sauti, G., Park, C., Fay, C. C. and King, G. C. (2015) "Nanomaterials for radiation shielding", *Mrs Bulletin*, 40(10), pp. 836–841.
33. Roco, M. C. (2007). "National nanotechnology initiative. Past, present, future", In Goddard III, W., Brenner, D., Lyshevski, S. and Iafrate, G. (eds.). *Handbook of Nanoscience, Engineering and Technology* (2nd ed.), Taylor and Francis Group, Boca Raton, FL, Chap 3, pp. 1–26.
34. Taylor-Smith, K. (2018). "What Nanomaterials Are Used in Space?", Available at: https://www.azonano.com/article.aspx?ArticleID=4983.
35. Nanotechnology in Space (2020). Available at: https://www.nanowerk.com/nanotechnology-in-space.php (Accessed: 20th April 2020).
36. Spillantini, P., et al. (2000) "Radiation shielding of spacecraft in manned interplanetary flights", *Nuclear Instruments and Methods in Physics Research Section A: Accelerators, Spectrometers, Detectors and Associated Equipment*, 443(2–3), pp. 254–263.
37. Cummings, B. C. (28 June 1994). "Radiation shielding for spacecraft components", U.S. Patent No. 5,324,952.
38. Haynes, H. and Asmatulu, R. (2013). "Nanotechnology safety in the aerospace industry", *Nanotechnology Safety*, Elsevier, pp. 57–72.
39. Hoyt, V. W. and Mason, E. (2008). "Nanotechnology: Emerging health issues", *Journal of Chemical Health and Safety*, 15(2), pp. 10–15.
40. Ray, P. C., Yu, H., and Fu, P. P. (2009). "Toxicity and environmental risks of nanomaterials: challenges and future needs".
41. Nasrollahzadeh, M. and Sajadi, S. M. (2019). "Risks of Nanotechnology to human life", *Chemical Society Reviews*, 48(18), pp. 4791–4822.
42. Morose, G. (2010). "The 5 principles of "design for safer nanotechnology", *Journal of Cleaner Production*, 18(3), pp. 285–289.
43. Olawoyin, R. (2018). "Nanotechnology: The future of fire safety", *Safety Science*, 110, pp. 214–221.
44. Zhang, Bangwei, et al. (2011). "Environmental impacts of nanotechnology and its products", Proceedings of the 2011 Midwest Section Conference of the American Society for Engineering Education.
45. Marchant, G. E., Sylvester, D. J. and Abbott, K. W. (2008). "Risk management principles for nanotechnology", *Nanoethics*, 2(1), pp. 43–60.
46. Oberdörster, G. (2010). "Safety assessment for nanotechnology and nanomedicine: concepts of nanotoxicology", *Journal of Internal Medicine*, 267(1), pp. 89–105,
47. Liu, X., Wang, D. and Li, Y. (2012). "Synthesis and catalytic properties of bimetallic nanomaterials with various architectures", *Nano Today*, 7(5), pp. 448–466.
48. An, K. and Somorjai, G. A. (2015). "Nanocatalysis I: synthesis of metal and bimetallic nanoparticles and porous oxides and their catalytic reaction studies", *Catalysis Letters*, 145(1), pp. 233–248.
49. Nanotechnology and the Environment (2020). Available at: https://www.nanowerk.com/nanotechnology-and-the-environment.php (Accessed: 21st April 2020).

50. AZoNano (2009). "Nanotechnology – What are the Environmental Benefits of Nanotechnology", Available at: https://www.azonano.com/article.aspx?ArticleID=2354 (Accessed: 21st April 2020).
51. Ray, U. (2019). "The Environmental Impact of Nanotechnology", Available at: https://www.azonano.com/article.aspx?ArticleID=5114 (Accessed: 21st April 2020).
52. Rothblatt, M. (2014). "Aviation regulation as a model for nanotech regulation", *Journal of Geoethical Nanotechnology*, 9(1), pp. 74–78.
53. Castranova, V., Schulte, P. A. and Zumwalde, R. D. (2013). "Occupational nanosafety considerations for carbon nanotubes and carbon nanofibers", *Accounts of Chemical Research*, 46(3), pp. 642–649.
54. Asmatulu, R., Nguyen, P. and Asmatulu, E. (2013). "Nanotechnology safety in the automotive industry", *Nanotechnology Safety*, Elsevier, pp. 57–72.
55. Khan, W. S. and Ramazan, A. (2013). "Nanotechnology emerging trends, markets, and concerns", *Nanotechnology Safety*, Elsevier, pp. 1–16.
56. Schulte, P. A. and Salamanca-Buentello, F. (2007). "Ethical and scientific issues of nanotechnology in the workplace", *Environmental Health Perspectives*, 115(1), pp. 5–12.
57. Schulte, P. A., Geraci, C. L., Hodson, L., Zumwalde, R., Castranova, V., Kuempel, E., and Murashov, V. (2010). "Nanotechnologies and nanomaterials in the occupational setting", *Archive of Issues*, (2).
58. Burger, M. (2010). "Nanotechnology and The Future of Advanced Materials", Available at: https://www.nanowerk.com/spotlight/spotid=16047.php (Accessed: 20th April 2020).
59. Benefits and Applications, Available at: https://www.nano.gov/you/nanotechnology-benefits (Accessed: 20th April 2020).
60. Brown, M. (2018). "How Nanotech Will Help Us Explore Other Planets", Available at: https://www.engineering.com/DesignerEdge/DesignerEdgeArticles/ArticleID/17828/How-Nanotech-Will-Help-Us-Explore-Other-Planets.aspx.
61. (2019). "Nanotechnology in Space", Available at: https://www.understandingnano.com/column-space.htm (Accessed: 19th April 2020).
62. Kumar, B. (2017). "Nanorobotics: The modern era of robotics", *International Research Journal of Management Science and Technology*, 8(10).
63. Chui, B. and Kissner, L (2000). *Nanorobots for mars eva repair (No. 2000-01-2478).* SAE Technical Paper.
64. Edwards, B. C. and Westling, E. A. (2003). *The space elevator*. BC Edwards.
65. Aithal, P. S. (2016). "Nanotechnology Innovations & Business Opportunities: A Review", *International Journal of Management, IT and Engineering*, 6(1), pp. 182–204.
66. Gebhardt, C. (2019). "For Mars Colonization, New Water Map May Hold Key of Where to Land", Available at: https://www.nasaspaceflight.com/2019/12/mars-colonization-new-water-map-hold-key-land/.

5 Nanotechnology Applications in the Sectors of Renewable Energy Sources

Parul Gaur

5.1 INTRODUCTION

Renewable energy sources (RESs) such as solar, geothermal, wind, and ocean thermal energies are very popular nowadays for the generation of clean energy. Initially, energy was generated using the non-RESs, which imposed serious implications on the environment such as global warming, biosphere and geosphere destruction, and ozone layer depletion. Therefore, the generation of energy using the non-RESs can be considered very harmful in terms of its harsh impact on the environment and population. However, RESs are the sources of clean energy, having no bad impact on the environment. Global demand for clean energy is increasing day by day. Due to a huge global demand for this energy, RESs are most widely used nowadays [1]. RESs are the clean sources of energy in comparison with nuclear energy and fossil fuels. Moreover, RESs play a crucial role in reducing the emission of pollutants to the environment. Figure 5.1 depicts some of the uses of RESs.

With the advancement in technology, a new field of science known as nanotechnology has grown rapidly. Nanotechnology has been gaining more attention than others due to its technological and engineering applications. The term nanotechnology is used to describe the materials and structures at nanoscale, which means the devices and structures with the dimensions in the range of 1–100 nm. Generally, nanoscale range lies between 1 and 100 nm and the structures within the nanorange are known as nanostructures. Nanostructures also require lesser energy due to the reduction in size. Nanotechnology-based structures offer numerous advantages for renewable energy applications such as (i) increase in electrical storage capacity; (ii) generation of energy without polluting the environment; and (iii) reduction in size of the product. Considering all these factors, nanotechnology has become the prominent field in the applications of RESs [2,3]. Due to nanomaterials, the efficiency of the products is increasing largely while the production cost is decreasing considerably. Some of the examples of nanomaterials are illustrated in Figure 5.2.

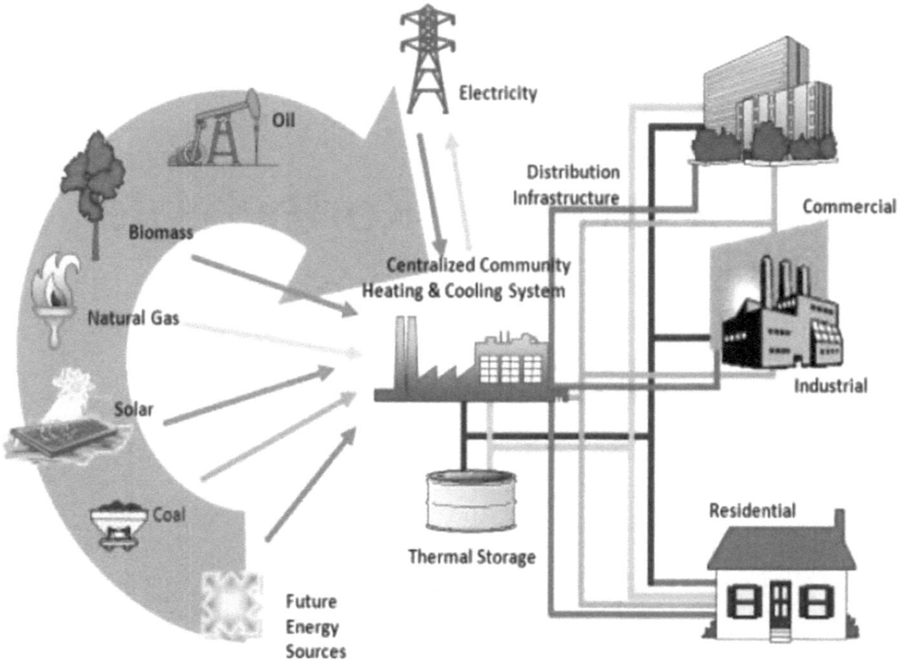

FIGURE 5.1 Applications of Renewable Energy Sources [1].

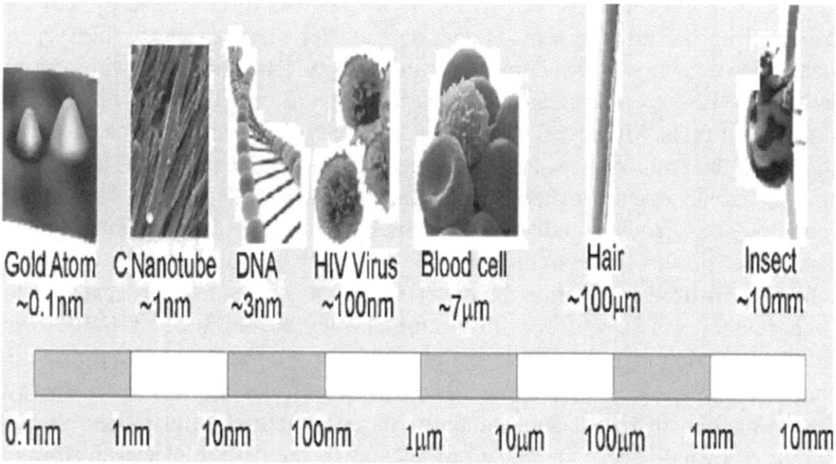

FIGURE 5.2 Length Scale and Nanomaterials [3].

Research is ongoing on the effect and significant applications of nanotechnology to enhance the growth of renewable energy industry. Nanomaterials are now being used in solar energy, bio energy, hydrogen energy, tidal/water energy, and geothermal energy [4,5]. Moreover, to improve the RESs, nanotechnology is finding a significant place for various improvements, e.g. the efficiency of wind energy is increased with the light and rotor blade strength can be improved using the nanomaterials. Corrosion in tidal energy equipment can be prevented using nanocoatings. To make drilling machines more resistant to fatigue in geothermal energy, nanocomposites are used. In fact, nanotechnology has made RESs more useful in terms of longer lifespan, increased efficiency, and overall improvement of the system. Some of the solar-based applications of nanomaterials include the manufacturing of ink-sensitized solar cell, improvement of the performance of solar water heater, and design of electrospun semiconducting nanofibers, etc. [6].

Nanotechnology is also very helpful to improve the economies in terms of increase in energy efficiency and development and implementation of new approaches, materials, and techniques based on RESs with numerous applications in different working areas. Nanotechnology is very effective for RESs. In fact, nanotechnology and RESs along with energy efficiency are the significant support for the sustainable energy. In this chapter, numerous significant nanotechnology applications in RESs are presented. Contributions of nanotechnology toward the implementation and development of RESs have been discussed. Nanotechnology promotes the use of more and more RESs for the betterment of mankind and environment [7]. Moreover, the solutions to the challenges such as how to increase the production and usage of energy without affecting the environment using the nanotechnology have been elaborated.

5.2 PRESENT SCENARIO OF RENEWABLE ENERGY SOURCES

RESs are now the major sources of power across the world. Around 1 GW renewable power capacity was deployed in 90 countries and more than 10 GW was deployed in 30 countries for the year 2018 [5]. In the past years, more and more renewable power capacity was deployed in comparison with nuclear power and fossil fuel. In fact, RESs are now responsible for above one-third of global power capacity. Main benefactor of renewable energy sector is hydropower and is increasing rapidly in the power sector as compared to any other RESs. Other renewable sources such as geothermal power, bio power, and solar power are also contributing to the power sector. In fact, technologies based on renewable energy have proven to be very reliable and efficient. Successful integration of RESs with the grid has also been done. As per 2018 report, at least nine countries have produced greater than 20% of electricity with the aid of RESs such as wind power and solar photovoltaic power [8]. Figure 5.3 demonstrates the additions in the capacity of renewable power annually from the year 2012 to 2018 as per 2019 global status report [5]. Presently, RESs are most widely used for meeting the worldwide energy demand. But, these RESs are expected to get extinct by the year 2100. Therefore, there will be a need of unconventional energy sources and to improve the present technology further. Nanotechnology field and the nanomaterials will be very beneficial to improve these RESs [9]. The renewable power capacities are discussed in Figure 5.3. In the subsequent sections, the importance and implementation of nanotechnology in sector of RESs are discussed.

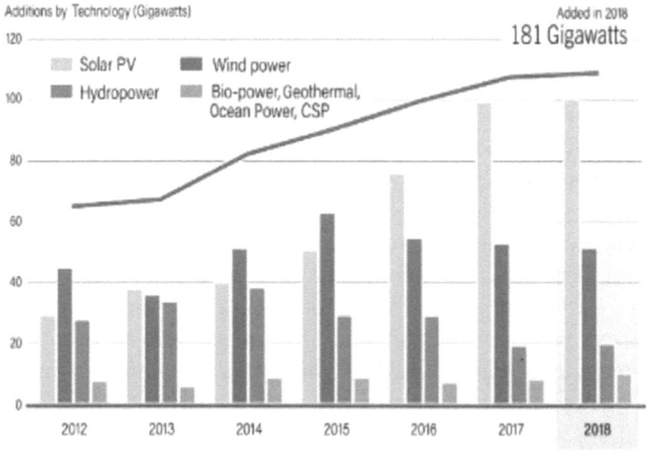

FIGURE 5.3 Renewable Power Capacities [5].

5.3 NANOTECHNOLOGY APPLICATIONS IN RENEWABLE ENERGY

To improve the performance and lifespan of RESs, the nanotechnology field is very beneficial. Using the nanostructures, more and more RESs have been enhanced, which will ultimately be helpful to the mankind and environment. The reason being these RESs are free of pollutants and result in a lesser emission in comparison with conventional sources of energy. Some of the applications of nanotechnology in the field of RESs are discussed in the later sections.

5.3.1 *Nanotechnology for Solar Energy*

One of the common and most widely used RES is solar energy. Solar energy offers many practical applications such as photovoltaic (PV) cells, solar power plants, and solar collectors. Solar cells are increasingly used in individual households and in industries to produce the electricity. The core of the solar cells is photovoltaic cells that convert the energy received from the sun into a usable electrical form. PV cells are manufactured from the numerous layers of structures, each having different properties. The development in the structures of PV cells increases the productivity and reduces the overall price and ultimately leads to the widespread application of solar panels in domestic, industrial, and grid level applications. PV technology is categorized into three generations depending upon the type of materials and manufacturing technology used. The first generation of PV cells made use of crystalline silicon with a very good quality. The manufacturing process of these solar cells is quite expensive. Second generation of PV cells used very slim film coatings with the semiconductor substance such as copper indium gallium selenide. The manufacturing cost is lesser in these generations of PV cells and there is a considerable increase in efficiency and performance. The third creation of PV cells include those classes of technologies, which are rising or are in the stages of development, e.g. nanostructured semiconductor substances, quantum dots, and amorphous silicon. Nanotechnology is very helpful in the design and manufacture of second generation, thin film PV cells. However, nanomaterials are widely used in the third creation of solar cell technologies, where novel technologies like radial junctions, nanowires, and quantum dots are increasing the efficiency of PV cells [10,11]. Solar cells are nowadays efficiently manufactured from nanostructures such as silicon and titanium dioxide. However, the development of these efficient solar cells involves some cost barriers, but due to the usage of low-cost raw materials, the price of commercial solar cells can be decreased. Schematic diagram of a nanomaterial-based PV cell is demonstrated in Figure 5.4. Generally, nanomaterials have the capacity to improve the productivity of each layer of a solar cell [12]. It further leads to the development of transparent coatings and better conductive electrodes for effective absorbers.

Solar cells are made cheaper, lighter, and more efficient using the nanostructures such as carbon nanotubes (CNT), quantum dots, and fullerenes. As an example, vertical laying CNTs in PV cells greatly increase the amount of light which can be collected. Basically, there is a significant increase in the efficiency of the PV cells, using the nanomaterials. Moreover, structural properties of PV cells can be improved using nanotechnology. Figure 5.5 represents some of the nanostructured cells.

Some of the advantages of the CNTs are listed below:

- Very small and fast components can be developed using CNTs.
- CNTs produce computers, consuming lesser energy.
- Very fast speed and better memory capacity are ensured.
- Circuits are more precise on the miniature scale.

5.3.2 *Nanotechnology for Wind Energy*

Another type of RES is wind energy in which the kinetic energy of the wind is converted into electrical or mechanical energy that can be further used for practical uses.

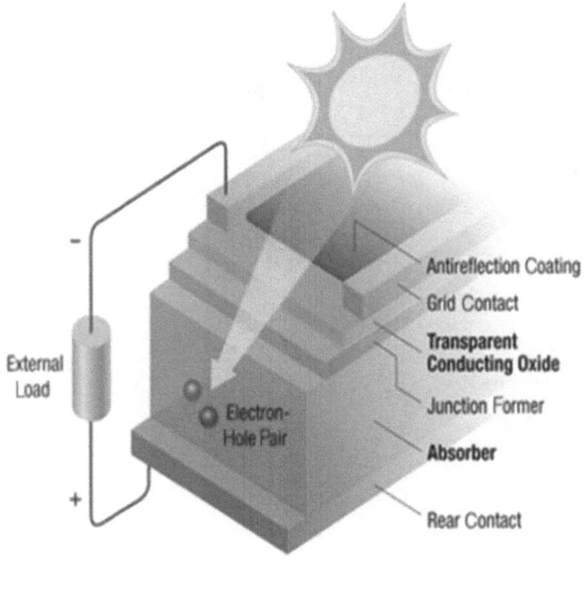

FIGURE 5.4 Schematic of a PV Cell.

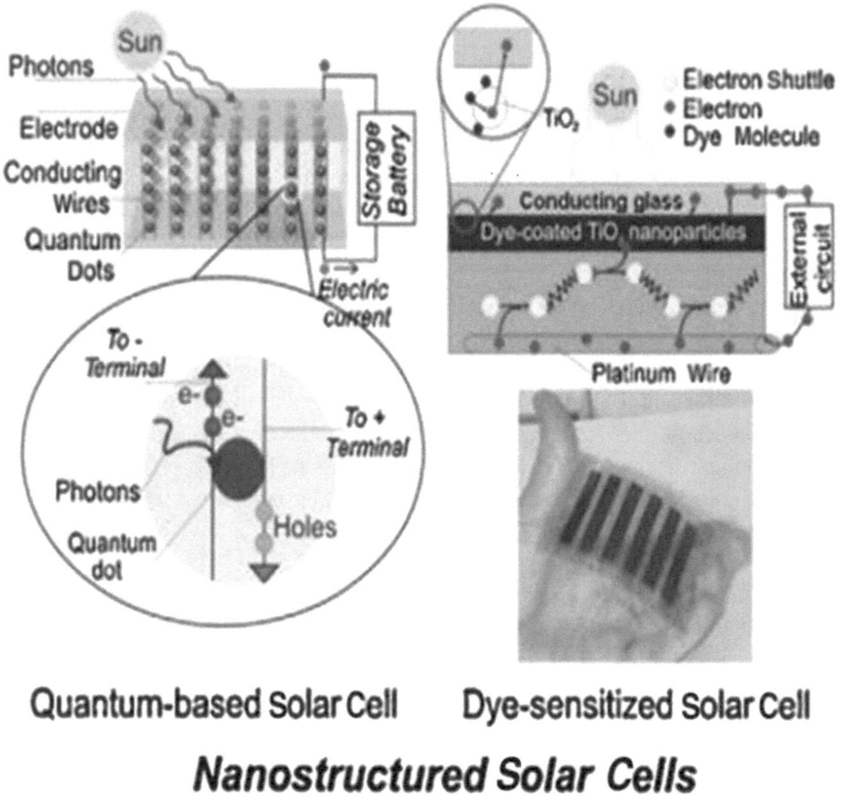

FIGURE 5.5 Nanomaterial-Based PV Cells [6].

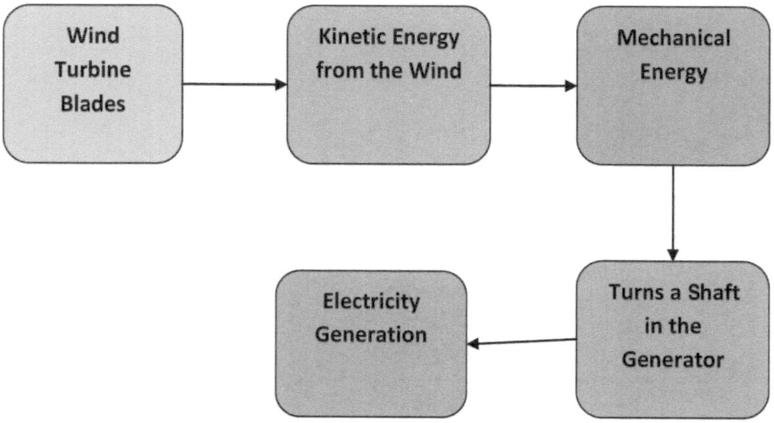

FIGURE 5.6 Wind Energy Systems.

Basically, wind energy and turbines are environmental friendly as they do not require fuel to burn. Figure 5.6 depicts the flowchart of a system involving wind energy.

Nanotechnology is also very helpful in wind-energy-based systems. Using the nanomaterials based on CNTs, high strength and light-weight rotor blades can be designed for the wind turbines. Composites of CNTs can be used in wind turbines, which results in a better conductivity. Efficiency of wind turbines can be improved using the nanocoatings, weight can be decreased by using fiber glass, and also nanopaints result in an increase in the lifetime of wind turbine systems. CNT-based wind turbine systems reduce the power loss in the transmission lines. Nano-optimized storing equipment allow the more efficient feeding of wind power to the grid [13,14]. In fact, nanotechnology has contributed toward the optimization of wind power using the nanomaterials. Some of the uses of nanotechnology in wind energy systems are represented in Table 5.1.

5.3.3 Nanotechnology for Hydrogen Energy

Nanotechnology also offers advantages in production and storage of hydrogen energy. Nowadays, nano fuel cells are widely used. Fuel cell is a device that converts a fuel directly into electricity in an electrochemical reaction. Fuel cell consists of an electrolyte layer in association with an anode and a cathode on either side. The electrodes anode and cathode are porous in nature and are fabricated with compressed carbon. The structure of a fuel cell is represented in Figure 5.7.

Anode is fed with hydrogen, where negatively charged electrons of hydrogen are separated with a catalyst as per below equation:

$$2H_2 \rightarrow 4H^+ + 4e^- \quad (5.1)$$

Air is fed at the cathode; therefore, oxygen is combined with electrons as given below:

$$O_2 + 4H^+ + 4e^- \rightarrow 2H_2O \quad (5.2)$$

TABLE 5.1.
Nanotechnology in Wind Turbines

Parameters	Applications
Weight	Development of more and longer robust blades can be done using the nanocomposite materials that provide better strength and stiffness
Blades	CNTs developed to make blades stronger and lighter improve the energy efficiency
Energy Losses	Low-friction coating improves the efficiency in the gearboxes and nanolubricant reduces the energy losses
Life Time	Nanopaints are used to increase wind turbines' lifetime

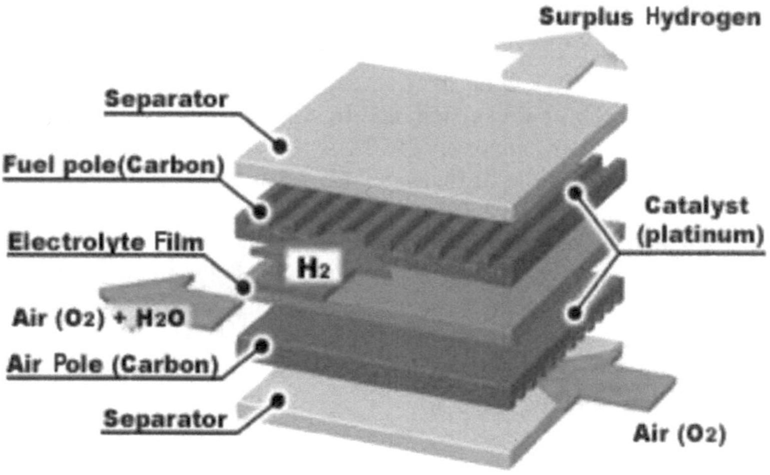

FIGURE 5.7 Structure of a Fuel Cell.

Electric current flows in opposite direction now, and the overall reaction becomes:

$$2H_2 + O_2 \rightarrow 2H_2O \tag{5.3}$$

There are some limitations of the fuel cell from reaching a widespread commercial use. Nanotechnology can improve the efficiency of fuel cell in several ways. Nanoparticles are used to increase the surface area to make the reaction more efficient. CNTs are used to enter the hydrogen into the fuel cell. The diameter of a nanotube is of the order of a few nanometers. CNTs make the hydrogen storage easy. In fact, nano-sized electrolyte particles dramatically increase the active surface area and therefore lead to an increase in the performance of the fuel cell.

Nano fuel cells are used in many applications such as transport, stationary, and portable formats. Figure 5.8 depicts some of the applications of the nano fuel cells. Nano fuel cells are widely used in light duty vehicles, ferries, and smaller boats, etc. In fact, nanotechnology regenerative fuel cells provide solutions for the problems, which are effective in internal combustion engines. Here, the development in fuel cells using nanotechnology is making it useful in numerous applications. Ultimately, our environment and RESs will be preserved. To compress more power into smaller volumes, researchers have begun to develop nano-based fuel cells.

5.3.4 *Nanotechnology for Water Energy*

Water is the one of the fundamental requirements of the life as it is used in different segments of social life such as environment, security, food, and energy. Due to the advantages of nanomaterials such as nanosize and unique behavior, these nanomaterials are emerging rapidly for solving the issues related to water energy quantity and quality. One of the applications of nanomaterials in water energy

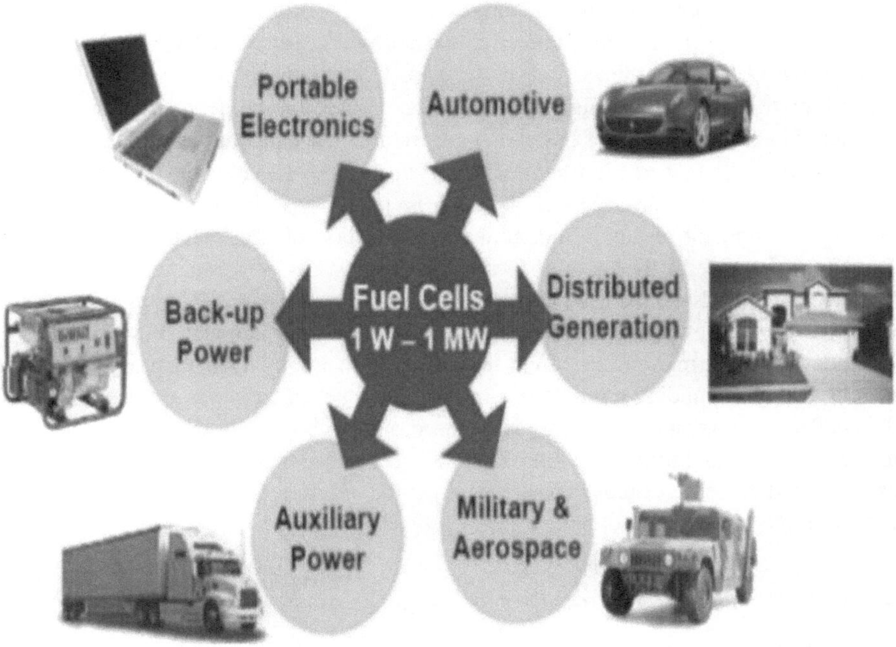

FIGURE 5.8 Applications of Nano Fuel Cells.

includes water purification using metal-free catalysts made up of nanomaterials with more surface area and better reactivity. Another application involves the development of stronger, durable, and reliable water piping components and systems using the improved strength to weight characteristics of nanomaterials. With the use of nanotechnology, more and more advancements in the next-generation water supply system can be explored [15]. Because of extraordinary features of nanomaterials such as photosensitivity, larger surface area, and magnetic and optical properties, they are useful for making advanced sensors for water quality monitoring and absorbents with good features and high performance membranes, etc. The advancement in nanotechnology should go in parallel with safety research and environmental health to develop a sustainable water management. Nanotechnology offers the following developments to water management system:

- To increase the water availability with the help of nanotechnology
- To enhance the water delivery efficiency using nanotechnology
- To enhance next-generation water tracking systems using nanotechnology

5.3.5 *Nanotechnology for Geothermal Energy*

Another form of energy is geothermal energy, which can be defined as the energy retrieved from the earth's crust that lies in the range of 5–10 km from the earth's crust. Temperature at these depths is very high. Nanofluids are used in these situations. These nanofluids act as cooling fluids, and purpose of these nanofluids is to cool the pipes that are exposed to very high temperature. Same nanofluids are also used to cool the various parts in the drilling machines such as sensors. Drilling machines are generally used under high temperature and high friction. Sources based on the geothermal energy are structured into three categories based on temperature: low temperature sources, medium temperature sources, and high temperature sources. The variation in the temperature between the earth's surface and its core is termed as the geothermal gradient. Geothermal gradient results in a continuous conduction of heat, which is thermal energy from the core to the earth's surface. Nanofluids are very beneficial in these situations. Nanofluids can be used to retrieve energy from the earth's core and to process it further to the power plant for the production of a huge amount of work energy. Nowadays, geothermal energy offers numerous applications. One such application is heating in which building are heated using the hot water in the pipes. However, one of the challenges in geothermal energy is the need of deep borings, which sometimes lead to tremors. Nanofluids are capable of absorbing huge amount of energy as compared to normal fluids. This can lead to the requirement of lesser deep borings for the usage of geothermal energy.

5.3.6 Nanotechnology for Bioenergy or Biomass

Although products and materials based on nanotechnology are being utilized in numerous fields of social and commercial life, yet the use of nanotechnology in bioenergy field is limited due to the challenges involving technical and economic issues that occur in the bioenergy sector. All organic materials that stem from the plants are called biomass. Green plants convert the sunlight into plant material via the process of photosynthesis and biomass is produced. Presently, biomass contributes 15–20% of the world's energy. Bioenergy is the better source of energy. Some of the bioenergy sources are biogas, biofuels, biodiesel, biooil, and vegetable oil. Nanotechnology is playing a vital role to improve these sources of energy further. Growth in the biofuel industry is very fast with a favorable role for producing renewable and dealing with any variations in climate. To attain cost-effective and procedure-efficient biofuel industry, nanotechnology is playing a very significant role. Enhancement and utilization of biofuel production have been done using nanomaterials having unique characteristics. The main motive is to design and implement the biofuel systems at a large scale based on nanotechnologies. Nanofibers, nanotubes, nanosheets, and metal nanoparticles are nowadays finding direct and indirect applications in the biofuel production such as biodiesel and bioethanol. As these biofuels are RESs and ecofriendly in nature, they are attracting a lot of attention at an industrial scale as a good option of energy sources. Some of the fascinating approaches such as the utilization of magnetic nanoparticles have also offered by nanotechnology. These magnetic nanoparticles acts as carriers, which are used to immobilize the enzymes applied in biodiesel or bioethanol production. Generally, nanoparticles possess large surface areas and exhibit greater activities as compared to the bulk materials. These nanoparticles also exhibit good stability, reliability and are more cost potent with a high recycling potential. Therefore, nanotechnology is also very helpful in biomass energy sector.

5.4 OTHER APPLICATIONS OF NANOTECHNOLOGY

Apart from these applications, nanotechnology is finding importance in other fields also, e.g. nanomedicine, nanofabrication, nanotechnology in memory and storage, nanotechnology for flexible electronics, and some industrial applications of nanotechnology such as textile and military. One of the medical field applications of nanotechnology is known as nanomedicine. Basically, the nanomedicine branch deals with the medical applications of nanomaterials along with nanoelectronic biosensors and also some of the upcoming applications of molecular nanotechnology. Nanotechnology is now being used in treating cancer through molecular imaging and therapy. Nanofabrication is another significant field of nanotechnology which deals with energy. Nanofabrication involves a process, which deals with the designing and implementation of the devices based on the nanoscale. Development of such type of nanodevices, having dimensions smaller than 100 nm help to seize, store, and transfer energy in a better form. In fact, nanomaterials play a very crucial role for the designing and implementation of flexible electronics. Flexible electronics components can also be developed and designed by changing the nanoscale structure of particles. Figure 5.9 illustrates the role of nanomaterials in numerous applications.

One of the important applications of nanotechnology is in the domestic area. Self-cleaning ceramic glasses can be easily cleaned using the nanomaterials. Heat resistance and smoothness of household appliances, e.g. flat iron, can be enhanced using the nanoparticles. Stain or water-repellent clothes are already designed using the engineered nanofibers. Nanotechnology-finish-based textiles can be washed easily at lower temperatures. Nanotechnology has been proven to be very beneficial to integrate the small carbon particle membrane and is successful to provide the full area protection from electrostatic charges. Nanotechnology is also helpful in military applications. Military sector would be capable to develop sensor systems for the detection of biological agents. To protect the soldiers from the dangers such as chemical threats, excessive temperatures, and impacts, nanomaterials can be inserted onto a soldier's uniforms. This also makes the uniform more durable.

One of the significant applications of nanotechnology is in the mobile technology. A nanotechnology-based device, known as Morph is designed and developed by University of Cambridge and Nokia Research Center. The Morph is super aquaphobic, which makes this a good dust repellent. Its surface is covered by the nanowire grass having PV cells, that makes it capable to charge itself using the light sources. Nokia has predicted that a mesh of nanofibers will allow the mobiles to be stretched, bent, and folded into numerous required shapes.

Another use of nanotechnology is in personal computers. Transistor-based CNTs can be easily installed in the personal computers instead of silicon transistors. In the near future, nanorods technology will be used for the purpose of displays because of advantages such as minimum consumption of electricity and lesser heat emission. Size of the microprocessors can be reduced to a larger extent using nanomaterials.

5.5 NANOTECHNOLOGY: KEY GOALS, CHALLENGES, AND SOLUTIONS

Nanoscience research and nanotechnology will be the emerging technology at a large scale in the coming years. Some of the examples of key goals in which nanotechnology is playing a very significant role are:

- Generation of solar power at a larger scale
- Development of economic catalysts for the conversion of electricity or sunlight into fuels
- Electrical storage systems for grid and transportation applications
- Design of nanomaterials to improve lighting efficiency
- Development of nanomaterials for economic energy conversion

Lots of light-weight, stronger, and easily programmed structures can be developed using the nanotechnology, and this will lead to the requirement of lesser amount

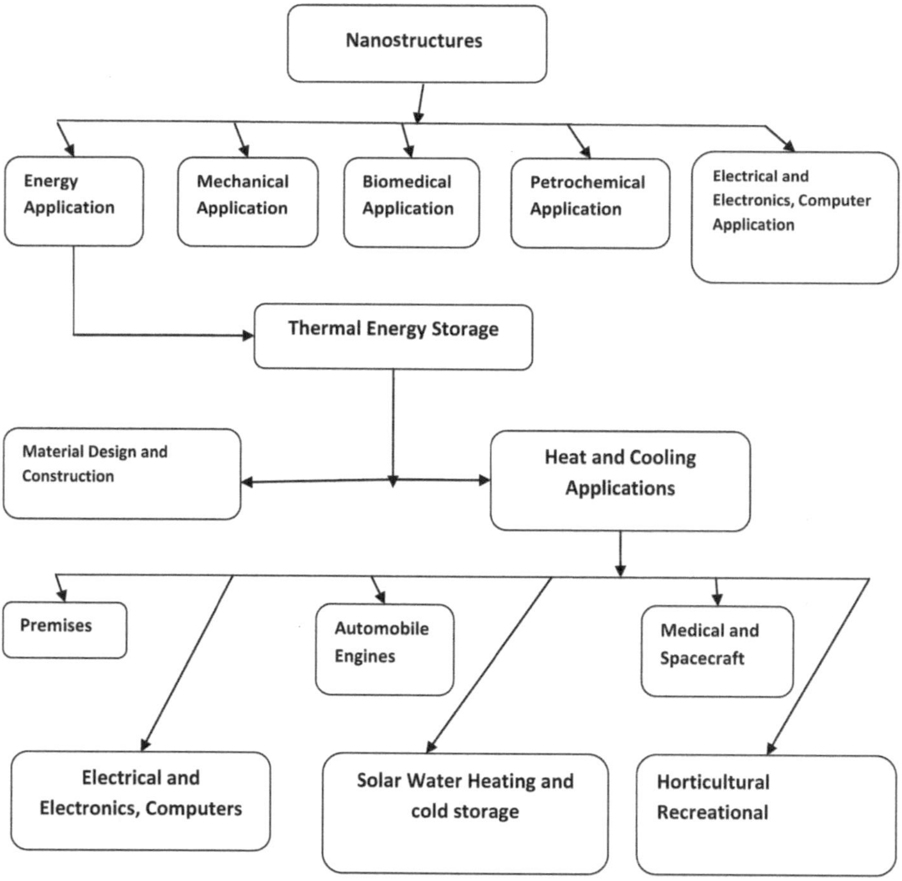

FIGURE 5.9 Nanotechnology and Its Impact on Various Fields.

of energy for the further production of conventional materials. These materials will be efficient to provide maximum fuel efficiency in the applications such as aircrafts, space vehicles, ships, and land transportation. Another upcoming technology is nanorobotics. These nanorobots will be able to perform human tasks efficiently as well as the tasks that human beings could never accomplish. However, nanoscience research offers some challenges. The most immediate challenge in nanotechnology is that we need to learn more about the nanomaterials and their properties at nanoscale [16–18]. Research is ongoing about the behavior of the particles and how the materials fit together to form the larger structures. Materials at nanoscales behave differently than they do in their bulk form. Hence, there is a concern that some nanomaterials could be toxic. Basically, nanoparticles are so small, they could easily cross the blood–brain barrier of the body of an human being. Therefore, there is a need to be sure that if nanoparticles are in use, they should not poison us [19,20].

There are some hefty social concerns about nanotechnology too. In fact, nanotechnology may also allow us to create more powerful weapons, both lethal and non-lethal. Nanotechnology is being used in medical science also. Medical nanotechnology could make us smarter, stronger and give us other abilities ranging from rapid healing to night vision. Nowadays, nanotechnology is being used in almost every field [21–23].

5.6 CONCLUSIONS

Nanotechnology is generating a lot of attention these days and therefore building great expectations in renewable energy challenges with nanosciences in the today's scientific world. For renewable energy, sources are solar, hydrogen, etc. and new generation batteries and supercapacitors are described as the most significant examples of the contributions of nanotechnology in the energy sector. A comprehensive overview and the applications of nanotechnology in the sector of RESs such as solar energy, wind energy, hydrogen energy, tidal energy and geothermal energy are discussed in this chapter. In fact, nanotechnology has the capacity to reorganize the energy system. Nanotechnology is found everywhere from fuel cells to mobile phone batteries, and also in space equipment. By providing a clean and cheap energy, nanotechnology and nanomaterials are playing a significant role in the human life and society. Nanotechnology may help to improve the efficiency of electricity transmission wires. Now there are conventional wires for transmission electricity such as Aluminum Conductor Steel Reinforced (ACSR) wire. Developing a nanomaterial-based metal matrix overhead conductor known as the aluminum conductor composite reinforced wire may provide more than twice the transmission capacity of conventional conductors of similar size and high performance. Although applications of nanotechnology are found everywhere, yet more research has to be done and lots of barriers have to crossed to make nanotechnology practicable at residential and industrial scales.

REFERENCES

1. Hussein, A. K. (2015) "Applications of nanotechnology in renewable energies – A comprehensive overview and understanding", *Renewable and Sustainable Energy Reviews*, 42, pp. 460–476.
2. Echiegu, E. A., (2016) "Nanotechnology as a tool for enhanced renewable energy applications in developing countries", *Journal of Fundamental of Renewable Energy and Applications*, 6, pp. 1–2.
3. Rouvimov, S., Mitchell,D. and Solanki, R., (2011) "Nano-materials for renewable energy: Toward the integration of education with research and internship", *11th IEEE International Conference on Nanotechnology, USA.*
4. Volkov, A. G., Shtein, D. A., Zharkov, M. A. and Klassen, S. V. (2019) " Comparative analysis of power generation systems for renewable energy using electric energy storage devices", *20th International Conference of Young Specialists on Micro/Nanotechnologies and Electron Devices, Russia.*
5. Renewables (2019) *Global Status Report.*
6. Sahan, K. M., Mohammed, H. J., Jalal, N. M. and Mahmood, R. S. (2013) "Manufacturing of ink sensitized solar cell by NANO technology", *International Conference & Exhibition on the Applications of Information Technology to Renewable Energy Processes and Systems, Jordan.*
7. Khan, I., Saeed, K. and Khan, I. (2019) "Nanoparticles: Properties, applications and toxicities", *Arabian Journal of Chemistry*, 12, pp. 908–931.
8. Pandiyan, G. K. and Prabaharan,T. (2020) "Implementation of nanotechnology in fuel cells", *Materials Today: Proceedings*, pp. 1–5.
9. Nasrollahzadeh, M., Sajadi, S. M., Sajjadi, M. and Issaabadi, Z. (2019) "Applications of nanotechnology in daily life", *Interface Science and Technology*, 28, pp. 113–143.
10. Bryant, S. T., Straker, K. and Wrigley, C. (2020) "The rapid product design and development of a viable nanotechnology energy storage product", *Journal of Cleaner Production*, 244, pp. 1–20.
11. Markovic, D. S., Zivkovic, D., Cvetkovic, D. and Popovic, R. (2012) "Impact of nanotechnology advances in ICT on sustainability and energy efficiency", *Renewable and Sustainable Energy Reviews*, 16, pp. 2966–2972.
12. Abdin, Z., Alim, M. A., Saidur, R., Islam, M. R. and Wadi, A. (2013) "Solar energy harvesting with the application of nanotechnology", *Renewable and Sustainable Energy Reviews*, 26, pp. 837–852.
13. Kar, S., Dey, S., Chakraborti, S. and Majumdar, G. (2020) "Nanomaterials for alternative energy", *Encyclopedia of Renewable and Sustainable Materials*, 3, pp. 606–618.
14. Oke, A. E., Aigbavboa, C. O. and Semenya, K. (2017) "Energy savings and sustainable construction: Examining the advantages of nanotechnology", *Energy Procedia*, 142, pp. 3839–3843.
15. Hussain, A., Muhammad Arif, S. and Aslam, M. (2017) "Emerging renewable and sustainable energy technologies: State of the art", *Renewable and Sustainable Energy Reviews*, 71, pp. 12–28.
16. Pathakoti, K., Manubolu, M. and Hwang, H. M. (2018) " Nanotechnology applications for environmental industry", *Handbook of Nanomaterials for Industrial Applications*, pp. 894–907, chapter 48.
17. Orue, I. G., Pedraz, J. L., Hernandez, R. M. and Igartua, M. (2017) "Nanotechnology based delivery systems to release growth factors and other endogenous molecules for chronic wound healing", *Journal of Drug Delivery Science and Technology*, 42, pp. 2–17.
18. Muzammil, W. K., Rahman, M. M., Fazlizan, A., Ismail, M. A., Phang, H. K. and Elias, M. A. (2018) "Nanotechnology in renewable energy: Critical reviews for wind energy", *Nanotechnology: Applications in Energy, Drug and Food*, pp. 49–71.

19. Fromer, N. A. and Diallo, M. S., (2013) " Nanotechnology and clean energy: Sustainable utilization and supply of critical materials", *Journal of Nanoparticles*, pp. 289–303.
20. Manjon, A. M. and Moldenhauer, K. (2011) "Nano-energy research trends: bibliometrical analysis of nanotechnology research in the energy sector", *Journal of Nanoparticle Research*, 13, pp. 3911–3922.
21. Idrees, M. (2015) "Role of nanotechnology in medical sciences: A review", *International Journal of Innovative Drug Discovery*, 5, pp. 14–24.
22. Patil, M., Mehta, D. S. and Guvva, S. (2008) "Future impact of nanotechnology on medicine and dentistry", *Journal of Indian Society of Periodontology*, 12, pp. 34–40.
23. Shrivastava, S. and Dash, D. (2009) "Applying nanotechnology to human health: Revolution in biomedical sciences", *Journal of Nanotechnology*, 2009, pp. 1–14.

6 Nano/Microelectromechanical Systems (NEMS/MEMS)

Prasantha R. Mudimela and Rekha Chaudhary

6.1 INTRODUCTION

A process technology that combines electrical and mechanical components together to create an integrated device is known as MEMS. The fabrication of MEMS devices is done using integrated circuit (IC) batch processing techniques [1]. A device is known as a MEMS device if the characteristic length of it is in the range of 100 nm to 1 mm; and if the characteristic length of the device is less than 100 nm, the device is known as a NEMS device [2]. Both MEMS and NEMS devices integrate electrical and mechanical devices on microscale and nanoscale, respectively. In Europe, MEMS is also known as Microsystems Technology (MST) while in Japan, it is known as Micromachines. Figure 6.1 shows that a MEMS device consists of mechanical microstructures, microactuators, microsensors, and microelectronics, and all are integrated onto the same chip of silicon [3–5]. The following are the specifications of the three units: (i) Microsensors: This unit senses the change in the system's ambience by measuring mechanical, thermal, magnetic, chemical, or electromagnetic information. (ii) Microelectronics: This unit processes the information gathered and triggers the microactuators unit to react. (iii) Microactuators: When the microelectronics unit sends any information, the microactuators unit gathers the information and reacts accordingly. MEMS devices like pressure sensors, accelerometers, and inkjet printer heads became more popular in mid-1990s [6–8].

IBM developed the first MEMS device, a micromechanical pressure sensor in the 1970s. Later in 1979, HP developed micronozzles. In 2000, IBM developed the first NEMS device, an array of Automatic Force Microscopy (AFM) tips [9].

MEMS has numerous advantages as a manufacturing technology. Firstly, MEMS is an interdisciplinary technology. It can be used in diverse applications. Secondly, the components that are fabricated using batch fabrication methods have increased performance, reliability, reduced size, and affordability. Thirdly, MEMS provides the basis for the manufacture of products that cannot be made by other methods. However, several challenges are also associated with miniaturization, which should be addressed and eradicated.

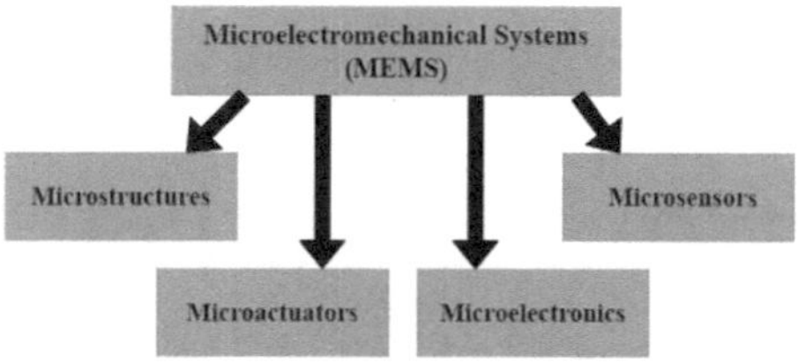

FIGURE 6.1 An Illustration of MEMS Components.

In MEMS, the whole system is not designed at microscale. For some applications, to incorporate the benefits of high sensitivity, better linearity, better responsivity, and so on, only the sensors/actuators are designed at microscale. But the efforts to shrink the complete system at microscale are still in progress.

All these characteristics of MEMS technology have resulted in the use of different MEMS devices in different applications. For automobile applications, MEMS accelerometer production has been done by several renowned companies. For medical and automotive applications, pressure sensors have gained attention and micromirrors are used in digital projection displays [10]. NEMS industry is still young and growing. M/NEMS technology has also played an important role in microfluidic applications. From the last few years, bio-MEMS/bio-NEMS devices have emerged in use rapidly [11]. M/NEMS switches have been fabricated and used at radio frequency (RF). RF M/NEMS switches have shown a superior performance than the already existing conventional switches [12]. The size of molecules, cells, and diffusion length for molecules are in the range of micro- and nanometer. M/NEMS devices can also be used for medical diagnostics, pharmaceuticals, and gene and DNA analysis [13,14]. NEMS devices also include transducers, optoelectronic devices, and energy devices [15,16].

6.1.1 *Background*

MEMS technology has seen an evolution arising in different places, owing to the knowledge and hard work of some researchers. In MEMS technology, new devices are still emerging for different applications. Following is a timeline which shows efforts by different inventors, leading to MEMS development [17–21]. Table 6.1 gives a brief look at the history of the MEMS technology.

R. Feyman first triggered the interest in MEMS while talking about it in a meeting held in 1959. According to him, there is an enormous scope of micron-size devices in many applications. It leads in making a device with better efficiency, cost-effectiveness, and size reduction [23]. The history of NEMS technology is given in Table 6.2.

Every day, new applications and better technologies are evolving in the field of M/NEMS. MEMS devices have evolved from measuring the pressure in engines to controlling the communication systems, automobiles, monitoring the blood pressure, and so on. The growth of M/NEMS is boundless and M/NEMS will continue to find its way in different applications.

TABLE 6.1
Background of MEMS Technology [22]

Decade	Device	Inventor
1940–1950	Germanium transistor	Shockley
1950–1960	The first integrated circuit, piezoresistive effect	Smith, Kilby, and Noyce
1960–1970	Surface micromachining	Nathanson
1970–1980	Silicon pressure sensor, accelerometer	Peterson Kulite
1980–1990	Polysilicon MEMS device, rotary drive motors, comb drive structure	Howe and Muller, Fan et al., Tang et al.
1990–2000	Polysilicon hinges, multiuser MEMS process, digital micromirror device demonstration	Pister et al., MEMSCAP, Texas Instruments

TABLE 6.2
History of NEMS Technology

Reference	Year	Device	Inventor
24	1960	The first MOSFET with 100 nm-thick gate oxide	M. Atalla and D. Kahng
25	1962	M–S junction transistor with 10 nm-thick gold layer	M. Atalla and D. Kahng
26	1987	The first MOSFET with 10 nm-thick gate oxide	Bijan Davari (IBM)
27	1998	FinFET with channel length less than 17 nm	University of California, Berkley

6.2 COMMON M/NEMS MATERIAL

M/NEMS devices are fabricated on a substrate. Single crystal silicon (SCS), fused quartz, and gallium arsenide are some materials that are used as substrates for M/NEMS fabrication. The devices can be fabricated by micromachining into substrates or by the deposition of material over substrates [28].

- For M/NEMS fabrication, silicon-based materials in different forms (SCS, amorphous silicon, polysilicon) are mostly used [29].
- Silicon dioxide always exists as native oxide over silicon substrate. Also, silicon wafer oxidation can be done either by wet oxidation method or dry oxidation method. The quality of oxide grown in dry oxidation is better than that in wet oxidation, but the oxidation rate in case of dry oxidation is slow.
- For the deposition of silicon nitride, chemical vapor deposition (CVD) method can be used.

Low pressure chemical vapor deposition (LPCVD) and plasma enhanced chemical vapor deposition (PECVD) are the two methods that are used for silicon nitride deposition.

- Quartz can be used in natural or synthesized forms as substrate material. Selective etching cannot be done in quartz because of poor edge definition [30].
- Silicon carbine, glass, diamond, and metals such as gold and alloy of nickel are also used for M/NEMS fabrication.
- Carbon nanotubes, quantum dots, nanowires, and so on are used as nanomaterials [31,32].

6.2.1 *MEMS Devices*

6.2.1.1 Established MEMS devices

Automotive air bag sensor

The first commercial MEMS device was the accelerometer that was used in an automotive air bag sensor. In this, a single chip contains a smart sensor called accelerometer that measures the rapid change in the speed of a vehicle when an object is hitting it. The change in the speed of vehicle is measured by the change in voltage. As the voltage changes, the control unit sends a signal to trigger and explode the air bag.

Before MEMS, the air bag technology used mechanical "ball and tube" type devices, which were complex, heavy, and costly. Those systems were mounted in the front of vehicles with separate electronics near air bag. But MEMS technology has enabled the same use by making a cost-effective device having a sensor (accelerometer) and the electronic circuitry integrated into a single silicon chip that is installed within the steering wheel column.

The success of the air bag sensor in the MEMS technology is very important. The air bag sensor has proven its reliability, and more than 100 million of such devices are sold. For example, the BMW 740i has over 100 MEMS devices including anti-lock braking systems, active suspension, appliance and navigation control systems, vibration monitoring, fuel sensors, noise reduction, rollover detection, seatbelt restraint and tensioning, etc. The automobile industry has become the main as a result, the automotive industry has become one the drivers for the development of MEMS technology [33,34].

Accelerometers are used for some other applications like earthquake detection, pacemakers, virtual reality video games, and weapon systems arming.

Pressure sensor

Another successful MEMS device is the pressure sensor. This is a miniaturized disposable device, used in hospitals to monitor blood pressure. These MEMS pressure sensors are cheaper than the alr eady available blood pressure sensors. MEMS pressure sensor measures the blood pressure with a saline-filled tube and diaphragm arrangement that has to be connected to an artery with a needle. To separate the saline solution from sensing element, a gel is used.

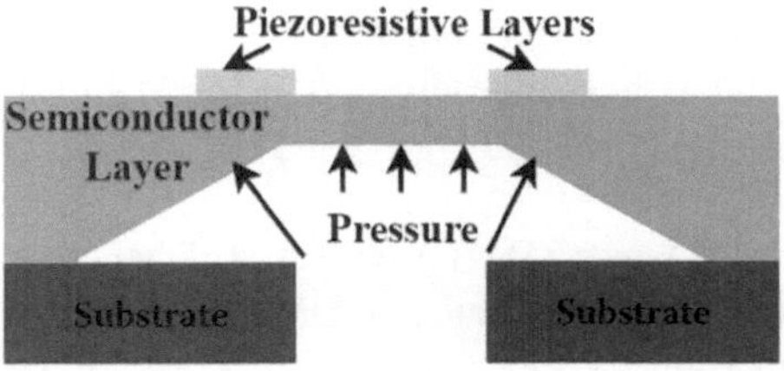

FIGURE 6.2 Piezoresistive Pressure Sensor.

In this, a silicon substrate is etched and a membrane is produced as shown in Figure 6.2. The membrane is placed over a substrate. At the edges of the membrane, a piezoresistive layer is deposited to convert the mechanical stress into electrical signal. When the pressure is applied, the membrane deflects and piezoresistive layer produces voltage. This sensing element is mounted on a plastic/ceramic base with a plastic cap over it and fits into the manufacturer's housing. In MEMS technology, pressure sensors are the biggest medical application [35,36].

Inkjet printer head

Another successful application of MEMS is the inkjet printer head. In this, a series of nozzles is used to spray ink directly onto a printing medium. The droplet of ink can form depending on the type of inkjet printer (thermally or piezoelectrically). Inkjet printer head was invented by Hewlett-Packard in 1979. In this method, thermal expansion of ink vapor is used. An array of small resistors also known as "heater" is used in the printer. An electronic pulse with a time period of less than 3 μsec is used to fire the heaters, and the whole circuitry is controlled by a microprocessor. When the heaters are fired and ink flowing over each heater heats up and gets vaporized, ink bubbles are formed. As soon as the bubble expands, the ink is thrown out of the nozzle, lands on the paper, and solidifies instantaneously as shown in Figure 6.3. In this case, there is no moving part in the system which means not all MEMS devices are mechanical.

To force the ink out of the nozzle, a piezoelectric element can be used. For that, a piezoelectric crystal is used and is positioned at the back of the ink reservoir of each nozzle. When a small electric current is received by the crystal, it starts vibrating. When the vibration is occurring inside the reservoir, it forces the ink out of the nozzle. When the crystal vibrates back out, it fills the reservoir with the ink again.

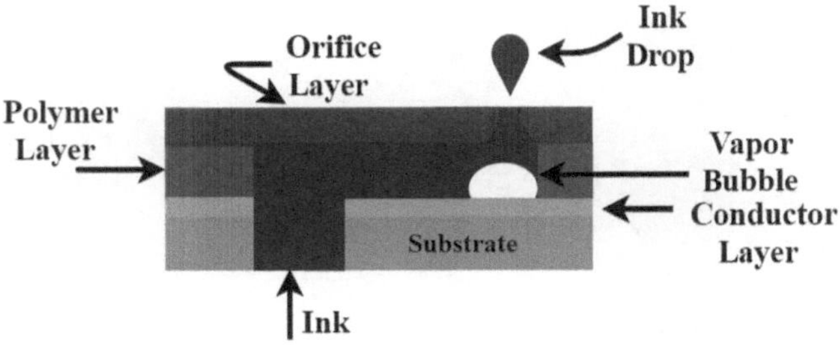

FIGURE 6.3 Thermal Ink Jet Technology.

This technology is patented by Epson and used by some other printer companies. Enabling more and more heaters and crystals is possible only due to MEMS [37].

Overhead projection display

For display applications, Digital Micromirror Device (DMD) was used. DMD was developed by Texas Instruments. Figure 6.4 illustrates that in a DMD, millions of micromirrors are used to display. All the micromirrors are organized in a rectangular array that resembles the pixels in the image to be displayed. Between the on–off state, the micromirrors can be rotated by ±10°. When the light from the bulb of projector is reflected into the lens, pixels become bright on the screen and this is called on state. But when the light is absorbed by the heat sink, pixels become dark. Aluminum is used to make mirrors and the dimensions of a single mirror is 16 μm*16 μm. DMDs are used for displays applications like PC projectors, high definition televisions (HDTVs), and for large venues such as digital cinemas [38].

6.2.1.2 New MEMS device

Apart from the basic MEMS applications, MEMS technology has emerged to be used in different new applications like in biomedical field and wireless communication.

Bio-MEMS

Bio-MEMS is an abbreviation for biomedical and microelectromechanical systems. Bio-MEMS generally applies to biological systems, and specially to human health. The study of Bio-MEMS started after 1967 when S.B. Carter invented pallidum islands for cell attachment. It took around 20–25 years of study, then in 1985 a commercialized bio-MEMS application, i.e. a pregnancy test kit was developed [39]. After that in 1991, the first oligonucleotide chip was developed that was used for genetic testing and forensic research [40]. For drug delivery, a microneedle was developed in 1998 [41]. In 1999, the first demonstration of heterogeneous laminar flow was done [42]. In bio-MEMS, very innovative products have been developed in the past few years. But still some products like micromachined pumps, flow sensors, and chemical sensors are under development. These devices can enable very fast analysis of small volume of liquids specially for home-based medical applications such as urine analysis and blood analysis.

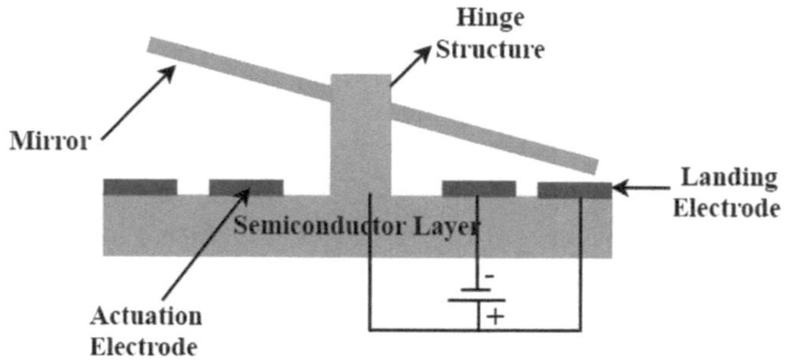

FIGURE 6.4 Basic Micromirror Device.

Microtiterplate is a new bio-MEMS device in which the cavities are filled accurately and repeatedly due to capillary forces. This is the simplest MEMS micromachined device with a plastic piece and microchannels. This product is classified as a "lab-on-chip" product.

One example of a new bio-MEMS device is the microtiterplate on which a number of cavities can be simultaneously filled accurately and repeatably by capillary force. This is a relatively simple MEMS product in the form of a piece of plastic with dimensions (20 mm x 37 mm x 3 mm) micromachined microchannels (96) and is classified as a 'lab-on-a-chip' product [44,45].

In lab-on-a-chip technology, the awaiting MEMS devices can include implantable "pharmacy-on-a-chip" devices. To carefully release the drug into the body, these devices can be used, eradicating the use of needles/injections.

In microfluidics, MEMS technology has played an important role. One of the amazing applications is "Pac-Man"-like microstructure. This structure interacts with red blood cells. This structure is developed by Sandia National Laboratories, USA, and it consists of a silicon microtooth that opens and closes like a jaw and releases a single red blood cell. It is pumped through a channel of 20 μm. The use of this structure is to puncture cells and inject them with DNA, proteins, or pharmaceuticals to counter biological or chemical attacks, gene imbalances, and natural bacterial or viral infections.

MOEMS

MOEMS stands for microoptoelectromechanical systems, also known as optical MEMS. MOEMS is the combination of MEMS and microoptics. In this, an optical signal is sensed at microscale using an integrated mechanical, optical, and electrical system. MOEMS technologies have enabled the miniaturization of critical optical systems. The applications of microoptics that cannot be addressed alone are possible to implement using MEMS called MOEMS.

The term MOEMS was coined by Dr. M.E. Motamedi in 1991–93 [45]. He clarified that optical MEMS deals with bulk optics while MOEMS is a microtechnology. In MOEMS, batch processing is done just like ICs.

MOEMS devices include waveguides, filters, attenuators, optical switches, multiplexers, modulators, and so on. These devices have features like size reduction, low cost, low power consumption, mechanical durability, high accuracy, high switching density, and low-cost batch processing. These features solve the various control and switching problems of the optical signal in communication network. In MEMS, mass fabrication of these devices is possible in a cost-effective way [47,48].

RF MEMS

A MEMS system in which electronic components consist of sub-mm-sized parts that provide RF functionality is called RF MEMS [48]. A variety of RF technology can be used to implement RF functionality. Each RF technology provides a tradeoff between cost, power handling, size, lifetime, etc. RF MEMS technology is emerging rapidly. RF MEMS devices are specifically the electronics components that are used in mobile phones and wireless communication systems such as antenna, RADAR, and satellite systems. Using MEMS technology, along with the size reduction, the performance parameters of these devices have improved. Nowadays, RF MEMS components have replaced the already existing components in mobile phones. The phones have become small in size and cost-effective using less power consumption. RF MEMS devices include circuit tuning elements like switches, capacitors, and varactors.

NEMS devices

In MEMS, the critical structural length is in micrometer while in NEMS it is at or below 100 nm. NEMS devices are lighter, and surface area to volume ratio is high as compared to MEMS. NEMS devices are foreseen in sensing, drug delivery, energy harvesting, and imaging applications. Some NEMS devices are already available in the market, and for some devices a research prototype is developed. The fundamental frequency range of NEMS-based devices is in microwave range (100 GHz) [49].

- The mechanical quality factor is of the order of tens of thousands
- Active mass is in femtogram [50], mass sensitivity up to atto-gram [51]
- Heat capacities around yocto calorie [52], power consumption 10 attowatts [53], etc.

These features of NEMS devices lead to some emerging applications like force sensors, chemical sensors, ultra-high frequency resonators. The NEMS devices are discussed in the following section.

Carbon nanotubes

A macromolecule of carbon discovered in 1991 by S. Lijima is known as carbon nanotube (CNT). CNT falls in the family of fullerene structures [54]. The properties of CNTs are determined by their atomic arrangement, length, and diameter. CNTs are light in weight, stiff but flexible, chemically inert, and thermally stable. The "twist" of the tube defines whether it is conducting or not. The twist is also known as "chirality/helicity". CNTs can exist either as single-walled nanotubes (SWNTs) or as multiwalled nanotubes (MWNTs) [55]. The basic structure of a CNT is shown in Figure 6.5.

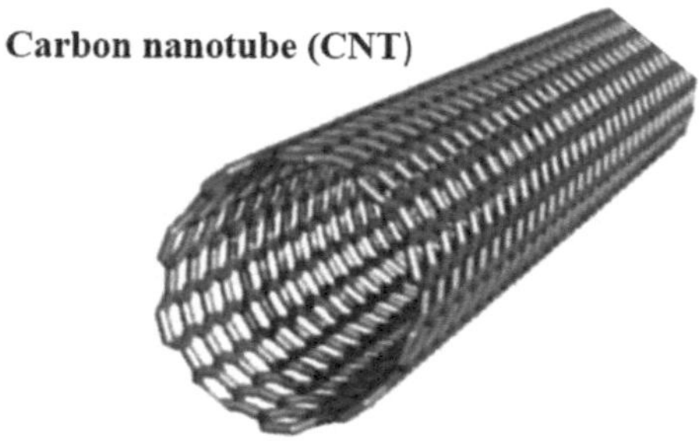

FIGURE 6.5 Basic Structure of a CNT.

Electric arc-discharge [56], catalytic CVD [57], and laser ablation [58] methods are used for CNT synthesis.

In the last decade, the mechanical and electrical properties of CNT have been investigated intensely. Some researchers have provided the comprehensive review about electronics of CNTs [59], while some others discussed the experimentation and modelling [60].

Fabrication methods

The fabrication techniques of NEMS devices can be categorized by two methods: top-down method and bottom-up method. In the top-down method in order to fabricate a device from bulk substrate, the manufacturing of NEMS structures utilizes sub-micron lithography method like e-beam lithography. In the bottom-up method, atoms and molecules are sequentially assembled in order to fabricate nanoscale devices. The resolution of e-beam lithography and etching roughness limits the size in the top-down method. Till now, most of the reported nanodevices are fabricated using both top-down and bottom-up methods (hybrid) [61]. The most challenging issue in CNT is the positioning of nanotube at desirable location.

CNT-based device

Non-volatile RAM [48], nanotweezers [62], feedback-controlled nanocantilever [63], rotational motors [64], tunable oscillators [65], nano relays, [66] etc., are some devices based on CNT. CNT can be used in gas sensors [67] and humidity sensors [68].

One of the most important NEMS device is the NEMS switch. The detailed information of a NEMS switch is as follows.

RF M/NEMS switch

Another most important M/NEMS device is the RF M/NEMS switch. The conventional mechanical and semiconductor switches have some shortcomings like they are heavy in weight, costly, and render poor performance at high frequency [69]. But all of these shortcomings are overcome by MEMS switches. M/NEMS switches offer benefits like high speed, are light in weight, provide high isolation, have low insertion loss, and are cost effective [70]. M/NEMS switch is a basic switch structure in which two states On and Off are achieved by actuation mechanism. There are four different actuation mechanisms used for M/NEMS switch working: Electrostatic [72,73], thermal [73], piezoelectric [74], electromagnetic [75]. Out of these four methods, the electrostatic method is preferred due to low power consumption, small electrode size, easy fabrication, etc.

M/NEMS switch configuration and principle of operation

M/NEMS is categorized into two basic configurations: ohmic switch and capacitive switch. Ohmic switches are mainly implemented as a series switch while the capacitive switch is mainly implemented as a shunt switch. To achieve the desired functioning of the switch, a cantilever or bridge structure made of conductive material is used. An actuation electrode is also used at which voltage is applied. The placement of cantilever or bridge can be done as discussed below.

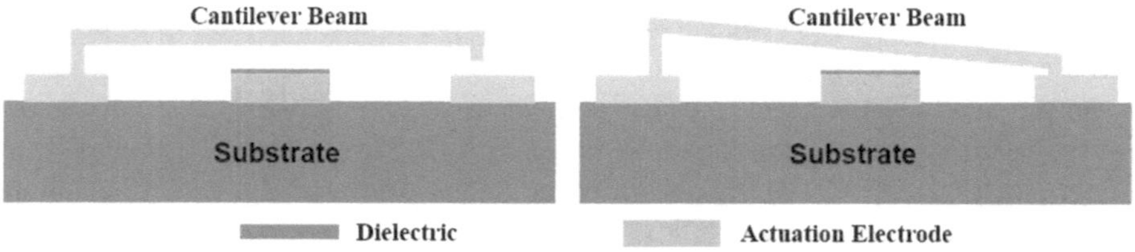

FIGURE 6.6 On and Off States in a Series Contact Switch.

Series contact switch/Ohmic switch

The schematic diagram of a series contact switch is shown in Figure 6.6. In an Ohmic switch, a metal cantilever fixed at one end is used. This cantilever is suspended at some height over a metal electrode which is covered with a dielectric. When no voltage is applied to the actuation electrode, the cantilever remains in the up-state. But when the voltage equal to actuation voltage is applied at the bottom electrode, the cantilever snaps down and touches the bottom electrode. This state is known as the down state. This switch configuration is known as series switch because it is placed in series with the signal line when used at RF.

Shunt capacitive switch

In a shunt capacitive switch, a conductive bridge or suspended beam is used which is fixed at both ends. This conductive beam is positioned at some height over the actuation electrode. In this, the voltage is applied at actuation electrode and bridge is kept at 0 V. When the applied voltage is 0 V, the bridge remains in the on state. But when the applied voltage is increased, the bridge starts deflecting toward the bottom actuation electrode. At a certain voltage, called actuation voltage, the bridge touches the bottom electrode. This state is known as the off state. As the bridge is located perpendicularly over the signal line, the switch structure is known as the shunt switch as shown in Figure 6.7.

When the suspended beam touches the bottom electrode, capacitance is formed known as off-state capacitance. In the on state, as the gap between the bridge and bottom electrode is large, small capacitance exists.

Substrate material

Materials like Quartz (3.78), Silicon (11.72), Alumina (9.75), Sapphire (11.72), and GaAs (12.91) are used as substrate materials in a RF M/NEMS switch.

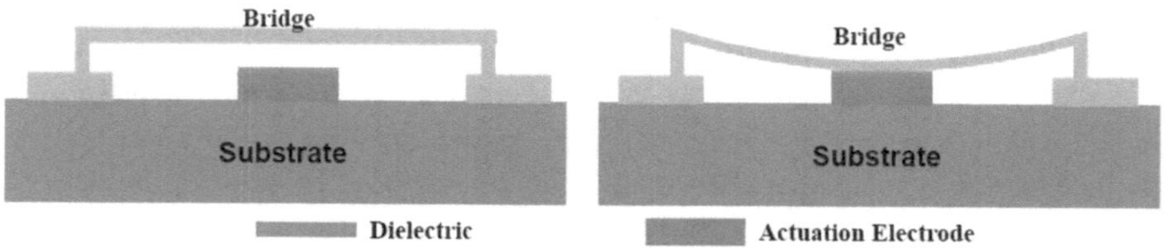

FIGURE 6.7 On and Off States in a Shunt Capacitive Switch.

TABLE 6.3
Material Properties for Beam Structure

Type of switch	Material	Young's Modulus (GPa)	Electrical Conductivity (S/m)	Resistance (μΩ*cm(ρ))
Metallic switches	Copper	117	29 E7	1.69
	Gold	79	45.2 E6	2.2
	Aluminum	69	37.7 E6	2.65
Carbon switches	CNT	1000	10^6 to 10^7	10
	Graphene	1000	10^8	10

Cantilever/bridge material

On the basis of materials used for cantilever/bridge structure, RF M/NEMS switches are categorized into two parts: Metallic switch and Carbon M/NEMS switch. Metals like copper, aluminum, and gold are used for metallic switches, and CNT and graphene are used in carbon-based switches. The electrical and mechanical properties of carbon-based switches are superior than metal-based switches. These materials reduce the size of material, i.e. from micro to nano [76–79]. The material properties are given in Table 6.3.

6.3 M/NEMS SWITCH FABRICATION

Metallic MEMS can be fabricated by two techniques: surface micromachining and bulk micromachining. In surface micromachining, the sacrificial layer is deposited over substrate surface and etching of sacrificial layer is done rather in order to release the bridge structure [80–82]. The process flow of cantilever and bridge RF MEMS switch is shown in Figure 6.8.

The switch fabrication starts by taking a quartz substrate. Then in order to form a coplanar line (CPW), aluminum metal is deposited. E-beam patterning in done to form CPW conductors. To avoid the short circuiting, a dielectric layer is deposited over the actuation electrode. Then sacrificial layer (photoresist) is deposited using spin coating and is patterned by lithography. The cantilever/bridge structure is deposited using gold sputtering method. Then at last, the sacrificial layer is removed and suspended cantilever/bridge structure is released.

In bulk micromachining, the etching of substrate takes place. But the etching depends upon the etch rate and etching profile [83].

Carbon-based RF M/NEMS switches are fabricated using three major steps [85,86]: patterning the CPW line, growth of CNT or graphene by CVD, and pattern metal contact onto two edges of beam [86].

6.4 DESIGN PARAMETERS

- **Actuation voltage:** The applied voltage at which the suspended beam/ cantilever snaps down and touches the actuation electrode is called actuation

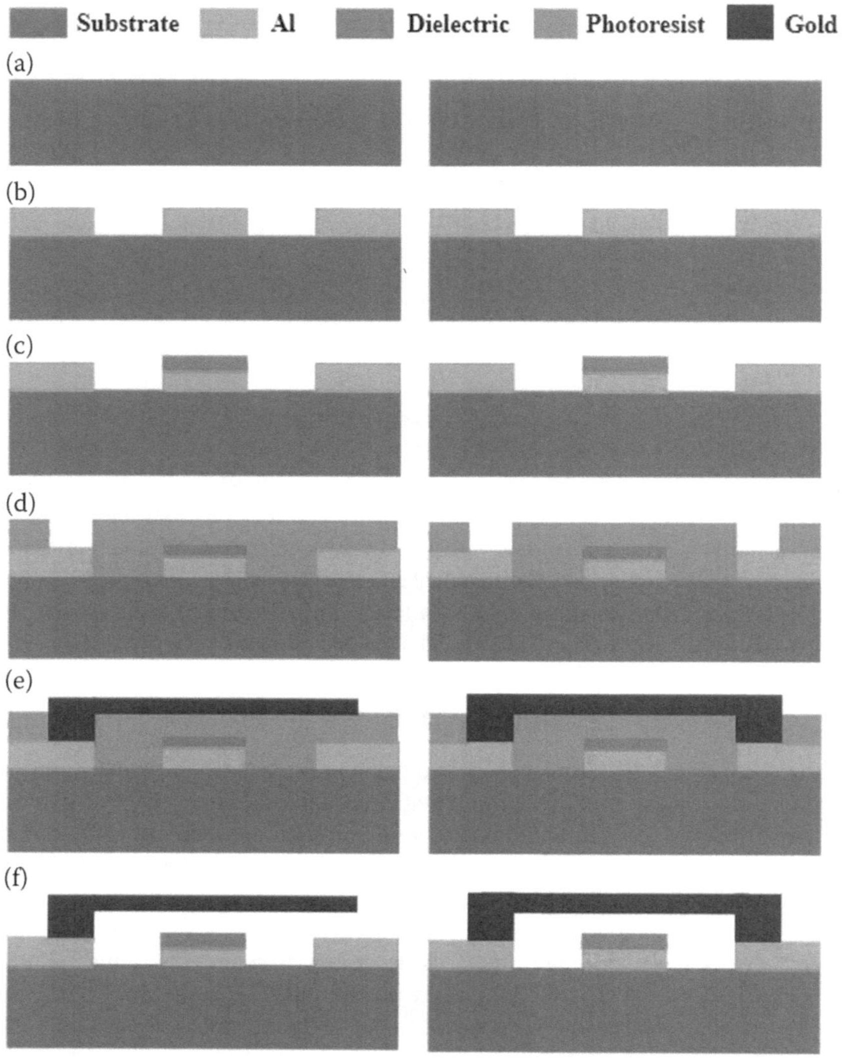

FIGURE 6.8 Fabrication Process Flow of Cantilever and Bridge Structure.

voltage. The actuation voltage can be reduced by reducing spring constant, air gap, increasing the length of beam, reducing the thickness of beam, or by making perforations/using meander structure [87].

- **RF parameters:** When the M/NEMS switch is used at RF, two factors are considered: isolation and insertion loss. The loss that occurs when the switch is inserted in the transmission line is known as the insertion loss. Low insertion loss is desirable. On inserting the switch in the transmission line, the process by which input and output ports are isolated is known as isolation. High isolation is desirable.

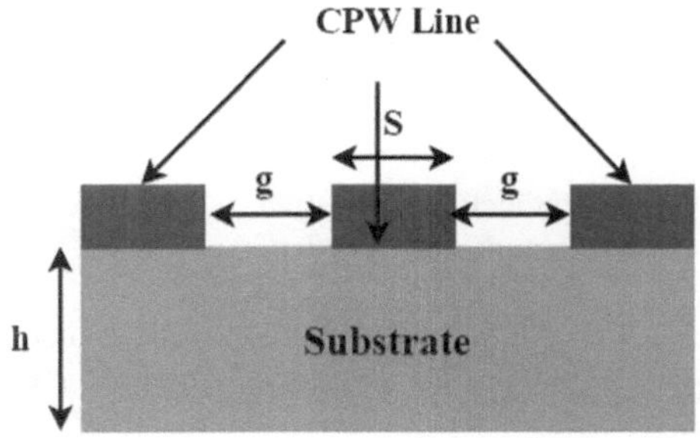

FIGURE 6.9 CPW Line Characteristics.

- **Transmission line characteristics:** For RF performance, insertion loss is measured in the on state, and isolation is measured in the off state. The mismatch between the characteristic impedance of the line and the switch leads to the insertion loss [88]. The characteristics of CPW line depend upon the width, conductor spacing, height of substrate, and permittivity of substrate to get desired characteristics impedance. Figure 6.9 shows the CPW line configuration. CPW of desired characteristics impedance can be designed by wisely choosing these parameters.

6.5 CONCLUSION

M/NEMS technology deals with the simulation, fabrication, and characterization of micro/nano-sized devices. In this technology, electrical and mechanical components are integrated together on a single chip. The performance of the systems increases when both electrical and mechanical systems work together, i.e. M/NEMS. The performance of M/NEMS devices is highly dependent upon the selection of material, design parameters, fabrication process, and the characterization of the device. M/NEMS technology has designed and fabricated the devices like mechanical sensors and actuators, microoptical systems, chemical sensors, bio-MEMS, etc., with superior performance. These devices have emerged to be used in various applications like communications, national security, automotive industry, health care, and environmental monitoring. With the help of significant features of the M/NEMS technology, novel future technologies like picoelectromechanical systems (PEMS) and femtoelectromechanical systems (FEMS) are emerging.

REFERENCES

1. Maluf, N. and Williams, K. (2004) *Introduction to Microelectromechanical Systems Engineering*. Artech House, London.
2. Bhushan, B. (ed.) (2017) *Springer Handbook of Nanotechnology*. Springer, Berlin.
3. Bryzek, J. (Aug. 1996) "Impact of MEMS technology on society", *Sensors and Actuators A: Physical*, 56(1–2,), pp. 1–9.
4. National Research Council (1998) *Microelectromechanical Systems: Advanced Materials and Fabrication Methods*. National Academies Press, Washington.
5. Madou, M. J. (2002) *Fundamentals of Microfabrication: The Science of Miniaturization*. CRC Press, New York.

6. Du, H. and Bogue, R. (Jan. 2007) "MEMS sensors: Past, present and future", *Sensor Review*, 27(1,), pp. 7–13.
7. Paul, W. and Pearson, G. L. (Jun. 1955) "Pressure dependence of the resistivity of silicon", *Physical Review*, 98(6), p. 1755.
8. Pfann, W. G. and Thurston, R. N. (1961) "Semiconducting stress transducers utilizing the transverse and shear piezoresistance effects", *Journal of Applied Physics*, 32(10), pp. 2008–2019.
9. Vettiger, P., Despont, M. and Drechsler, U. et al. (May 2000) "The Millipede – more than one thousand tips for future AFM data storage", *IBM Journal of Research and Development*, 44(3), pp. 323–340.
10. Crone, W. C. (2008) *A Brief Introduction to MEMS and NEMS*. Springer, New York.
11. Ziaie, B., Baldi, A., Lei, M., Gu, Y. and Siegel, R. A. (Feb. 2004) "Hard and soft micromachining for BioMEMS: Review of techniques and examples of applications in microfluidics and drug delivery", *Advanced Drug Delivery Reviews*, 56(2), pp. 145–172.
12. Jaafar, H., Beh, K. S., Yunus, N. A. M., Hasan, W. Z. W., Shafie, S. and Sidek, O. (Dec. 2014) "A comprehensive study on RF MEMS switch", *Microsystem Technologies*, 20(12), pp. 2109–2121.
13. Craighead, H. G. (Nov. 2000) "Nanoelectromechanical systems", *Science*, 290(5496), pp. 1532–1536.
14. Beeby, S., Ensel, G., White, N. M. and Kraft, M. (2004) *MEMS Mechanical Sensors*. Artech House, London.
15. Gammel, P., Fischer, G. and Bouchaud, J. (2005) "RF MEMS and NEMS technology, devices, and applications", *Bell Labs Technical Journal*, 10(3), pp. 29–59.
16. Goddard III, W. A., Brenner, D., Lyshevski, S. E. and Iafrate, G. J. (2012) *Handbook of Nanoscience, Engineering, and Technology*. CRC Press, New York.
17. Rai-Choudhury, P. (2000) *MEMS and MOEMS Technology and Applications*. SPIE Press, Washington.
18. Nathanson, H. C. and Wickstrom, R. A. (1965) "A resonant-gate silicon surface transistor with high-q band-pass properties", *Applied_Physics Letters*, 7(4), pp. 84–86.
19. Wilfinger, R. J. (1971) *U.S. Patent No. 3,614,677*. Washington, DC: U.S. Patent and Trademark Office.
20. Wilfinger, R. J., Bardell, P. H. and Chhabra, D. S. (Jan. 1968) "The resonistor: A frequency selective device utilizing the mechanical resonance of a silicon substrate", *IBM Journal of Research and Development*, 12(1), pp. 113–118.
21. Bergveld, P. (Oct. 1985) "The impact of MOSFET-based sensors", *Sensors and Actuators*, 8(2), pp. 109–127.
22. Allen, J. J. (2007) *Introduction to MEMS (Microelectromechanical Systems)*. Sandia National Lab.(SNL-NM), Albuquerque, NM (United States).
23. Ventra, M., Evoy, S. and Heflin, J. R. (2006) *Introduction to Nanoscale Science and Technology*. Springer Science & Business Media, Moscow.
24. Sze, S. M. (2008) *Semiconductor Devices: Physics and Technology*. John Wiley & Sons, India.
25. Sattler, K. D. (2010) *Handbook of Nanophysics: Nanoelectronics and Nanophotonics*. CRC Press, London.
26. Davari, B., Ting, C.-Y., Ahn, K. Y., Basavaiah, S., Hu, C.-K., Taur, Y., Wordeman, M. R., Aboelfotoh, O., Krusin-Elbaum, L., Joshi, R. V., Polcari, M. R. (1987) "Submicron tungsten gate MOSFET with 10 nm gate oxide", 1987 Symposium on VLSI Technology. Digest of Technical Papers: pp. 61–62.
27. Colinge, J. P. (2008) *FinFETs and Other Multi-Gate Transistors*, Vol. 73. Springer, New York.
28. Chhowalla, M., Jena, D. and Zhang, H. (Aug. 2016) "Two-dimensional semiconductors for transistors", *Nature Reviews Materials*, 1(11), pp. 1–15.

29. Nagy, D., Indalecio, G., García-Loureiro, A. J., Elmessary, M. A., Kalna, K. and Seoane, N. (Feb. 2018) "FinFET versus gate-all-around nanowire FET: performance, scaling, and variability", *IEEE Journal of the Electron Devices Society*, 6, pp. 332–340.
30. Senturia, S. D. (2007) *Microsystem Design*. Springer Science and Business Media, New York.
31. Lange, P., Kirsten, M. and W. Riethmüller (Jun. 1996) "Thick polycrystalline silicon for surface-micromechanical applications: Deposition, structuring and mechanical characterization", *Sensors and Actuators A: Physical*, 54(1–3), pp. 674–678.
32. Holzinger, M., Le Goff, A. and Cosnier, S. (Aug. 2014) "Nanomaterials for biosensing applications: A review", *Frontiers in Chemistry*, 2, p. 63.
33. Hulteen, J. C. and Martin, C. R. (1997) "A general template-based method for the preparation of nanomaterials", *Journal of Materials Chemistry*, 7(7), pp. 1075–1087.
34. Chakarvarti, S. K. (Mar. 2006) "Science and art of synthesis and crafting of nano/microstructures and devices using ion-crafted templates: A review", *Smart Structures and Materials 2006: Smart Electronics, MEMS, BioMEMS, and Nanotechnology*, 61702, p. 61720G.
35. Peterson, K. E. and Christel, L. A. (1993) *U.S. Patent No. 5,231,301*. Washington, DC: U.S. Patent and Trademark Office.
36. Ramsey, M. (1972) *U.S. Patent No. 3,648,687*. Washington, DC: U.S. Patent and Trademark Office.
37. Bolash, J. P., Edwards, M. J., James III, E. H., Parish, G. K. and White, D. H. (2000) *U.S. Patent No. 6,161,915*. Washington, DC: U.S. Patent and Trademark Office.
38. Gulick, P. E. (1994) *U.S. Patent No. 5,337,103*. Washington, DC: U.S. Patent and Trademark Office.
39. Grayson, A. C. R., Shawgo, R. S. and Johnson, A. M. (Nov. 2004) "A BioMEMS review: MEMS technology for physiologically integrated devices", *Proceedings of the IEEE*, 92(1), pp. 6–21.
40. Tang, X. R., Zhang, J. S., Zhao, H., Gong, Y. H., Wang, Y. Z. and Zhao, J. L. (Apr. 2007) "Detection of hepatitis B virus genotypes using oligonucleotide chip among hepatitis B virus carriers in Eastern China", *World Journal of Gastroenterology: WJG*, 13(13), pp. 1975.
41. Kubby, J. A. (2013) Review of Introduction to BioMEMS. Albert Folch, Berlin.
42. Fodor, S., Read, J., Pirrung, M., Stryer, L., Lu, A. and Solas, D. (Feb. 1991) "Light-directed, spatially addressable parallel chemical synthesis", *Science*, 251(4995), pp. 767–773.
43. Kopp, M. U., de Mello, A. J. and Manz, A. (May 1998) "Chemical amplification: Continuous-flow PCR on a chip", *Science*, 280(5366), pp. 1046–1048.
44. Takayama, S., McDonald, J. C., E. Ostuni. (May 1999) "Patterning cells and their environments using multiple laminar fluid flows in capillary networks", *Proceedings of the National Academy of Sciences*, 96(10), pp. 5545–5548.
45. Motamedi, M. E. (2005) *MOEMS: Micro-opto-electro-mechanical Systems*, Vol. 126. SPIE Press, Washington.
46. Chuang, W. C., Lee, H. L., Chang, P. Z. and Hu, Y. C. (Jun. 2010) "Review on the modeling of electrostatic MEMS", *Sensors*, 10(6), pp. 6149–6171.
47. Motamedi, M. E. (1993) "Merging micro-optics with micromechanics: Micro-opto-electro-mechanical (MOEM) devices", *Diffractive and Miniaturized Optics: A Critical Review*, 10271, p. 102710G.
48. Rebeiz, G. M. and Muldavin, J. B. (Dec. 2001) "RF MEMS switches and switch circuits", *IEEE Microwave Magazine*, 2(4), pp. 59–71.
49. Pelesko, J. A. and Bernstein, D. H. (2002) *Modeling MEMS and NEMS*. CRC Press, New York.
50. Lucyszyn, S. (Mar. 2004) "Review of radio frequency microelectromechanical systems technology", *IEEE Proceedings–Science, Measurement and Technology*, 151(2), pp. 93–103.

51. Rueckes, T., Kim, K., Joselevich, E., Tseng, G. Y., Cheung, C. L. and Lieber, C. M. (Jul. 2000) "Carbon nanotube-based nonvolatile random access memory for molecular computing", *Science*, 289(5476), pp. 94–97.
52. Ilic, B., Craighead, H. G., Krylov, S., Senaratne, W., Ober, C. and Neuzil, P. J. (Apr. 2004) "Attogram detection using nanoelectromechanical oscillators", *Journal of Applied Physics*, 95(7), pp. 694–3703.
53. Davis, Z. J., Abadal, G., Kuhn, O., Hansen, O., Grey, F. and Boisen, A. (Mar. 2000) "Fabrication and characterization of nanoresonating devices for mass detection", *Journal of Vacuum Science & Technology B: Microelectronics and Nanometer Structures Processing, Measurement, and Phenomena*, 18(2), pp. 612–616.
54. Roukes, M. L. (Mar. 1999) "Yoctocalorimetry: Phonon counting in nanostructures", *Physica B: Condensed Matter*, 263, pp. 1–15.
55. Ekinci, K. L. and Roukes, M. L. (Jun. 2005) "Nanoelectromechanical systems", *Review of Scientific Instruments*, 76(6), p. 061101.
56. Iijima, S. (1991) "Synthesis of carbon nanotubes", *Nature*, 354, pp. 56–58.
57. Journet, C., Maser, W.K. and Bernier, P. (Aug. 1997) "Large-scale production of single-walled carbon nanotubes by the electric-arc technique", *Nature*, 388(6644), pp. 756–758.
58. Ebbesen, T.W. and Ajayan, P. M. (Jul. 1992) "Large-scale synthesis of carbon nanotubes", *Nature*, 358(6383), pp. 220–222.
59. Li, W. Z., Xie, S. S. and Qian, L. X. (Dec. 1996) "Large-scale synthesis of aligned carbon nanotubes", *Science*, 274(5293), pp. 1701–1703.
60. Thess, A., Lee, R. and Nikolaev, P. (1996) "Crystalline ropes of metallic carbon nanotubes," Science, 273(5274, July), pp. 483–487.
61. McEuen, P. L., Fuhrer, M. S. and Park, H. (2002) "Single-walled carbon nanotube electronics," IEEE Transactions on Nanotechnology, 1(1, Aug), pp. 78–85.
62. Qian, D., Wagner G. J. and Liu W. K.. (Nov. 2002) "Mechanics of carbon nanotubes", *Applied Mechanics Reviews*, 55(6), pp. 495–533.
63. Husain, A., Hone, J. and Postma, H. W. C. (Aug. 2003) "Nanowire-based very-high-frequency electromechanical resonator", *Applied Physics Letters*, 83(6), pp. 1240–1242.
64. Kim, P. and Lieber, C. M. (Dec. 1999) "Nanotube nanotweezers", *Science*, 286(5447), pp. 2148–2150.
65. Ke, C. (Jan. 2009) "Resonant pull-in of a double-sided driven nanotube-based electromechanical resonator", *Journal of Applied Physics*, 105(2), p. 024301.
66. Fennimore, A. M., Yuzvinsky, T. D., Han, W. Q., Fuhrer, M. S., Cumings, J. and Zettl, A. (Jul. 2003) "Rotational actuators based on carbon nanotubes", *Nature*, 424(6947), pp. 408–410.
67. Sazonova, V., Yaish, Y., Üstünel, H., Roundy, D., Arias, T. A. and McEuen, P. L. (Sep. 2004) "A tunable carbon nanotube electromechanical oscillator", *Nature*, 431(7006), pp. 284–287.
68. Kinaret, J. M., Nord, T. and Viefers, S. (Feb. 2003) "A carbon-nanotube-based nanorelay", *Applied Physics Letters*, 82(8), pp. 1287–1289.
69. Mudimela, P. R., Scardamaglia, M. and González-León, O. (Jun. 2014) "Gas sensing with gold-decorated vertically aligned carbon nanotubes", *Beilstein Journal of Nanotechnology*, 5(1), pp. 910–918.
70. Mudimela, P. R., Grigoras, K. and Anoshkin, I. V. (Jun. 2012) "Single-walled carbon nanotube network field effect transistor as a humidity sensor", *Journal of Sensor*, 496546, pp. 1–7.
71. Sharma, P., Perruisseau-Carrier, J., Moldovan, C. and Ionescu, A. M. (Nov. 2013) "Electromagnetic performance of RF NEMS graphene capacitive switches", *IEEE Transactions on Nanotechnology*, 13(1), pp. 70–79.

72. Jhanwar, P., Bansal, D., Pandey, S., Verma, S. and Rangra, K. J. (Oct. 2015) "Design aspect of high power handling applications: Metal contact switches", *Microsystem Technologies*, 21(10), pp. 2083–2087.
73. Persano, A., Quaranta, F., Martucci, M. C., P., Siciliano and Cola, A. (Aug. 2015) "On the electrostatic actuation of capacitive RF MEMS switches on GaAs substrate", *Sensors and Actuators A: Physical*, 232, pp. 202–207.
74. Kalafut, D., Bajaj, A. and Raman, A. (Oct. 2017) "Multistability of cantilever MEMS/NEMS switches induced by electrostatic and surface forces", *International Journal of Non-Linear Mechanics*, 95, pp. 209–215.
75. Shojaei-Asanjan, D., Bakri-Kassem, M. and Mansour, R. R. (Jan. 2019) "Analysis of thermally actuated RF-MEMS switches for power limiter applications", *Journal of Microelectromechanical Systems*, 28(1), pp. 107–113.
76. Zaghloul, U. and G. Piazza (May 2014) "Sub-1-volt piezoelectric nanoelectromechanical relays with millivolt switching capability", *IEEE Electron Device Letters*, 35(6), pp. 669–671.
77. Chen, Z., Tian, W., Zhang, X. and Wang, Y. (Oct. 2017) "Effect of deposition parameters on surface roughness and consequent electromagnetic performance of capacitive RF MEMS switches: A review", *Journal of Micromechanics and Microengineering*, 27(11), p. 113003.
78. Dresselhaus, M. S., Dresselhaus, G. and Eklund, P. C. (1996) *Science of Fullerenes and Carbon Nanotubes: Their Properties and Applications*. Elsevier, San Diego, CA.
79. Dubois, S. M., Zanolli, Z., Declerck, X. and Charlier, J. C. (Nov. 2009) "Electronic properties and quantum transport in graphene-based nanostructures", *The European Physical Journal B*, 72(1), pp. 1–24.
80. Bolotin, K. I., Sikes, K. and Jiang, Z. (Jun. 2008) "Ultrahigh electron mobility in suspended graphene", *Solid State Communications*, 146, pp. 351–355.
81. Teo, K. B. K., Chhowalla, M. and Amaratunga, G. A. J. (Sep. 2001) "Uniform patterned growth of carbon nanotubes without surface carbon", *Applied Physics Letters*, 79(10), pp. 1534–1536.
82. Song, Y. T., Lee, H. Y. and Esashi, M. (Dec. 2006) "Low actuation voltage capacitive shunt RF-MEMS switch having a corrugated bridge", *IEICE Transactions on Electronics*, 89(12), pp. 1880–1887.
83. Giacomozzi, F., Mulloni, V. and Colpo, S. (Jan. 2011) "A flexible fabrication process for RF MEMS devices", *Romanian Journal of Information Science and Technology*, 14(3), pp. 259–268.
84. Bahadorimehr, A. and Majlis, B. Y. (Jan. 011) "Fabrication of glass-based microfluidic devices with photoresist as mask", *Informacije MIDEM*, 41(3), pp. 193–196.
85. Gad-el-Hak, M. (ed.) (2005) *MEMS: Design and Fabrication*. CRC Press, New York.
86. Acquaviva, D., Arun, A. and Esconjauregui, S. (Dec. 010) "Capacitive nanoelectromechanical switch based on suspended carbon nanotube array", *Applied Physics Letters*, 97(23), p. 233508.
87. Cassell, A. M., Franklin, N. R., Tombler, T. W., Chan, E. M., Han, J. and Dai, H. (Sep. 999) "Directed growth of free-standingsingle-walled carbon nanotubes", *Journal of the American Chemical Society*, 121(34), pp. 7975–7976.
88. Zulkefli, M. A., Mohamed, M. A. and Siow, K. S. (Aug. 2017) "Three-dimensional finite element method simulation of perforated graphene nano-electro-mechanical (NEM) switches", *Micromachines*, 8(8), p. 236.

7 A Study on the Prevention of Hot Corrosion of Boiler Steel with a High-Velocity Oxy-Fuel Spray-Coating Process

Jaswinder Singh, Hitesh Vasudev, and Sharanjit Singh

7.1 INTRODUCTION

Material degradation is a serious problem faced by every industry. India is a growing country with a huge amount of coal resources, which are used as a fuel in boilers. (1) When coal burns, sulphur is produced. This sulphur comes in contact with metal surfaces and erodes them. (2) Low-grade coal contains sulfur content, which produces SO_2 because of combustion, which is partially oxide SO_3. This SO_3 further reacts with NaCl and water vapor to give Na_2SO_4 at combustion temperature. (3) Moreover, a small quantity of vanadium is present in coal, which on combustion gives V_2O_5. This might further react with the Na_2SO_4 to form vanadrates and have a low melting point. These vanadrates are highly in corrosive in nature.

So, high-temperature degradation in the boiler tube is a major concerned due to hot corrosion and erosion. The erosion factor is usually responsible for the downtime of the boiler for 60–70% of the total maintenance time. Minimizing high-temperature erosion and corrosion is a big challenge for researchers. Surface modification is a method that helps minimize the problems related to high-temperature oxidation. Surface modification can be done by a number of ways, such as laser cladding, weld over lays, chemical vapor deposion (CVD), physical vapor deposition (PVD), thermal spraying and heat treatments.

Amongst all of these processes stated above, thermal spraying has gained popularity for protection surfaces from erosion and corrosion at high temperatures because of its versatility and possibility for onsite application when compared with other alternatives of surface modification.

Thermal spray coating is a general term used for a number of coating processess where coating is deposited on the substrate material by applying a steam of particles,

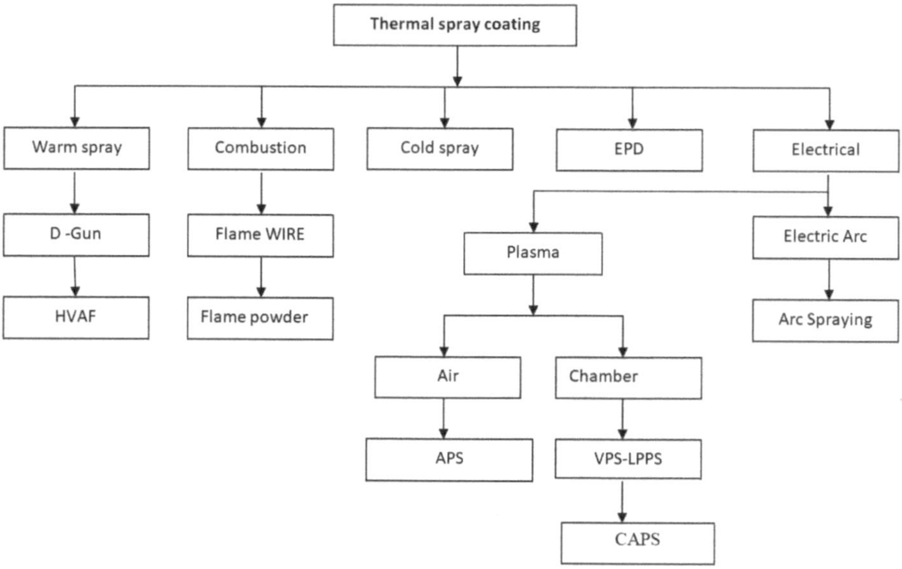

FIGURE 7.1 Classifications of Thermal Spray Coating.

metallic or ceramic, and forming splats. Several layers of these splats from the coating strike with high velocity and form bonds with the surface, which helps to give the coating its final thickness. Figure 7.1 shows the classifications of thermal spray coating.

In this chapter, we will discuss how the HVOF process has gained worldwide popularity in the field of thermal spray techniques due to its effectiveness and flexibility. The HVOF process produces dense and hard coatings, which help minimize the corrosion and wear that occurr at higher temperatures. In this process, heated powder particles, coming from a thermal spray gun with ultrasonic velocity in molten and semi-molten forms strike on the substrate material and develop a dense coating. The coating generated from the HVOF spray-process produces better coatings than many other spray-coating processes.

7.2 STUDY ON THE HVOF THERMAL SPRAY PROCESS

In a study, the authors conducted a hot corrosion study on uncoated surface and also on a specimen sprayed with HVOF after exposing them to molten salt at 900 °C under cyclic conditions NiCr, Cr_3C_2-Nicr,WC-Co and Stellite-6 coating applied on boiler tube steel ASTM SA213-T11, by the HVOF spray process [1, 2]. LPG was used as the fuel gas. Fe_2O_3 was identified and coatings provided better corrosion resistance, while on the other hand, the WC-CO coating on the substrate material provided the lowest protection and cracking and peeling of coating.

Researchers have examined the performance of NiCr coating on T-91boiler steel substrate material, and adopted the HVOF method for substrate material coating [3]. The substrate is placed for 15 cycles where each cycle consists of 100 hour cycle and 1 hour cooling in ambient conditions. The authors observed that bare T-91 steel forms porous oxide, and a higher gain in weight as compared to coated steel. X-Ray Diffraction (XRD) analysis showed that bare steel had a higher content of ferrous oxide, where coated steel had a higher content of chromium oxide, which protects steel from corrosion. Cross-sectional analysis gives evidence that bare steel had cracks and pores; on the other hand, coated steel showed a continuous dense coating without any degradation [4].

Researchers have also compared the overall weight gain of bare metal coated with NI-20Cr by different thermal spraying processes. The weight gain data of the various coatings are presented in Table 7.1.

From the above table, researcher show that when the substrate material ASTM A213 347 H is coated with Ni 20Cr, following the process High-Velocity Oxy Fuel, the overall weight gain is reduced at 900 °C under the stimulated environment conditions.

Authors have studied the behavior of 75% Cr_3C_2-25NiCr coating applied on T91steel at different operating conditions. The coating was applied on substrate material by adopting the high-velocity oxy-fuel method. The coating applied on the specimen was homogeneous and thick with less than 2% porosity. The sample was placed in a corrosive environment of Na_2SO_4-60%V_2O_5 for 50 cycles, each cycle consisting of 1 hour heating at different temperatures i.e. 550 °C, 700 °C, 800 °C in a furnace and cooling for 20 minute at room temperature. The results were obtained using visual analysis, thermo gravimetric technique, XRD (X-Ray

TABLE 7.1
The Weight Gain Data of Various Coatings

S.NO	Coating Technique	Bare material	Weight gain (mg/cm^2)
1.	Plasma Spray Technique	SA210 Grade A1	25.78
		SA213 T11	21.6
		SA213 T22	76.746
2.	Plasma Spray Technique	Superni75	13.98
		Suprni600	11.42
		Superni601	10.59
		Superni718	14.03
		Superni800H	10.63
3.	HVOF Technique	Superni75	7.121
		Suprni600	7.16
		Superni601	6.97
		Superni718	4.72
		Superni800H	4.33
4.	HVOF Technique	ASTM SA210 GradeA1	10.56
		ASTM SA213 T11	13.96
		ASTM SA213 T22	19.9
5.	Cold Spray Technique	SA 516 steel	34.1
6.	HVOF Technique	ASTM A213 347 H	0.3

diffraction), scanning electrons microscopy/Energy Dispersive and cross-sectional analysis technique. The unquoted specimen shows higher weight gain as compared with the coated specimen at all operating temperatures. It was also observed that bare specimen had an irregular-scale crack; on the other hand, the coated specimen had negligible crack. The reasons behind this are spinels of nickel chromium. Hence it was observed that coating gives more protection to the surface of the metal than the uncoated metal surface [5].

Researchers examined the coating behavior of NiCr and Cr_3C_2-NiCr, on T-91 boiler steel at a temperature of 750 °C. The high-velocity oxy-fuel method is utilized for coating on a sample of a boiler steel substrate. The substrate was placed inside a molten salt environment at 750 °C for 50 cycles. Each cycle consists of 1 hour of heating and 20 min of cooling in ambient conditions. The results were obtained by weight change, X-Ray Diffraction (XRD), and scanning electrons microscopy/Energy Dispersive (SEM/EDS) analyses. From the experiment, it was noticed that the uncoated specimen gained more weight upon the formation of an iron oxide layer on the surface of the metal. On the other hand, it was also observed that the specimen coated with NiCr on T-91steel was superior to Cr_3C_2-NiCr with the high-velocity oxy fuel technique. But both coatings show better corrosion-resistance results [3].

Authors investigated the outcome of NiAl and Tio_2 coating on the T-91 boiler at the temperature of 900 °C. The high-velocity oxy fuel method is used to apply the coating on the sample of T-91 boiler steel in a stimulated boiler environment at a temperature of 900 °C. High velocity oxy fuel was used to apply the coating on the sample of boiler steel T-91. The specimen was placed in the environment of molten salt for cycles. The oxide scale formed on the surface was examined by using the (XRD) X-Ray Diffraction technique. It was found that the uncoated specimen was Fe_2O_3, Fe_3O_4, Cr_2O_3 as the main phase; on the other hand, the coated specimen has Nio, Al_2O_3 as a major face. At the same time, Fe_2O_3, Fe_3O_4 are minor parts of the samples. Tio_2 is more protective than the $NIAlO_3$ as Nio has a loose structure; as a result of this, more pores lead to increased corrosion [6].

The authors investigated the coating behavior of $Cr_3C_2$25NiCr coating on a T-91 boiler tube under actual boiler conditions at a temperature of 900 °C [7]. A high-velocity oxy fuel process was used for coating the T-91 sample. Coated and uncoated samples were placed inside the steel boiler for cycles of 100 hours of heating and 1 hour of air cool. The results were examined by X-Ray Mapping, SEM/EDS, and cross-sectional analysis technique. It was observed that internal oxidation attack inside the substrate and corrosion scale formation results in metal loss in uncoated T-91 steel samples. In case of a coated metal surface, there are no internal cracks and formation of corrosion takes place. It indicates that coating helps prevent hot corrosion.

The performance of thermal spray coating of NiCrAlY coating on boiler steel T-91 was studied [8]. The high-velocity oxy fuel method is adopted for coating the bare sample. The bare sample and the coated sample were placed in an SIC furnace for 50 cycles. Each cycle contained one hour of heating and 20 minute of cooling in ambient environment. The results were evaluated by using the SEM/EDS and X-Ray Diffraction techniques. It was observed that the uncoated sample shows evidence of increase weight, spalling and peeling offscale. Fe_2O_3 is formed on the surface of the uncoated samples. EDS analysis shows that Fe and O are chief elements that form Fe_2O_3. On the other hand, coated samples illustrate negligible weight gain and formation of Cr_2O_3, which shows a major presence of chromium oxide and prevents corrosion. It shows that Ni,Cr, Al, were the chief elements where as Fe was the minor element in the coated sample. Therefore, the NiCrAlY coating plays an important role in avoiding hot corrosion in a high-temperature environment.

Researchers studied the coating effect of Al_2O_3 + COCrAlTay on the bare metal of Ti-31 boiler steel. The high-velocity oxy fuel method is used for coating the bare sample. The experiment was conducted in salt environment conditions: 50%$NaSO_4$-V_2O_5 at a temperature of 800 °C. The results were examined by using XRD, SEM/EDS and weight change technique. It was observed that the bare sample gains weight and a large amount of oxide content; on the other hand, the coated sample had a less change in weight measurement and a high percentage of chromium oxide layer provided protection from corrosion [9].

The authors studied the effect of 93(WC-Cr_3C_2)-7Ni, 75Cr_3C_2-25NiCr, 83WC-17CO and 86WC-10CO-4CR coating on T-91 steel. Coating was applied on the substrate by using the high-velocity oxy fuel technique [10]. The coated and uncoated substrates were placed inside the coal-fired boiler for 10 cycles, each consisting of 100 hr of heating at 900 °C and 1 hour of cooling in atmospheric air. The results were obtained by using visual examination, SEM/EDS, Weight measurement technique, X-Ray Diffraction. With the help of SEM/EDS, it was noticed that the uncoated T-91 Sample consisted of chromium oxide and iron oxide, which fails to stop corrosion as iron oxide moves inside the substrate and causes corrosion. On the other hand, side-coated samples had a major part nickel, chromium, tungsten, cobalt, but no iron oxide, which confirm that coating protects the surface from corrosion. From the results of the experiment, it could be decided which coating material provides maximum protection against corrosion and prevents internal oxidation attack on the substrate and corrosion.

Authors have examined the effect of Cr_3C_2-25 (Ni-20Cr) and Ni-20Cr coatings on T-22 boiler steel tube material in boiler. In boiler, the temperature reached around 900 °C and to protect the material of boiler tubes, they have tested two types of samples coated using the High Velocity Oxy Fuel (HVOF) process in the molten salt environment (Na_2So_4-V2O5) for 50 Cycles at 900 °C, applying a 30 μ thick coating. The experimentation is done in a boiler of silicon tube furnace. Analysis was done by using XRD techniques shows that formation of NiO and Cr_2O_3 on the surface of specimen. Uncoated specimen T-22 tested gives the result as Fe_2O_3 forms at minor peaks of the surface and Cr_2O_3 at major peaks. Coating prevents this oxidation, which erodes the material even at elevated temperatures of 900 °C and above [11].

The authors performed an experiment to study the performance of high-velocity oxy-fuel and plasma-spray process and find which coating process provides better corrosion resistance in high-temperature environments [12]. In this experiment, T-22 boiler steel is used as a substrate material for coating Ni-20Cr by adopting two different coating methods: one is the high velocity oxy fuel and other is the plasma spray method. The test was conducted in an actual boiler environment. It was noticed that the uncoated boiler steel showed a spalling oxide layer during the molten salt environment at the temperature of 900 °C. While on the other hand, both techniques, high velocity oxy fuel and plasma spray, used for coating the Ni-20Cr on boiler steel, provided a protective layer that helps control high temperature corrosion and erosion without any spalling. Ni-20Cr-coated specimens were exposed to molten salt environment at 900 °C under cyclic conditions. The results were obtained using XRD AND EDS techniques and the presence of Nio and Cr_2O_3 was examined to form protective oxides of Nickel, Chromium, and mixed. The high-velocity oxy-fuel sprayed coating shows better corrosion resistance than the plasma sprays coating coated with Ni-20Cr on T-22 steel, and weight gain for bare specimen was reduced by 75% with high velocity oxy fuel and 61% with plasma spray.

Authors studied the behavior of the NiCrBSi coating on the substrate material Suprni600, Superni601, Superfer 800 H, and the coating was successfully applied by using high velocity oxy fuel technique and obtained thickness of coating is 250–300 μm with a porosity less than the 1.4%. It was also observed that the coating of NiCrBSi was also helpful to increase micro hardness than the uncoated substrate material when the uncoated and coated substrates were exposed to a molten salt environment. The uncoated superfer 800 H Super alloy show high spalling and peeling, whereas spalling and peeling was less in case of the uncoated Suparni 600 and suparni 601 alloys. On the other hand, in case of the coated substrate, the coating was found to effective and decreased the corrosion rate in the molten salt environment. It is observed that the NiCrBsi coating formed oxides of chromium, Nickel and silicon and spinal of Nickel and chrome. The peeling and sapallation oxide scale was insignificant for the NiCrBsi coating [13].

The authors investigated the coating resistance behavior of Cr_3C_2-25(Ni-20Cr) and Ni-20Cr coating on T 91boiler steel at the temperature of 900 °C. For coating, the HVOF method was employed. High temperature oxidation was performed on uncoated and HVOF T 91 boiler steel sample. The coating thickness was in the range of 250–300 μm. The uncoated and coated samples were exposed to a molten salt environment ($NaSO_4$-60%V_2O_5) at the temperature of 900 °C under cyclic conditions. Each cycle consists of 1 hour of heating in the tube furnace and allow cooling for 20 minutes in ambient temperature. The results were analyzed by using the weight change and XRD techniques. SEM/EDS were used to analyze the formation of corrosion. The uncoated T 91 boiler steel experienced a high rate of corrosion as compared to coated T 91 boiler steel in the molten salt environment. While on the other side, the loss of corrosion is more in Ni-20Cr as compared to the Cr_3C_2-25(Ni-20Cr). The rate of corrosion for uncoated and coated T 91 boiler steel specimen in environment of molten salt is as follows.

Cr_3C_2-25(Ni-20Cr)>Ni-20Cr>bare substrate T 91 boiler steel. [14]

The authors studied the coating behavior of the alloy-718/NiCrALY bi-layer coating that was successfully applied on the GCI (Grey cast iron) substrate material using the high-velocity oxy fuel technique [15]. To recognize the correlation of structural properties, micro, structural and mechanical analyses were done. From the coating, the micro structure obtained was very dense with low porosity, and coating with material alloy-718/NiCrAlY showed higher values of micro hardness as compared to the uncoated sample. Oxidation test was conducted in ambient air at 900 °C and demonstrated the formation of thick and unstable scale of FeO, FeO_3, FeO_4, on the uncoated sample of grey cast iron substrate. While coated alloy-718/NiCrALY showed a lower rate of oxidation with insignificant gain in weight. It showed that the alloy-718/NiCrAlY coating may contribute to the formation of a protective layer of $NiCrO_4$, Al_2O_3, Cr_2O_3 and TiO_2, correspondingly. The outstanding erosion performance of alloy-718/NiCrALY contributes to the development of a stable phase of Al_2O_3 and Cr_2O_3. Due to this, alloy-718/NiCrAlY coating illustrates the highest oxidation and erosion resistance for the component working under severe condition at higher temperature conditions. The HVOF process plays a significant role in minimizing hot corrosion resistance [16–20]. The use of composite coatings has synergistics effects in combating erosion as weel as corrosion [17–24]. Nickel-based alloys provide protection against high-temperature oxidation resistance [25–32].

7.3 CONCLUSION

In this chapter, detailed literature reviews have been provided for the oxidation behavior of thermal spray coating on boiler steel at higher temperature and the following conclusion are made:

At higher temperatures, oxidation is a serious concern in erosion and corrosion of boiler tubes. In recent years, lots of methods have been developed to reduce higher temperature oxidation on surface, which is affected by higher temperature oxidation but thermal spray coating is the one of the cheap methods which help minimize the effect of high temperature oxidation. Thermal spray coating is a general term that includes a group of coating process, but in this chapter we have discussed the thermal spray coating process, high velocity oxy fuel and found that the high-velocity oxy fuel process produces a dense coating with less porosity, which helps reduce high-temperature oxidation on the surface of the metal to some extent, not 100%. So it means that there is a future scope to carry out research work in this area to minimize these defects.

REFERENCES

1. Sidhu, T. S., Prakash, S. and Aggarwal, R. D. (2006). "Hot corrosion studies of HVOF sprayed Cr3C2-NiCr and Ni–20Cr coatings on nickel-based superalloy at 900 °C", *Surface & Coatings Technology*, 201, pp. 792–800.
2. Sidhu, H. S., Sidhu, B. S. and Prakash, S. (2007). "Hot corrosion behavior of HVOF sprayed coatings on ASTM SA213-T11 steel", *Journal of Thermal Spray Technology*, 16(3), pp. 349–354.
3. Chatha, S., Sidhu, H. and Sidhu, B. (2012). "High temperature hot corrosion behaviour of NiCr and Cr_3C_2–NiCr coatings on T91 boiler steel in an aggressive environment at 750 °C", *Surface & Coatings Technology*, 2, pp. 3839–3850.
4. Kaushal, G., Singh, H. and Prakash, S. (2011). "High temperature corrosion behavior of HVOF-sprayed Ni-20 Cr coating on boiler steel in molten salt environment at 900 °C", *International Journal of Surface Science and Engineering*, 5, pp. 415–433.
5. Bhatia, R., Singh, H. and Sidhu, B. S. (2013). "Hot corrosion studies of HVOF-sprayed coating on T-91 boiler tube steel at different operating temperatures", *Journal of Materials Engineering and Performance*, 23, pp. 493–505.

6. Singh, S., Goyal, K. and Goyal, R. (2016). "Performance of Ni_3Al and TiO_2 coatings on T91 boiler tube steel in simulated boiler environment at 900 °C", *Journal of Thin Films, Coating Science Technology and Application*, 3, pp. 27–34.
7. Chatha, S., Sidhu, H. and Sidhu, B. (2016). "Performance of 75Cr3C2-25NiCr coating produced by HVOF process in a coal-fired thermal power plant", *Advanced Materials Research*, 1137, pp. 88–100.
8. Singh, G., Bala, N. and Chawla, V. (2016). "High temperature oxidation behaviour of HVOF thermally sprayed NiCrAlY coating on T-91 boiler tube steel", 6th International Conference of Materials Processing and Characterization, Vol. 4, pp. 5259–5265.
9. Jagadeeswaran, N., Ramesh, M. and Bhat, K. (2013). "Hot corrosion studies on as-received and HVOF SprayedAl2O3+CoCrAlTaY on Ti-31 alloy in salt environment", International Conference On Design and Manufacturing, Procedia Engineering, Vol. 3, pp. 1013–1019.
10. Sidhu, V., Goyal, K. and Goyal, R. (2017). "An investigation of corrosion resistance of HVOF coated ASME SA213 t91 boiler steel in an actual boiler environment", *Anti-Corrosion Methods and Materials*, 64(5), pp. 499–507, published online.
11. Singh, S., Goyal, K. and Goyal, R. (2016). "Performance of Cr3C2-25 (Ni- 20Cr) and Ni-20Cr coatings on T-22 boiler steel tube material in stimulated boiler environment", *Journals of Thin Films, Coatings Science Technology and Applications*, 3, pp. 19–26.
12. Mangla, A., Chawla, V. and Singh, G. (2017). "Comparative hot corrosion behavior of HVOF and plasma sprayed Ni-20Cr coated T-22 steel in actual coal field boiler environment", *Journals of Engineering Science and Researches*, ISSN 2348-8034.
13. Sidhu, T. S., Prakash, S. and Aggarwal, R. D. (2006). "Hot corrosion behaviour of HVOF-sprayed NiCrBSi coatings on Ni-and Fe-based superalloys in Na2SO4–60% V2O5 environment at 900 °C", *Acta Materialia*, 54, pp. 773–784.
14. Singh, S., Goyal, K. and Goyal, R. (2016). "Performance of Cr3C2-25(Ni-20Cr) and Ni-20Cr coatings on T91 boiler tube steel in simulated boiler environment at 900 °C", *Chemical and Materials Engineering*, 4(4), pp. 57–64.
15. Vasudev, H., Thakur, L., Bansal, A., Singh, H. and Sunny, Z. (2019). "High temperature oxidation and erosion behaviour of HVOF sprayed bilayer alloy-718/ NiCrAlY coating", *Surface and Coatings Technology*, 393, pp. 366–380.
16. Edris, H., Mc-Cartney, D. and Sturgeon, A. G. (1997). "Micro-structural Characterization of HVOF Sprayed Coatings of Inconel 625", *Journal of Materials Science*, 32, pp. 863–868.
17. Singh, H., Grewal, M. S., Sekhon, H. S. and Rao, R. G. (2008). "Sliding wear performance of high velocity-oxy-fuel spray Al_2O_3/TiO_2 and Cr_2O_3 coatings", *Engineering*, 222, pp. 601–610.
18. Singh, G., Mangla, A. and Chawala, V. (2017). "Comparative study of hot corrosion behavior of HVOF and plasma sprayed Ni20Cr coating on SA213(T22) boiler steel in Na2SO4-60%V2O5 environment", International Journal of Engineering Sciences & Research Technology, 6(10), pp. 674–686.
19. Sidhu, T. S., Prakash, S. and Agrawal, R. D. (2006). "Hot corrosion behaviour of HVOF sprayed NiCrBSi coating on Ni and Fe based super alloy in Na_2SO_4-60%V2O5 environment", *Acta Materialia*, 54, pp. 773–784.
20. Sidhu, H. S., Sidhu, B. S. and Prakash, S. (2006). "Hot corrosion behavior of HVOF sprayed coatings on ASTM SA213-T11 steel", *Thermal Spray Technology*, 6(3), pp. 349–354.
21. Sidhu, T. S., Prakash, S. and Agrawal, R. D. (2006). "A comparative study of hot corrosion resistance of HVOF sprayed NiCrBSi and stellite-6 coated Ni based super alloy at 900 °C", *Material Science and Engeering*, 445–446, pp. 1–9.

22. Sidhu, T. S., Prakash, S. and Agrawal, R. D. (2006). "Hot corrosion resistance of high-velocity oxy-fuel sprayed coatings on a Nickel-Base super alloy in molten salt environment", *Thermal Spray Technology*, 15(3), pp. 387–399.
23. Sidhu, T. S., Prakash, S. and Agrawal, R. D. (2006). "Characterization of HOVF sprayed NiCrBSi coating Ni- and Fe based super alloy in molten salt environment", *Thin Solid Film*, 515, pp. 95–105.
24. Sidhu, H. S., Sidhu, B. S. and Prakash, S. (2006). "Evaluation of hot corrosion behavior of LPG assisted HVOF NiCr wire sprayed boiler tube steel in molten salt environment", *ISIJ International*, 46(10), pp. 1067–1074.
25. Kaushal, G., Singh, H. and Prakash, S. (2011). "Comparative high temperature analysis of HVOF sprayed and detonation gun sprayed Ni–20Cr coating in laboratory and actual boiler environments", *Journal of Oxidation*, 76, pp. 169–191.
26. Somasundara, B., Kodali, R. and Ramesh, R. M. R. (2014). "Hot corrosion behavior of HVOF sprayed Cr3C2–35% NiCr+5%Si coating in the presence of Na_2SO_4–60% V2O5 at 700 °C", *Transactions of the Indian Institute of Metals*, 68, pp. 1–10, https://doi.org/10.1007/S12666-014-0453-0.
27. Kaur, M., Singh, H. and Prakash, S. (2012). "High temperature behavior of high velocity oxy-fuel sprayed Cr3C2–NiCr coating", *Metallurgical and Material Transaction*, 43-A, pp. 2979–2993.
28. Shukla, V. N., Jayaganthan, R. and Tewari, V. K. (2016). "Degradation behaviour and microstructural characterisation of HVOF-sprayed Cr3C2-NiCr coatings in molten salt environment", *International Journal of Materials and Product Technology*, 53, pp. 15–27.
29. Bala, N., Singh, H., Prakash, S. and Karthikeyan, J. (2012). "Investigations on the behavior of HVOF and cold sprayed Ni-20Cr coating on T22 boiler steel in actual boiler environment", *Thermal Spray Technology*, 21(1), pp. 144–158.
30. Shukla, V. N., Jayaganthan, N. and Tewari, V. K. (2012). "Hot corrosion studies of HVOF-sprayed Cr_3C_2-NiCr coating on 310S stainless steel in an actual environment of a coal fired boiler", *Advanced Materials Research*, 585, pp. 483–487.
31. Kaushal, G., Singh, H. and Prakash, S. (2011). "Comparative high temperature analysis of HVOF sprayed and detonation gun sprayed Ni–20Cr coating in laboratory and actual boiler environment", *Oxidation of Metals*, 76, pp. 169–191.
32. Kaur, M., Singh, H. and Prakash, S. (2012). "High-temperature behavior of a high-velocity oxy-fuel sprayed Cr_3C_2-NiCr coating", Metallurgical and Materials Transactions, 43, pp. 2979–2993.

8 Nanocomposite Coatings

HVOF Spray Processing, Microstructural Evolution and Performance

Gaurav Prashar and Hitesh Vasudev

8.1 INTRODUCTION

Composite coatings, composed of Ni-based superalloys such as Inconel-625, 718 and thermally stable reinforcing particles, deposited by the HVOF technique have been established as high-performance protective coatings for applications requiring both corrosion and erosion resistance at elevated temperatures, especially waste-to-energy boilers [1–8]. These coatings include metal-matrix, polymer-matrix and ceramic-matrix varieties of composites [9–15]. Thermal spray methods present a progressive approach for the deposition of these coatings with respect to materials, medium of deposition and the thickness achieved when compared to other deposition processes.

Any material can be deposited, from soft to hard metals, alloys and ceramics, with a wide range of velocities and processing temperatures. Therefore, any composition can be prepared and then combined to form a composite with optimized properties. For example, hard ceramic (Al_2O_3), having a high melting point, can be combined with a ductile material like Ni-based superalloys. The thickness achieved in nanocomposite coatings can vary from 50 μm to several millimeters, compared with PVD or CVD methods, where the thickness achieved is less than 5 μm [16]. The schematic of the thermal spray process is illustrated in Figure 8.1. During the process, a stream of high-temperature particles (molten or in semi-molten state) is directed towards the substrate with a specific velocity, and upon impact, these particles are flattened to a disc-like shape, known as splats.

The major thermal spraying methods are high-velocity oxy-fuel (HVOF) [17], cold spray [18], vacuum plasma spray [19], magnetron sputtering [20], sol-gel method [21], laser cladding [22], electro deposition [23], and plasma spraying [24].

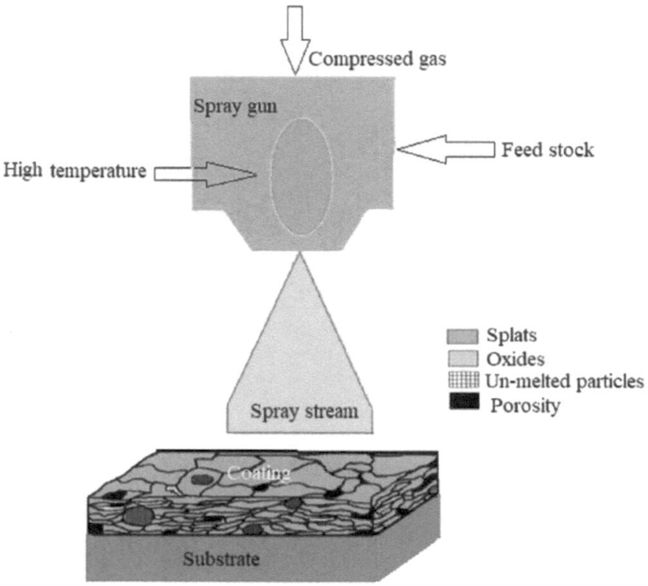

FIGURE 8.1 Schematic of the Thermal Spray Process.

Out of all the above-mentioned techniques, HVOF is the one that produces thick coatings, approximately upto 300 m, with minimum porosity levels, superior bond strength and high hardness at a relatively low cost. By using mixtures of oxygen and combustion fuel, the powder particles in molten or semi-molten state are deposited onto the substrate at supersonic velocities of approximately 1000 m/s. This process has applications in almost all fields where engineering components are exposed to corrosion and erosion conditions [25,26]. The focus of the current article is to review nanocomposite coatings that are deposited by HVOF with respect to processing, performance and deposition mechanism. The feedstock used is in the form of powder/wire or liquid, and the section 'Feedstock Materials' of this article is dedicated specifically to the characteristics and production of these materials.

8.2 HIGH-VELOCITY OXY-FUEL (HVOF)

One of the major drawbacks associated with the plasma-spraying method is that often, the temperature of in-flight particles is higher than the feedstock melting-temperature, which makes it difficult to achieve partial melting of the agglomerated particles. Therefore, development of the HVOF process is aimed at reducing the operating temperature of particles ($<2000\,°C$) and increasing their velocity [27]. HVOF systems can generate high particle velocities, as compared to plasma jets, essentially due to the convergent-divergent nozzle, which accelerates the low-temperature HVOF gases. Third-generation HVOF systems like JP5000, DJ2700 and DJ2600 have a chamber pressure of 1Mpa and can attain velocities upto 650 m/s against 450 m/s of the first- and second-generation systems. Another parameter that plays a major role is torch design. To check the effect [28], a series of experiments were conducted with same powder and sintered and agglomerated WC-Co having particle size between 10 m and 45 m. Different HVOF systems were employed for powder spraying: Jet kote, Top Gun, DJ2600 and DJ2700, JP5000 and Top Gun-K. It was found that the degree of the phase transformations will depend upon the manufacturing route of the spray powder, the flame temperature of the fuel used and the heat transfer rate to the particles in the respective spray systems. Phase transformations in the Top Gun system were more, because in this, injection of powder takes place in the region where the flame temperature is the highest. Vice-versa phase transformation is less when injection of powder takes place in the region where flame temperature is less i.e, for JP5000 and Top Gun systems, in which powder is injected downstream, or when flame temperature is lowered by the cooling air, like for DJ2600 and DJ2700 systems [29].

HVOF is the candidate of choice instead of the plasma systems when feedstock material is nanometer-sized agglomerated powder [30]. The formation of nanozones solely depends upon control of heat propagation within the oxide particles, which requires less heat propagation within oxide particles [31]. Marple and Lima [32] successfully demonstrated that when nanometer-sized particles of TiO_2 were deposited by HVOF, more semi-molten particles existed as compared to the plasma spray process, which has a higher temperature of conventional particles (Al_2O_3-TiO_2) and less velocity. Furthermore, HVOF endowed TiO_2 coatings with excellent wear resistance compared to the plasma process.

HVOF can also be employed for suspension spraying [33–35]. Killinger et al. [33,34] were among the first researchers who highlighted this process. They named it HVSFS (high-velocity suspension flame spraying).

8.3 FEEDSTOCK MATERIALS

Feedstock materials that can be used to manufacture nanocomposite coatings are typically in the form of (i) powder; (ii) solution or suspension; and (iii) wire [16]. Among all, powder feedstock is used commonly due to its compatibility with almost all feeding systems and spray processes. However, when the particles are nanosized, they can create problems like handling and feeding. Therefore, it is necessary to processes nanoparticles to micronsize, i.e. to 3D morphology, before using them as feedstock material for thermal spraying. Wire feedstock is commercially available in the form of cored wire, and the core is composed of agglomerated nanoparticles. Suspension or liquid feedstock is still in the R&D phase but is becoming a popular route for the production of nanocomposite coatings, without the need for extensive manufacturing steps that were required in production of powder and wire feedstock materials.

In this study, we will focus on the HVOF technique, and the feedstock material used for HVOF is mainly powder. Therefore, the next section, 'Feedstock Materials,' will discuss the preparation of different types of feedstock material for HVOF.

8.3.1 Preparation of Feedstock Material

Feedstock materials are an integral part of the coating system. Nanostructured coating powders for HVOF spraying can be developed through the following three main routes: (i) mechanical processing; (ii) thermal or physical processing; and (iii) chemical processing. The mechanical method involves crushing/milling large particles mechanically to the nanoscale. This is the a commonly employed method by researchers to produce feedstock material. However, a major issue related to mechanical milling is that the shape and size of the nanoparticles obtained are not consistent and particles of size less than 100 nm block the nozzle during thermal spraying [30]. Therefore, these particles are agglomerated to micron-size by the spray drying method [30,36], but it is an expensive route [37–40].

Chemical processing means nucleating/precipitating the nanoparticles from slurry or solution, and it can be carried out with or without a chemical reaction. The drawback of this method is that it needs expensive raw materials. Thermal processing involves the condensation of nanoparticles by rapid cooling of supersaturated vapour to produce high-purity, fine particles, but it requires high capital investments.

As mentioned earlier, the as-collected nanoparticles will not be suitable for thermal spray feedstock directly, due to the following technical issues: (i) difficulty in handling and related health concerns; (ii) poor flowability, resulting in blocking of injection line; and (iii) due to insufficient momentum and inertia, nanoparticles will not be able to enter the core of the thermal spray jet [41]. A universal solution to overcome these drawbacks is manual agglomeration of nanoparticles using an organic binder, which is better than the complex and costly spray-drying method. Singh et al. carried out manual agglomeration of nanosized (80 nm) Al_2O_3 using 3 wt% PVA (polyvinyl alcohol binder) having molecular weight 14000. Manual agglomeration will result in a wide range of sizes, which were further consolidated to micronsize by sieving them through sieve shakers of different sizes [42]. Lastly, agglomerated Al_2O_3 powder was then dried in an oven for 3 h before using as feedstock material for thermal spraying.

Another common approach is to introduce nanotubes or nanoparticles directly into micron-sized particles to prepare feedstock for HVOF spraying but Thakur et al. modified nanostructured WC-Co-Cr HVOF feedstock powder by adding a small quantity (2 wt%) of MWCNT (multi-walled carbon nano tubes) in the binder matrix and mixing them properly by jar milling for 24 hrs in order to examine their effect on slurry erosion resistance [43].

Other common methods like sol-gel [44,45] and freeze drying [46] are also used to produce nanocomposite powders for feedstock. However, the use of the aforementioned techniques can produce particles of irregular morphology, angular shapes and poor flowability.

8.4 NANOCOMPOSITE COATINGS

8.4.1 Ni-Reinforced Nanocomposites

Nickel-based alloys are preferred as better candidates to be sprayed by HVOF for the protection of structural components in power plants that are made up of low-alloyed steel. Ni can be reinforced with elements such as Ti, Al, Cr, B and Si in order to improve tribological and mechanical properties. Ni-Al, NiCrBSi, Ni-Cr and NiCrAlY are the most common Ni-base alloys that are used in corrosion- and erosion-resistant applications.

8.4.2 Ni-Al_2O_3 Coatings

The HVOF process is used to deposit dense Al_2O_3 coatings with improved mechanical properties whereas the properties of plasma spray coatings are not adequate. Although coatings the deposited by HVOF are dense as compared to plasma spray coatings, the properties of the coatings are still inferior as compared to bulk ceramics due to the presence of pores and cracks, which adversely affects the properties of coatings, i.e. wear resistance, hardness and toughness.

One strategy to improve these properties is to decrease the grain size of the ceramic phase and add toughening elements (Ni) to the microstructure, which will resist crack formation.

Hannula et al. developed Ni-Al_2O_3 nanocomposite coatings to examine the effect of adding Ni to the nano Al_2O_3 matrix. Ni was added upto 10%. It was found that with increase in Ni content, the length of the cracks reduces and toughness increases. On the other hand, the hardness and wear resistance of the composite reduces [47]. The authors recommended that the properties of coatings strongly depend upon spraying parameters and to obtain a desired composite structure, coatings that contain 5% Ni exhibit higher toughness and good wear resistance [48].

8.4.3 NiCrBSi-Al_2O_3 Coatings

NiCrSiB is another nickel-based alloy used for wear- and hot corrosion-resistant applications. Most specifically, NiCrSiB coatings have a low environmental impact compared with other coatings that have a similar set of properties [49–52]. The properties, to great extent, can be due to the presence of hard phases that are influenced by Cr, boron (B) and silicon (Si), which are then dispersed in the nickel (Ni) matrix. More importantly, self-fluxing characteristics of boron and silicon lower the melting temperature, allowing for lower energy usage [53,54].

Despite excellent oxidation- and corrosion-resistant properties of NiCrBSi coatings, their low hardness as compared to ceramics and carbides makes them unsuitable for certain industries. Therefore, reinforcement in the form of a hard phase is needed to improve the erosion-corrosion resistance of NiCrSiB coatings. In the context, Praveen et al. deposited two weight compositions, 1.4 wt% and 0.17 wt %, of nano Al_2O_3 with NiCrSiB by the HVOF technique. With the addition of 1.4 wt% nano Al_2O_3, microhardness increases from 576 to 748 Hv, which in turn improves the erosion resistance of the composite coating [55].

In literature it has been observed that for Cr_3C_2-NiCr coatings there is a 20.5% increase in hardness value (846 Hv to 1020 Hv) when shifting from conventional sizes to nanostructured sizes [56–58]. This increase in hardness is attributed to a uniform microstructure and the presence of nanophase, and this increase in hardness value to some extent is also contributed by the low thermal and high kinetic energy of HVOF.

It has also been reported that for nanostructured coatings that undergo heat-treatment, there is a remarkable increase in hardness value (1020–1240 Hv) [58]. Also, the rate of work hardening for nanocrystalline grains is high because of the restricted deformation of nanoscale grains, which slow down dislocation movements.

Ramanathan et al. demonstrated the successful application of the nano-structured Cr_3C_2–25(Ni-20Cr) coating sprayed by the HVOF method for a high-temperature erosion-oxidation application. The fracture toughness, young's modulus and microhardness values of both the as-received and nanostructured coatings were compared, and it was found that the nanostructured coatings exhibit higher values due to their dense and homogeneous structure [59]. The microhardness value of the nanostructured coatings was high due to the precipitation of fine oxide particles (Cr_2O_3) in the Ni-20Cr binder phase. At the temperature of 800 °C, the E-O resistance of the nanocoating was found to be 52% higher than the as-received coating. The hardness values for some WC-Co nanostructured and conventional coatings deposited by HVOF are shown in Table 8.1.

Commercially available coating powders Cr_3C_2, Ni and Cr with an average particle size of approximately 40–100 m were first mechanically mixed for six hours to prepare a conventional coating (27%Cr_3C_2- 23%Ni- 50%Cr) and then ball milled for 20 hours in a ball miller to obtain a nanocomposite coating of the same composition with an average particle size of 50 nm. Both the mixed powders were thermally sprayed onto the SA-210 Gr carbon steel substrate by using the DJ2600 HVOF thermal spray gun. Nanostructured coatings exhibit a highly dense appearance with less pores as compared to conventional coatings. The coating thickness

TABLE 8.1
Hardness Values for Some WC-Co Nanostructured and Conventional Coatings Deposited by HVOF

Coatings (reference)	Hardness value (Gpa)	reference
Conventional	11.10	[60]
Nano	11.90	[60]
Conventional	10.6	[61]
Nano	12.2	[61]
Conventional	12.12	[62]
Nano	15.38	[62]
Nano*	12.07	[63]
Nano*	12.73	[63]
Conventional**	10.67	[64]
Nano**	11.25	[64]
Conventional**	12.41	[64]
Nano**	12.80	[64]

* Co-Co matrix, ** Co-Cr matrix

for the nano-coating was in the range of 280–320 μm, while for the conventional coating, it was approximately 290–325 μm. Erosion experiments were performed at 450 °C with impact angles of 30°, 60° and 90°. It was concluded that the erosion resistance of the nanocomposite coating was better than the conventional and uncoated substrates due to the presence of a Cr_2O_3 layer, which acts as a protective barrier against incoming erodent particles [65]. Less porosity of the nanocomposite was also found to be a reason for low erosion rates, as an interconnected network of pores could destroy the effectiveness of the coating. At oblique angles, the erosion rate was higher for all materials showing ductile behavior. Moreover, both nanocomposite and conventional coatings provide 7.5 times and 3.5 times better erosion resistances, respectively, at 30° impact angle as compared to the uncoated substrate.

Picas et al. deposited nanocrystalline powders of Cr_2C_3 75%+NiCr20 25% and Cr_2C_3 60%+NiCr20 40% onto a steel substrate by the HVOF method. SEM analysis was used to characterize the morphology of powders and the coating microstructure. Microhardness and surface roughness tests were done on coatings. A pin-on-disc tribometer was used to evaluate tribological properties. It was found that the surface finish increases with decrease in the size of the feedstock powder [66]. The wear rates and the friction coefficient of the nanostructured CrC60–NiCr40 coating were found to be better than the nanostructured CrC75–NiCr25 coating.

A coating of nanocrystalline Alloy-718 was deposited onto stainless steel substrate using the HVOF thermal-spraying technique by Tellkamp et al. [67].

8.5 HVOF PROCESS: FORMATION MECHANISM, DEPOSITION AND PROPERTIES

8.5.1 Conventional Approach (Formation and Deposition Mechanism)

HVOF-sprayed nanocomposite coatings via the conventional approach use feedstock material in the form of micro-meter size agglomerates of nanoparticles. Two types of approaches are involved in this: first, micron-sized particles are crushed down to nanoscale – known as the top-down approach – and then agglomerated to micron-sized particles to be used as feedstock material for deposition of nanocomposite coatings (the bottom-up approach). The top-down and bottom-up approaches for the fabrication of nanocomposites are illustrated in Figure 8.2. Once the particles enter into the core of the thermal spray jet, melting of particles starts from the outer surface of the particle. But the thermal transport properties of agglomerated particles are different from conventional ones due to a porous structure and low density of agglomerated powder particles. The pores present in particles retard the heat transfer rate [68], and as a result, heat conduction is lower compared to the dense particles of an equal diameter.

This effect enables partial melting of feedstock particles for effective deposition. Moreover, the nanostructure characteristics of feedstock particles are also retained due to this effect. It is emphasized that parameters employed to spray conventional feedstock will not be used for agglomerated feedstock particles as it will destroy nano-features during the spraying process. Hence, partial melting will result in loss

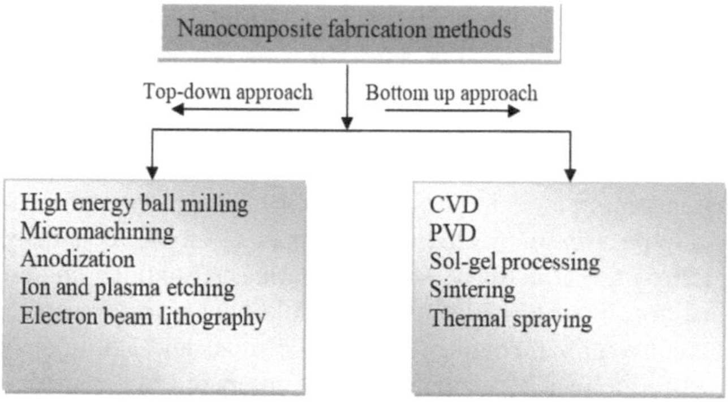

FIGURE 8.2 Top-down and Bottom-up Approach for Nanocomposite Fabrication.

of nanofeatures to some degree. Such a coating architecture is known as a bi-modal structure [30], as shown in Figures 8.3 and 8.4.

8.5.2 Properties

Mechanical Properties

Four important criteria often used to describe the mechanical properties of HVOF-sprayed coatings are (a) hardness, (b) fracture toughness, (c) bond strength, and (d) elastic modulus.

A 20% increase in hardness was observed in nanostructured Cr_3C_2–25(Ni20Cr) HVOF sprayed coatings as compared to their conventional counterpart. This increase in hardness is attributed to the reduced grain size in nanocomposites. However, in

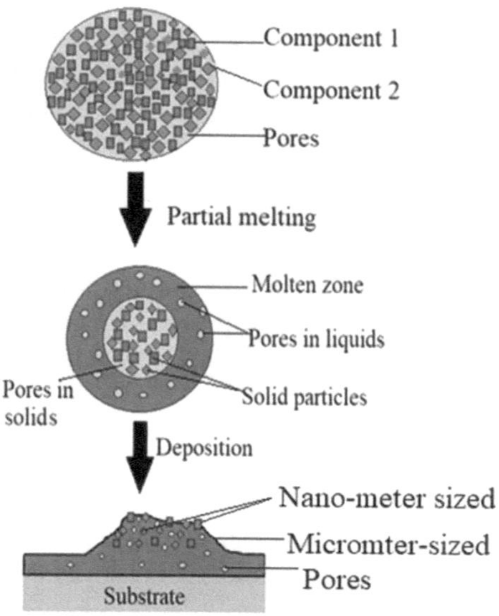

FIGURE 8.3 Agglomerated Nanoscale Particle Melting & Deposition Process.

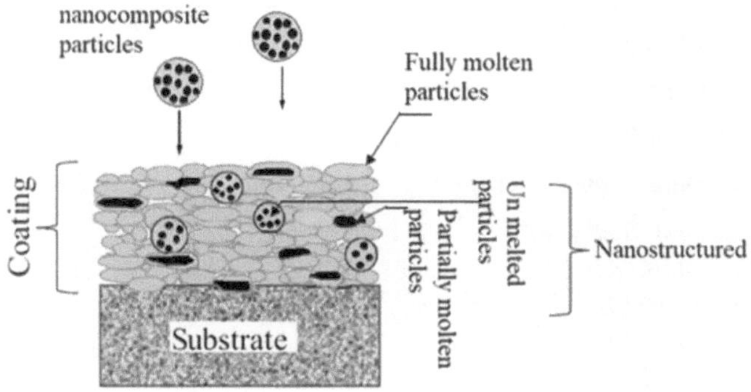

FIGURE 8.4 Nanocomposite Microstructures Deposited by HVOF Process Using Agglomerated Feedstock.

bimodal structure coatings, hardness depends upon microstructural variations rather than grain size [69,70]. Different hardness values were observed in the fully melted and partially melted (nanostructured) areas of the coatings. As compared to fully melted zones, the partially melted zones exhibit a lower hardness value.

Failure takes place due to crack initiation and will depend upon the fracture strength of the material. Greater the fracture toughness value, lesser will be the wear rate. When surface stresses reach a critical value due to the impact of solid particles, micro-cracks start to initiate. The formation of cracks on the surface leads to the growth of the cracks on the subsurface region of a substrate. Fracture toughness can be calculated by the indentation method with a maximum load of 10 kg and a dwell time of 15 sec [71]. For the measurement of crack length, a Vickers optical microscope is used. In conventional coatings, long and well-defined splat boundaries provide an easy path for crack propagation, periodic disruptions of the splat boundaries by partially melted areas (nanostructured) arrest crack deflection and help in improving fracture toughness. A homogeneous distribution of the particles also increases the fracture toughness by enhancing the interlamellar strength. Table 8.2 shows the different relations to calculate the fracture toughness of the coatings.

The capacity of a layer to remain attached to the base metal under operating conditions is termed as bond strength. Failure of coating adhesion to the substrate results in interfacial bonding, known as cracking for brittle material. The cohesion strength between the splats and adhesion among substrate and the coating govern bond strength. Due to refinement of the splat size in nanostructured coatings, the contact between the splats enhances and this ultimately improves cohesion strength. Singh et al. used the ASTM C-633 adhesion test to measure the bond strength of the nanostructured Cr_2O_3-TiO_2 coating. The coating layer was glued onto a pull rod by using an epoxy adhesive, which was cured for 24 hr at a temperature of 40 °C. A material-testing machine was used to conduct bond strength tests under ambient conditions [42]. The authors reported that the adhesion strength was 25.8% better than the bare substrate, which indicates excellent intersplat bonding.

TABLE 8.2
Different Relationships to Calculate the Fracture Toughness of the Coatings

Fracture toughness relations	reference
$Kc = 0.16\ H_v a^{1/2} (c/a)^{-3/2}$	[72]
$Kc = \beta\ (H_v P/21)^{1/2}$	[73]
$Kc = 0.0711 (H_v a^{1/2})\ (E/H_v)^{2/5} (c/a)^{-3/2}$	[74]
$Kc = 0.0193 (H_v D)\ (E/H_v)^{2/5} (a)^{-1/2}$	[75]

The various properties and microstructure of the developed coatings mainly depend on the material or combination of materials i.e. the composite and the process utilized for the fabrication of the coating [76–83].

8.6 FUTURE PERSPECTIVE AND CHALLENGES

The method proposed (HVOF) above is still undergoing research in different fields. Every field has its own challenges. Nanocomposite coatings are preferred due to their enhanced physical properties as compared to their conventional counterparts. Nano-sized feedstock material has low mass, due to which the problem of deposition occurs during processing, due to poor flowability. Therefore, feedstock needs to be agglomerated before feeding into the HVOF jet for deposition. This will increase operating costs from the consumable and the machine part configurations. Hence, a lot of R&D work is still required in this field to achieve optimal results.

8.7 CONCLUSION

In this article, nanocomposite coatings deposited by the HVOF method are explained comprehensively. During fabrication of HVOF-sprayed coatings, molten feedstock material in powder form piles up to form layers and upon solidification, a coating is obtained. Microstructural properties of the developed coating not only depend upon the composition of the feedstock material to be used in spraying but also on some other factors of that powder, like distribution of the particle size, velocity at which the particles were propelled towards the substrate, temperature of spray, substrate type, temperature of substrate and degree of the solidification of particles during the spraying. The major area of application of HVOF-sprayed nanocomposite coatings is in the field of wear-, erosion- and corrosion-resistant improvements. Studies conducted by authors/researchers using nanocomposite coatings of Ni plus various reinforcements and cermet coatings exhibit promising results for the improvement of erosion- and corrosion-resistant applications, which also shows their future prospects in a particular field. Hence, further R&D activities in this area can lead to better results and understanding of HVOF process characteristics along with a wider range of applications.

REFERENCES

1. Dooley, R. and Wiertel, E. (2009). "A survey of erosion and corrosion resistant materials being used on boiler tubes in waste to energy boilers". *Nawtec17- 2334*. pp. 37–41.
2. Zhang, D., Harris, S. J. and McCartney, D. G. (2003). "Microstructure formation and corrosion behaviour in HVOF-sprayed inconel 625 coatings", *Materials Science and Engineering A*, 344(1–2), pp. 45–56, https://doi.org/10.1016/S0921-5093(02)00420-3.
3. Prashar, G. and Vasudev, H. (2020). "Hot corrosion behavior of super alloys", *Materials Today: Proceedings*, 26, pp. 1131–1135, https://doi.org/10.1016/j.matpr.2020.02.226.
4. Vasudev, H., Bansal., A., Thakur, L. and Singh, H. (2020). "An investigation on oxidation behaviour of high velocity oxy-fuel sprayed Inconel718-Al2O3 composite coatings", *Surface and Coatings Technology*, 393, p. 125770, https://doi.org/10.1016/j.surfcoat.2020.125770.
5. Al-Fadhli, H. Y., Stokes, J., Hashmi, M. S. J. and Yilbas, B. S. (2006). "HVOF coating of welded surfaces: Fatigue and corrosion behaviour of stainless steel coated with Inconel-625 alloy", *Surface and Coatings Technology*, 200(16–17), pp. 4904–4908, https://doi.org/10.1016/j.surfcoat.2005.04.052.
6. Sampath, S., Jiang, X. Y., Matejicek, J., Prchlik, L., Kulkarni, A. and Vaidya, A. (2004). "Role of thermal spray processing method on the microstructure, residual stress and properties of coatings: An integrated study of Ni-5 wt. % Al bond coats", *Materials Science and Engineering A*, 364(1–2), pp. 216–231, https://doi.org/10.1016/j.msea.2003.08.023.
7. Bolelli, G., Lusvarghi, L. and Giovanardi, R. (2008). "A comparison between the corrosion resistances of some HVOF-sprayed metal alloy coatings", *Surface and Coatings Technology*, 202(19), pp. 4793–4809, https://doi.org/10.1016/j.surfcoat.2008.04.056.
8. Walsh, D. A., Li, L. E., Bakare, M. S. and Voisey, K. T. (2009). "Visualisation of the local electrochemical activity of thermal sprayed anti-corrosion coatings using scanning electrochemical microscopy", *Electrochimica Acta*, 54(20), pp. 4647–4654, https://doi.org/10.1016/j.electacta.2009.03.057.
9. Westfall, L. J. (1985). "The United States of America as represented by the Administrator of the National Aeronautics and Space Administration: 'Arc spray fabrication of metal matrix composite monotape", *United States Patent* (4,518,625).
10. Steffens, H. D. and Kaczmarek, R. (1991). "Metal matrix composites made by thermal spraying", *Powder Metallurgy International*, 23(2), pp. 105–107.
11. Legoux, J. G. and Dallaire, S. (1993). "Copper-titanium diboride coatings obtained by plasma spraying reactive micropellets", *Journal of Thermal Spray Technology*, 2(3), pp. 283–286, https://doi.org/10.1007/BF02650477.
12. Tiwari, R., Herman, H. and Sampath, S. (1992). "Vacuum plasma spraying of MoSi2 and its composites", *Materials Science and Engineering A*, 155(1–2), pp. 95–100, https://doi.org/10.1016/0921-5093(92)90316-S.
13. Kucuk, A., Lima, R. S. and Berndt, C. C. (2000). "Composite coatings of Si3N4-soda lime silica produced by the thermal spray process", *Journal of Materials Engineering and Performance*, 9(6), pp. 603–608, https://doi.org/10.1361/105994900770345449.
14. Sun, L., Berndt, C. C. and Gross, K. A. (2002). "Hydroyapatite/polymer composite flame-sprayed coatings for orthopedic applications", *Journal of Biomaterials Science, Polymer Edition*, 13(9), pp. 977–990, https://doi.org/10.1163/156856202760319135.
15. Yan, F. Y., Gross, K. A., Simon, G. P. and Berndt, C. C. (2004). "Mechanical and erosion properties of CaCO 3-EMAA thermal sprayed coatings", *Polymer Engineering and Science*, 44(8), pp. 1448–1459, https://doi.org/10.1002/pen.20141.
16. Gan, J. A. and Berndt, C. C. (2015). "Nanocomposite coatings: Thermal spray processing, microstructure and performance", *International Materials Reviews*, 60(4), pp. 195–244, https://doi.org/10.1179/1743280414Y.0000000048.
17. Mahesh, R. A., Jayaganthan, R. and Prakash, S. (2008). "Oxidation behavior of HVOF sprayed Ni-5Al coatings deposited on Ni- and Fe-based superalloys under cyclic

condition", *Materials Science and Engineering A*, 475(1–2), pp. 327–335, https://doi.org/10.1016/j.msea.2007.04.108.

18. Bala, N. and Singh, H. (2018). "Fundamentals of corrosion mechanisms in cold spray coatings", In Cold-Spray Coatings, pp. 351–371, https://doi.org/10.1007/978-3-319-67183-3_12.
19. Zhai, C., Niu, Y., Huang, L., Pan, H., Li, H., Zheng, X. and Sun, J. (2016). "Microstructure characteristics and oxidation behavior of vacuum plasma sprayed tungsten disilicide coating", *Ceramics International*, 42(16), pp. 18798–18805, https://doi.org/10.1016/j.ceramint.2016.09.024.
20. Rahman, A., Jayaganthan, R., Prakash, S., Chawla, V. and Chandra, R. (2009). "High temperature oxidation behavior of nanostructured Ni-Al coatings on superalloy", *Journal of Alloys and Compounds*, 472(1–2), pp. 478–483, https://doi.org/10.1016/j.jallcom.2008.04.091.
21. Teng, S., Liang, W., Li, Z. and Ma, X. (2008). "Improvement of high-temperature oxidation resistance of TiAl-based alloy by sol-gel method", *Journal of Alloys and Compounds*, 464(1–2), pp. 452–456. https://doi.org/10.1016/j.jallcom.2007.10.017.
22. Partes, K., Giolli, C., Borgioli, F., Bardi, U., Seefeld, T. and Vollertsen, F. (2008). "High temperature behaviour of NiCrAlY coatings made by laser cladding", *Surface and Coatings Technology*, 202(10), pp. 2208–2213, https://doi.org/10.1016/j.surfcoat.2007.09.010.
23. Srivastava, M., Balaraju, J. N., Ravisankar, B., Anandan, C. and William Grips, V. K. (2012). "High temperature oxidation and corrosion behaviour of Ni/Ni-Co-Al composite coatings", *Applied Surface Science*, 263, pp. 597–607, https://doi.org/10.1016/j.apsusc.2012.09.115.
24. Singh, H., Sidhu, B. S., Puri, D. and Prakash, S. (2007). "Use of plasma spray technology for deposition of high temperature oxidation/corrosion resistant coatings - A review", *Materials and Corrosion*, 58(2), pp. 92–102, https://doi.org/10.1002/maco.200603985.
25. Sidhu, T. S., Prakash, S. and Agrawal, R. D. (2005). "Studies on the properties of high-velocity oxy-fuel thermal spray coatings for higher temperature applications", *Materials Science*, 41(6), pp. 805–823, https://doi.org/10.1007/s11003-006-0047-z.
26. Wang, B. Q. and Luer, K. (1994). "The erosion-oxidation behaviour of HVOF Cr3C2-NiCr coating", Wear, 174, pp. 177–185.
27. Gärtner, F., Stoltenhoff, T., Schmidt, T. and Kreye, H. (2006). "The cold spray process and its potential for industrial applications", *Journal of Thermal Spray Technology*, 15(2), pp. 223–232, https://doi.org/10.1361/105996306X108110.
28. Schwetzke, R. and Kreye, H. (1998). "Microstructure and properties of tungsten carbide coatings sprayed with various HVOF spray systems", *Proceedings of the International Thermal Spray Conference*, 1(September), pp. 187–192.
29. Dobler, K., Kreye, H. and Schwetzke, R. (2000). "Oxidation of stainless steel in the high velocity oxy-fuel process", *Journal of Thermal Spray Technology*, 9(3), pp. 407–413, https://doi.org/10.1361/105996300770349872.
30. Lima, R. S. and Marple, B. R. (2007). "Thermal spray coatings engineered from nanostructured ceramic agglomerated powders for structural, thermal barrier and biomedical applications: A review", *Journal of Thermal Spray Technology*, 16(1), pp. 40–63, https://doi.org/10.1007/s11666-006-9010-7.
31. Ettouil, F. Ben, Mazhorova, O., Pateyron, B., Ageorges, H., El Ganaoui, M. and Fauchais, P. (2008). "Predicting dynamic and thermal histories of agglomerated particles injected within a d.c. plasma jet", *Surface and Coatings Technology*, 202(18), pp. 4491–4495, https://doi.org/10.1016/j.surfcoat.2008.04.032.
32. Lima, R. S., Moreau, C. and Marple, B. R. (2007). "HVOF-Sprayed coatings engineered from mixtures of nanostructured and submicron Al2O3-TiO2 powders: An enhanced wear performance", *Journal of Thermal Spray Technology*, 16(5–6), pp. 866–872, https://doi.org/10.1007/s11666-007-9092-x.

33. Killinger, A., Kuhn, M. and Gadow, R. (2006). "High-velocity suspension flame spraying (HVSFS), a new approach for spraying nanoparticles with hypersonic speed", *Surface and Coatings Technology*, 201(5), pp. 1922–1929, https://doi.org/10.1016/j.surfcoat.2006.04.034.
34. Gadow, R., Killinger, A. and Rauch, J. (2008). "New results in high velocity suspension flame spraying (HVSFS)", *Surface and Coatings Technology*, 202(18), pp. 4329–4336, https://doi.org/10.1016/j.surfcoat.2008.04.005.
35. Oberste Berghaus, J., Legoux, J. G., Moreau, C., Hui, R., Decès-Petit, C., Qu, W., Yick, S., Wang, Z., Maric, R. and Ghosh, D. (2008). "Suspension HVOF spraying of reduced temperature solid oxide fuel cell electrolytes", *Journal of Thermal Spray Technology*, 17(5–6), pp. 700–707, https://doi.org/10.1007/s11666-008-9249-2.
36. Tao, K., Zhou, X. lin, Cui, H. and Zhang, J. shan. (2009). "Oxidation and hot corrosion behaviors of HVAF-sprayed conventional and nanostructured NiCrC coatings", *Transactions of Nonferrous Metals Society of China (English Edition)*, 19(5), pp. 1151–1160, https://doi.org/10.1016/S1003-6326(08)60421-5.
37. Fauchais, P., Montavon, G. and Bertrand, G. (2010). "From powders to thermally sprayed coatings", *Journal of Thermal Spray Technology*, 19(1–2), pp. 56–80, https://doi.org/10.1007/s11666-009-9435-x.
38. Viswanathan, V., Rea, K. E., Vaidya, A. and Seal, S. (2008). "Role of spray drying of nanoagglomerates in morphology evolution in nanostructured APS coatings". *Journal of the American Ceramic Society*, 91(2), pp. 379–386, https://doi.org/10.1111/j.1551-2916.2007.02090.x.
39. Mukesh, C. G. (2009). http://www.pharmainfo.net/reviews/spray-dryingreview (accessed 28 September 2009).
40. Parihari, A. (2009). Performance study of spray dryer using various salt solutions. M.Tech thesis, Department of Chemical Engineering, National Institute of Technology, Rourkela, India.
41. Fauchais, P., Montavon, G., Lima, R. S. and Marple, B. R. (2011). "Engineering a new class of thermal spray nano-based microstructures from agglomerated nanostructured particles, suspensions and solutions: An invited review", *Journal of Physics D: Applied Physics*, 44(9), https://doi.org/10.1088/0022-3727/44/9/093001.
42. Singh, V. P., Sil, A. and Jayaganthan, R. (2012). "Tribological behaviour of nanostructured Al 2O 3 coatings", *Surface Engineering*, 28(4), pp. 277–284, https://doi.org/10.1179/1743294411Y.0000000076.
43. Thakur, L. and Arora, N. (2017). "A study of processing and slurry erosion behaviour of multi-walled carbon nanotubes modified HVOF sprayed nano-WC-10Co-4Cr coating", *Surface and Coatings Technology*, 309, pp. 860–871, https://doi.org/10.1016/j.surfcoat.2016.10.073.
44. Muoto, C. K., Jordan, E. H., Gell, M. and Aindow, M. (2010). "Phase homogeneity in MgO-ZrO2 nanocomposites synthesized by a combined sol-gel/thermal decomposition route", *Journal of the American Ceramic Society*, 93(10), pp. 3102–3109, https://doi.org/10.1111/j.1551-2916.2010.03821.x.
45. Wang, J., Jordan, E. H. and Gell, M. (2010). "Plasma sprayed dense MgO-Y2O3 nanocomposite coatings using sol-gel combustion synthesized powder". *Journal of Thermal Spray Technology*, 19(5), pp. 873–878, https://doi.org/10.1007/s11666-010-9496-x.
46. Jiansirisomboon, S., Mackenzie, K. J. D., Roberts, S. G. and Grant, P. S. (2003). "Low pressure plasma-sprayed Al2O3 and Al2O3/SiC nanocomposite coatings from different feedstock powders", *Journal of the European Ceramic Society*, 23, pp. 961–976.
47. Hannula, S. P., Turunen, E., Keskinen, J., Varis, T., Fält, T., Gustafsson, T. E. and Nowak, R. (2006). "Development of nanostructured Al2O3-Ni HVOF coatings", *Key*

Engineering Materials, *317–318*, pp. 539–544, https://doi.org/10.4028/www.scientific.net/kem.317-318.539.
48. Turunen, E., Varis, T., Gustafsson, T. E., Keskinen, J., Fält, T. and Hannula, S. P. (2006). "Parameter optimization of HVOF sprayed nanostructured alumina and alumina-nickel composite coatings", *Surface and Coatings Technology*, 200(16–17), pp. 4987–4994, https://doi.org/10.1016/j.surfcoat.2005.05.018.
49. Saaedi, J., Coyle, T. W., Arabi, H., Mirdamadi, S. and Mostaghimi, J. (2010). "Effects of hvof process parameters on the properties of Ni-Cr coatings", *Journal of Thermal Spray Technology*, 19, pp. 521–530.
50. Miguel, J. M., Guilemany, J. M. and Vizcaino, S. (2003). "Tribological study of NiCrBSi coating obtained by different processes", *Tribology International*, 36(3), pp. 181–187.
51. Serres, N., Hlawka, F., Costil, S., Langlade, C., Machi, F. and Cornet, A. (2009). "Dry coatings and eco design: I. environmental performances and chemical properties", *Surface and Coatings Technology*, 204(1–2), pp. 187–196.
52. Kawahara, Y. (2007). "Application of high temperature corrosion-resistant materials and coatings under severe corrosive environment in waste-to-energy boilers", *Journal of Thermal Spray Technology*, 16, pp. 202–213.
53. Simunovic, K., Saric, T. and Simunovic, G. (2014). "Different approaches to the investigation and testing of the Ni-based self-fluxing alloy coatings—a review. Part 1: general facts, wear and corrosion investigations", *Tribology Transactions*, 57, pp. 955–979.
54. Tobar, M. J., Álvarez, C., Amado, J. M., Rodriguez, G. and Yanez, A. (2006). "Morphology and characterization of laser clad composite NiCrBSi—WC coatings on stainless steel", *Surface and Coatings Technology*, 200(22–23), pp. 6313–6317.
55. Praveen, A. S. and Arjunan, A. (2019). "Effect of nano-Al2O3 addition on the microstructure and erosion wear of HVOF sprayed NiCrSiB coatings", *Materials Research Express*, 7(1), p. 15006. https://doi.org/10.1088/2053-1591/ab5bda.
56. Shukla, V. N., Jayaganthan, R. and Tewari, V. K. (2015). "Degradation behavior of HVOF-Sprayed Cr3C2-25%NiCr cermet coatings exposed to high temperature environment", *Materials Today: Proceedings*, 2(4–5), pp. 1805–1813, https://doi.org/10.1016/j.matpr.2015.07.048.
57. He, J., Ice, M. and Lavernia, E. J. (2000). "Synthesis and characterization of nanocomposite coatings", *Nanostructured Films and Coatings*, 57, pp. 131–148.
58. He, J., Ice, M., Lavernia, E. J., Shin, D. H. and Schoenung, J. M. (2001). "Thermal Stability of Nanostructured Cr3C2-NiCr Coatings", *Journal of Thermal Spray Technology*, 10(2), pp. 293–300.
59. Ramanathan, L. V., Cecílio, A. C., Olandir, V. C. and Isaac, J. S. (2017). "High temperature erosion-oxidation resistance of thermally sprayed nanostructured Cr3C2-25(Ni-20Cr) coatings", *Materials Research*, 20(4), pp. 994–1002.
60. Stewart, D. A., Shipway, P. H. and McCartney, D. G. (1999). "Abrasive wear behaviour of conventional and nanocomposite HVOF-sprayed WC-Co coatings", *Wear*, *225–229*(PART II), pp. 789–798, https://doi.org/10.1016/S0043-1648(99)00032-0.
61. Liu, Y., Hang, Z., Chen, H., Ceng, S., Gou, G., Wang, X., Tu, M. and Wu, X. (2016). "Erosion–Corrosion Property of CeO2-Modified HVOF WC-Co Coating", *Journal of Thermal Spray Technology*, 25(4), pp. 815–822, https://doi.org/10.1007/s11666-016-0391-y.
62. Guilemany, J. M., Dosta, S., Nin, J. and Miguel, J. R. (2005). "Study of the properties of WC-Co nanostructured coatings sprayed by high-velocity oxyfuel", *Journal of Thermal Spray Technology*, 14(3), pp. 405–413, https://doi.org/10.1361/105996305X59350.
63. Baik, K. H., Kim, J. H. and Seong, B. G. (2007). "Improvements in hardness and wear resistance of thermally sprayed WC-Co nanocomposite coatings", *Materials Science and Engineering A*, *449–451*, pp. 846–849, https://doi.org/10.1016/j.msea.2006.02.295.

64. Ghabchi, A., Varis, T., Turunen, E., Suhonen, T., Liu, X. and Hannula, S. P. (2010). "Behavior of HVOF WC-10Co4Cr coatings with different carbide size in fine and coarse particle abrasion", *Journal of Thermal Spray Technology*, 19(1–2), pp. 368–377, https://doi.org/10.1007/s11666-009-9433-z.
65. Premkumar, K. and Balasubramanian, K. R. (2018). "Investigation of erosion behaviour on nanocrystalline composite thermal spray coating under hot air jet condition", *Journal of Advanced Research in Dynamical & Control Systems*, 10(4), pp. 1061–1071.
66. Picas, J. A., Forn, A., Igartua, A. and Mendoza, G. (2003). "Mechanical and tribological properties of high velocity oxy-fuel thermal sprayed nanocrystalline CrC-NiCr coatings", *Surface and Coatings Technology*, *174–175*(03), pp. 1095–1100, https://doi.org/10.1016/S0257-8972(03)00393-1.
67. Tellkamp, V. L., Lau, M. L., Fabel, A. and Lavernia, E. J. (1997). "Thermal spraying of nanocrystalline inconel 718", *Nanostructured Materials*, 9(1–8), pp. 489–492, https://doi.org/10.1016/S0965-9773(97)00107-4.
68. Hurevich, V., Smurov, I. and Pawlowski, L. (2002). "Theoretical study of the powder behavior of porous particles in a flame during plasma spraying", *Surface and Coatings Technology*, *151–152*, pp. 370–376, https://doi.org/10.1016/S0257-8972(01)01594-8.
69. He, J., Ice, M. and Lavernia, E. J. (2000). "Synthesis of nanostructured Cr3C2-25(Ni20Cr) coatings", *Metallurgical and Materials Transactions A*, 31A, pp. 555–564.
70. Roy, M., Pauschitz, A., Bernardi, J., Koch, T. and Franek, F. (2006). "Microstructure and mechanical properties of HVOF sprayed nanocrystalline Cr3C2-25(Ni20Cr) coating", *Journal of Thermal Spray Technology*, 15(3), pp. 372–381, https://doi.org/10.1361/105996306X124374.
71. Chivavibul, P., Watanabe, M., Kuroda, S., Kawakita, J., Komatsu, M., Sato, K. and Kitamura, J. (2010). "Effect of powder characteristics on properties of warm-sprayed WC-Co Coatings", *ASM International*, 19, pp. 81–88.
72. Evans, A. G. and Charles, E. A. (1976). "Fracture toughness determination by indentation", *Journal of the American Ceramic Society*, 59(7–8), pp. 371–372.
73. Shetty, D. K., Wright, I. G., Mincer, P. N. and Clauer, A. H. (1985). "Indentation fracture of WC-Co cermets", *Journal of Material Science Letters*, 20, pp. 1873–1882.
74. Nihara, K., Morena, R. and Hasselman, D. P. H. (1982). "Evaluation of KIC of brittle solids by the indentation method with low crack-to-indent ratios", *Journal of Material Science Letters*, 1, pp. 13–16.
75. Nihara, K. (1983). "A fracture-mechanics analysis of indentation induced palmqvist crack in ceramics", *Journal of Material Science Letters*, 2(5), pp. 221–223.
76. Leyland, A. and Matthews, A. (2000). "On the significance of the H/E ratio in wear control: A nanocomposite coating approach to optimised tribological behaviour", *Wear*, 246(1–2), pp. 1–11, https://doi.org/10.1016/S0043-1648(00)00488-9.
77. Singh, G., Vasudev, H., Bansal, A., Vardhan, S. and Sharma, S. (2020). "Microwave cladding of Inconel-625 on mild steel substrate for corrosion protection," *Materials Research Express*, https://doi.org/10.1088/2053-1591/ab6fa3.
78. Singh, J., Vasudev, H. and Singh, S. (2020). "Performance of different coating materials against high temperature oxidation in boiler tubes – A review," *Materials Today: Proceedings*, 26, 972–978, https://doi.org/10.1016/j.matpr.2020.01.156.
79. Vasudev, H. (2020). "Wear characteristics of Ni-WC powder deposited by using a microwave route on mild steel: Microwave cladding of Ni-WC," *International Journal of Surface Engineering and Interdisciplinary Materials Science*, 8(1), pp. 44–54, doi: 10.4018/IJSEIMS.2020010104.
80. Vasudev, H., Singh, P., Thakur, L. and Bansal, A. (2020). "Mechanical and microstructural characterization of microwave post processed Alloy-718 coating," *Materials Research Express*, 6(12), p. 1265f5, https://doi.org/10.1088/2053-1591/ab66fb.

81. Bansal, A., Vasudev, H., Sharma, A. K. and Kumar, P. (2019). "Investigation on the effect of post weld heat treatment on microwave joining of the Alloy-718 weldment," *Materials Research Express*, 6(8), p. 086554, https://doi.org/10.1088/2053-1591/ab1d9a.
82. Vasudev, H., Singh, G., Bansal, A., Vardhan, S. and Thakur, L. (2019). "Microwave heating and its applications in surface engineering: a review," *Materials Research Express*, 6(10), p. 102001, https://doi.org/10.1088/2053-1591/ab3674.
83. Vasudev, H., Thakur, L., Singh, H. and Bansal, A. (2018). "Mechanical and microstructural behaviour of wear resistant coatings on cast iron lathe machine beds and slides," *Kovove Materialy*, 56(1) pp. 55–63, DOI: 10.4149/km2018155.

9 Application of Nanostructured YSZ Thermal Barrier Coatings for Gas Turbine Engine

Amrinder Mehta, Hitesh Vasudev, and Sharanjit Singh

9.1 INTRODUCTION

Thermal barrier coatings (TBCs) were used in those components of a gas turbine that operated in high temperatures and were used to enhance the efficiency of hot section components in the gas turbine. The high temperature in the surroundings of the gas turbine may cause many surface degradation to these components. The gas turbine is extensively used in the electricity generation and commercial aerospace industry [1]. The ceramic top coating helps to maintain the integrity of the underlying turbine components by decreasing heat transfer [2]. The state of the art material of TBCs presently concentrates on yttria-stabilized zirconia (YSZ) because of its less thermal conductivity and comparatively lesser coefficient of thermal expansion [3]. The nanostructured materials and technology have provided ground for important developments in the representation of existing materials depending on advancements in thermal and electrical features right from reduction in size by factors of 100 to 1000 times (to the size of grain), as showed in the modern ceramic materials. The nanomaterials have particle sizes that are lower than 100 nm in at least one dimension [4]. The Hall Petch empirical relationship equation is used to show the superior quality of the coating and the enhancement of the thermal characteristics by reducing the grain size of the powder. [5]. The general equation is

$$A = A_0 + kd^{1/2} \tag{9.1}$$

where A indicates the mechanical properties of the metal like yield strength and hardness; the index 0 relates to the materials, i.e. the endless-state size of grain; k represent a constant, which shows that this grain boundary as an impediment to the creation of elongation in the material; and d represents the size of the grain. Equation (9.1) represents that some thermal and mechanical properties of the metals can, more importantly, be enhanced when the dimensions of grain are reduced to the nanostructure level. This is the reason nanotechnology and science are one of the most highly researchable fields today and are giving way to more researches in material science. This technology is approximately used in whole types of materials, containing ceramic and metallic alloys. Additionally, carbon nanotubes are one of the nanostructured metals that are being used increasingly for higher temperature applications. This fact was found by Iijima in 1991 [6]. Nanostructured materials show an increase in mechanical, electrical, and thermal properties. It was observed that in the past decade, rapid growth in the area of thermal spray coatings had happened [7]. Plasma spray is one of the most important products in the field of thermal spray coating. It is very versatile as compared to other technologies and mostly acceptable in all kinds of environmental conditions. This is used at high temperatures and is able to work on all types of ceramic materials to be deposited on substrate metals. High-velocity oxy-fuel (HVOF) technology was improved during the past centenary for enhancing material velocity and it reduced the time of deposition on the coating materials. The realization of spray embedded at entirely hard-state, chill gas-dynamic spraying held recommending for embedded material substrate metal depends upon this plastic elongation sprinkle ceramic powder. Vacuum cold spray is developed as it further expedites the process of embedding the powder nanoparticle to solidify into a hard state.

9.2 THERMAL SPRAY COATINGS PROCESSED FROM CERAMIC POWDERS

9.2.1 *Nanostructured Agglomerated Ceramic Powders for Thermal Spray Coating*

The thermal spray method has been expanded to the study of nanostructured materials for the coating process. At present, there is an available extensive limit on the investigation possibilities to the nanostructured ceramic powder particles for coating.

A more superior thermal barrier coating in a thermal spray process, as compared to conventional process, has been invented. Powder feedstock plays a vital role in making a thermal spray coating. The traditional powder particle size varies from 10 to 100 μm, but nanostructured powder particle size is lower than 100 nm. These small nanoparticles that would create blockage the hoses pipe that helps transportation of powder particle from the powder feeder to spray gun.

SEM micrographs are represented in Figure 9.1(a), apparently show the manufactured YSZ nanostructure was inside that size of particles into this nanofield. It was also noted for nanostructured agglomerated powder further has smooth crystalline stucture; besides, all structures are uniform in size and shape [Figure 9.1(b)]. It was found that for the size of a particle, YSZ powder average varied from 40 to 50 nm. In the thermal spraying process of YSZ, nanoclusters are used as a feedstock. The nanoclusters were agglomerated by utilizing the spray drying process and obtaining micro-sized particles, as shown in reference [8]. In the 1990s, nano-sized agglomerated powders were commercially acceptable to the coating process [9]. Chemical reaction techniques are used for manufacturing nanostructured particle size powder.

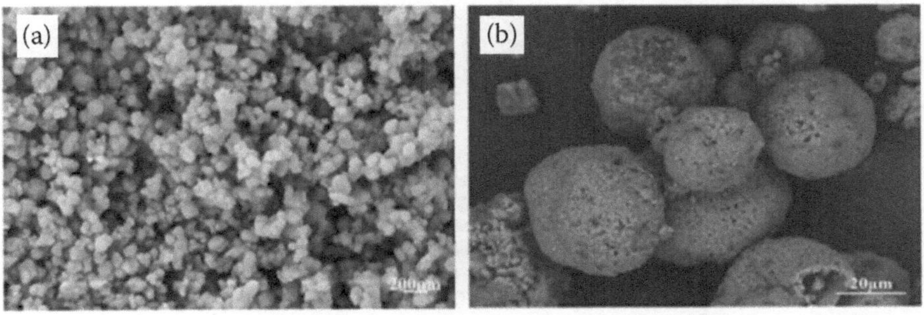

FIGURE 9.1 (a) SEM Micrographs of Nano YSZ Powder Particle Without Agglomerated, and (b) the Agglomerated and Sintered Powder Micro-Sized YSZ Particles [8].

The spray-drying method is used for agglomerated nanostructured powder particles before thermal spray [10]. The thermal spray method helps to melt the powder grains before they get deposited on the base material. It is excessively challenging to produce thermal spray coatings when some powder particles are not correctly melting, primarily related to ceramic materials. The melting temperature of powder particles is essential for adhesion and cohesion. The nanostructural properties of the powder get eliminated. When entire nanostructural grains completely melt into this spray gun, it generate hurdles in the working of the thermal spray process. It is essential to raise the temperature of powder particles carefully at the time of the thermal spray process and get a better quality result of the coating. The feedstock components have been used for controlling the feed rate of the nanostructured powder particles. In the thermal spray process, some critical optimization techniques are useful to achieve good-quality results, reducing the coating process time in developing spray parameters. It is feasible to see that the temperature values of moderate particles likely to be near to the melting point related nanostructured spray powder materials. They are required for protecting the nanostructured powder elements and maintain the original microstructure characteristics. The nanostructured powder particles are enabled to work at a higher melting point temperature than conventional powder particles. Spray powder particles use high-velocity oxygen fuel (HVOF) method at a high velocity. In this process, a lower dwell time is required for the powder particles and would contribute to generating obstruction entire nanostructured powder melts in the thermal spray jet.

9.2.2 Bimodal Microstructure of Nanostructured Agglomerated Ceramic Powders from Thermal Spray Coating

The nanostructured powder particles get deposited on the surface of the coating layer and essentially prevent powder particles from getting wholly melted. The bimodal structure is represented in Figure 9.2.

The semi-molten feedstock particles that help to prepare a microstructure coating, surrounded by full molten particles, work as a binder to control the quality of the coating surface. This type of coating layer is created from the mixture of powder grains that are in a partially-melted condition inside spray jet [11].

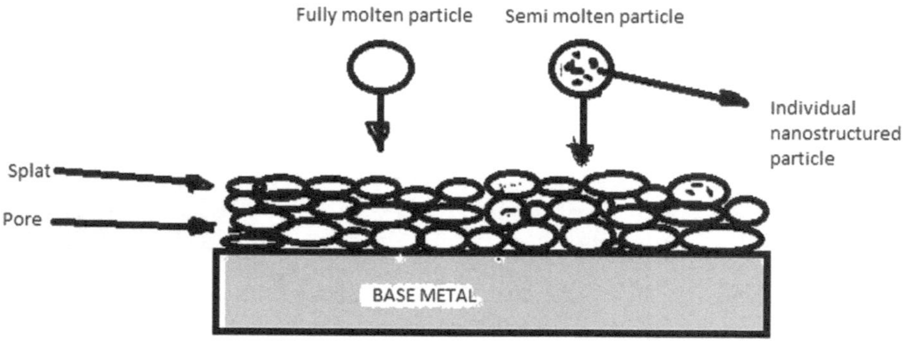

FIGURE 9.2 The Bimodal Microstructure of Nanostructured Agglomerated Ceramic Powders.

The semi-molten particles create the bimodal microstructure of nanostructured agglomerated ceramic powders.

The average particle size of spherical agglomerated and the sintered powder ranged approximately from 30 to 70 um in diameter, as shown in Figure 9.3(a). That manufactured from YSZ (8 wt% Y2O3-stabilized ZrO2) of nanostructured powder particles with standard chemical composition and average sizes 80 to 250 nm, is displayed in Figure 9.3(b).

The particles conducted hot spray utilizing air plasma spray (APS) gun (LE-15, a center of Dalian Maritime University). The diagnostic tool (DPV 2000, Tecnar Automation) was used for controlling the working temperature and velocity of the deposited powder particles in the coating.

This instrument works on the principle of optical pyrometry, and time of the flight particles is measured by the combination of the grain speed and heat. For effective results, there were some critical parameters used in the thermal spray process, such as spray temperature was 2563 °C, the speed of powder particles 208 m/s, and spray gun distance was 100 mm from the base metal [12]. The temperature is lower than the melting point of YSZ-8% powder particles, recorded to be near about 2700 °C.

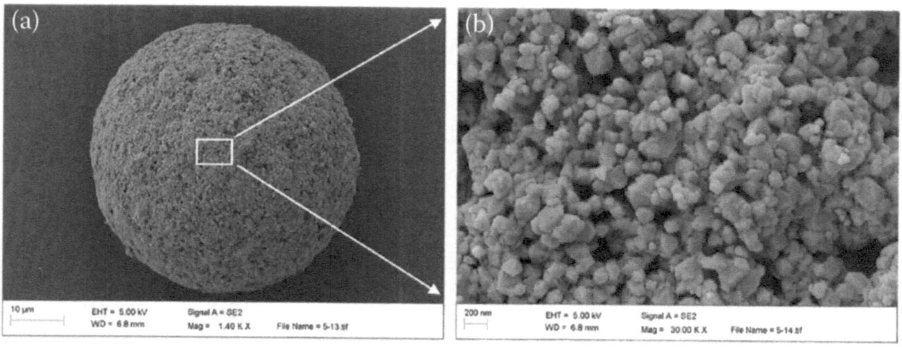

FIGURE 9.3 Morphology from Feedstock Powders (a) Spray-Dried Agglomerated and Sintered Spherical Powders and (b) Original Nanoparticle Detail [12].

The jet of spray embedded on this surface for base metal could be composed of complete melted, partially-melted, and not-melted powder grains, as shown in Figure 9.4. It is easy to differentiate the darker and lighter shaded regions in the surface morphologies of the bimodal microstructure in the coating shown in Figure 9.4(a). Figure 9.4(b) shows that the Scanning Electron Microscope (SEM) makes it possible to identify the similarity in this different kind of dark zone in nanostructures at higher level magnification. The lighter colored nanozone, as shown in Figure 9.4(a), is used for observe and identify the full molten region in nanostructured powder particles in thermal spray coating. Some important points are required for control in thermal spray coatings like that the size and surface morphology for increase various microstructural characteristics and mechanical property of the surface coating. The density of the agglomerated powder particles is the critical parameter in the nanozones, as shown in Figure 9.3. The thickness of the nanozones depends on the thermal spray conditions and feedstock parameters. When the partially melted agglomerated powder grains make no entry with filter into the nonmolten core at the time of thermal spray and hence porous nanozones are expected to be obtained. On the opposite side, the dense nanozones may be possible if the semi-molten and fully molten particles completely infiltrate in the miniature tubes in the without-melted area. Many researchers worked in this new area and met the desired requirements of the microstructure of the surface coating of the nanostructured agglomerated ceramic powder widely used in thermal spray coating for the industrial applications [14].

9.3 IMPROVED PROPERTIES OF CERAMIC COATING

9.3.1 *Hardness and Toughness*

It is generally considered that strong surface layers have outstanding wear-resistance characteristics. Many authors researching on APS nano-sized YSZ

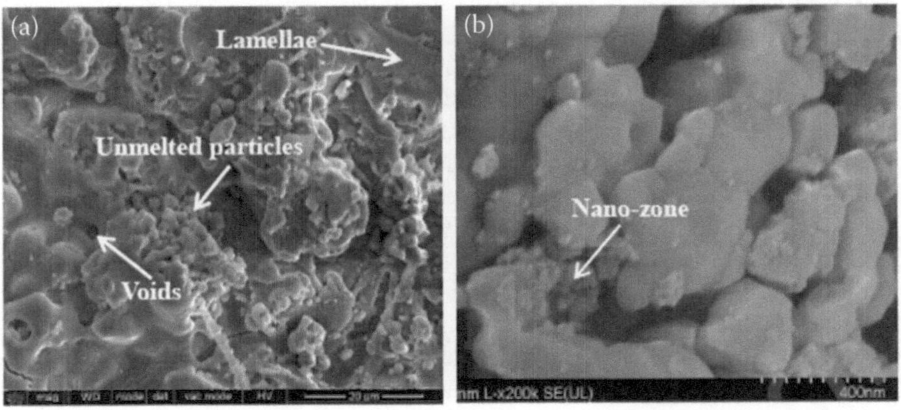

FIGURE 9.4 Surface Morphologies of (a) Nanostructured 8YSZ Coatings and Unmelted Feedstock Particles, (b) Nanozone of Feedstock [13].

coating observed that the abrasion resistance levels were necessarily higher than conventional ones. The Vickers hardness values of conventional coating are lower than the nanostructured coating [14]. The use of feedstock in a thermal spray for control the critical parameter of agglomerated nanostructured powder particles which embedded in the microstructure surface coating most of the whole nano-sized grains wholly molten into the jet of spray, then this coated layer did no show a meaningful nano-sized quality and layer tend to act being one conventionalized. It is noted that nanostructured thermal spray coatings show significantly more important crack propagation resistance as compared to the conventional thermal spray coatings [15]. The crack generation protection was assessed and analysed by applying the Vickers indentation technique. When applying to enough weights, on surface coating during Vicker indentation, cracks were formed and a Vickers indentation impact/crack propagated along a small distance. This smaller crack spread to a distance to an assigned weight, and greater crack spread the protection to the coated layer. Hence, that greater wear the protection from that nano-sized coatings usually characteristic on that more excellent crack spread protection. Estimated and presented few test proof for showing to the partially-melted nano-sized powder grains deposited on that coated morphology while a jet of spray tends for work essentially the crack arresters, whereby improving the toughness of the coating. Several authors have hypothesized and presented some experimental proof to show that the semi-molten nanostructured powder particles get deposited in the coating microstructure while thermal spraying tends to work as a crack arrester, whereby increasing coating toughness [15].

9.3.2 *Bond Strength*

Various authors have seen an increase in the strength of the bond in the nano-sized jet spray used for fatigue resistance purposes. Through practising that C633-01 standard, that change from the bond coat hardness proposed to occur directed through this adhesive force when that breakdown happens in this interface from the bond coated base metal and that cohesive force when the fracture is entirely inside this coated layer.

This failure picture for the YSZ TBC is displayed under Figure 9.5. This straight-pull test performed one fracture on this interface for the metal bond coated and then top-coated that indicated the adhesive fracture or breakdown [16]. Therefore, this bond the power within that related splatted do greater as compared to the without splatted. It was well understood that combining governed the adhesive strength the situation within sprinkling grains including that base material, because that controlled residual stress from that base material coated method [17]. This residual stress made from couple parts in that sprayed method likes quenched stress produced of that reduction from different splats and cooled stress obtained of that heat extension non-matched among that deposited to the base material while all cooled collectively subsequent deposited [18]. It was observed that greater bonded durability from that nano-sized coating was defined through the

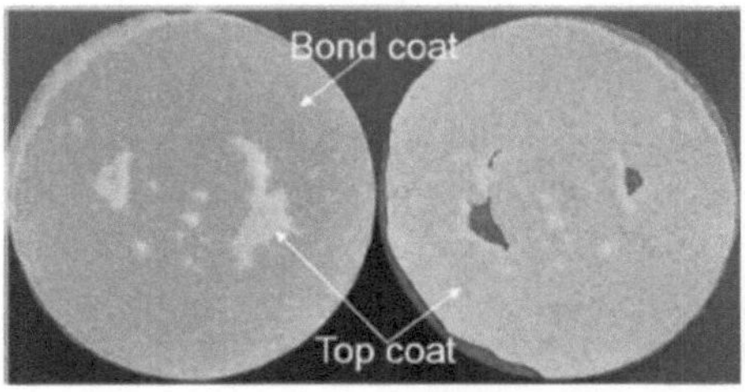

FIGURE 9.5 Tensile Fracture Region for the YSZ Coating [16].

more internal toughness obtained [19]. Traditional coated method observed that internal face within this powder grains held completely melted into a jet of spray and this base metal showed few small cracks. Nanostructured coated observed that those interfacial within this powder grains were a partially melted stage during this spraying process and this base metal happened to be adherents in the coating. Hence, the interface cracks within those nano-sized coated were prevented through the tough adherent compact nanostructure, through enhancing bond strength.

9.3.3 *Plasticity*

Many authors have done subsequent testing for the wear resistance that the damage mark for the nano-sized coated is more regular as compared to that traditional coating method. The greater flexibility for the nano-sized coating method was an aspect seen during APS nano YSZ while compared to conventional coatings sprayed from cladding, sintered, and pulverized grain size sequentially [20]. This longer covered the introduction of the damage marks from this nano-sized coating process and appeared to show this plastics elongation for that principal wear resistance system this happened throughout the wear process. While microfracture detected at that wear marks from this traditional coating process showed the brittle failures were this principal wear system. These variations within the microstructure for these erosion marks for the nano-sized and traditional coating process can be seen. This is the main reason to describe the behavior of surface coating material before selecting for the thermal spray process. This should be noted for the plastic elongation and fragmentation happening when rubbing the grain particles in thermal spray coatings [21]. When pulverized for the powder elements, one change for removing the metal tool from plastic deformation change toward breakable form happens. In the beginning, plastic draws very slow, turns to breakable crack, and after some significant increase, the crack deepness moves to the base metal. While significant parts for the powder grains do the right amount on this degree of hardness and strength of the surface coating. Hence, nano-sized and traditional method lead to show the equivalent value of hardness, as the nano-sized coating process become harder for the coating toughness. Hence, they analyse for the nano-sized coating process that further shows one large base crack on the surface layer of coating. The more crucial part of the coating is that the cutting ratio should turn in one more regular erosion mark, as seen through the work of many authors. The increased flexibility for the nano-sized coating process can be helpful through this grinding process of the powder grains. [22].

9.3.4 *Thermal Diffusivity*

Thermal diffusivity for the APS YSZ nano-sized and traditional coating process is done at 1200 ^{0}C throughout the process. [23]. This YSZ nano-sized and traditional coating process within this steady heat holds area 1.80–2.54 × 10^{-3} cm^2/s, sequentially for thermal diffusivity. Certain thermal diffusivity implications for the YSZ nanostructures, the coating is lesser than the listed within this article to YSZ traditional coating process leads to a similar heating ratio [24]. This may be linked to the presence of a nanoporosity arrangement in every individual nanozone while observing for the YSZ nanostructured coating. The globular and intersplat porosities perform an important part in thermal spray coatings. This permeable nanostructured expand coated layer morphology and into some normal interfacial porosities for the coating method. The nanostructured coating process can support the reduced thermal diffusivity for this surface coating further, overall. The coefficient of thermal expansion (CTE) from the YSZ nanostructured and traditional coating process was further evaluated as a similar heat ratio [25].

9.3.5 *Thermal Shock Resistance*

While the crack was made inside the coated surface, these leads were extended simultaneously with this small point for that nanostructured powder particles and stripped from the coating surface.

Many researchers explain that the nano-sized YSZ coated process does work at high-temperature situations [26].

The variation under sintered rate is visible in the molten grain and the unmelted regions inside spray jet during the coating process. This reduction for the nanozone area is noticed, through finishing in enhanced permeability and advanced ability to withstand a hot temperature of the surface coating method. That aspect is seen within the existing research, being presented under arrow-1 that represent microcrack inside the bond coat in Figure 9.6. It also is given that the sintered impact mainly generates one huge crack inside this non-zone and the small region of entirely molten grains obtained. Figure 9.6 shows that maximum cracks equal into this coated layer is finished within this inadequately molten microstructured area, in arrow-2. Besides, larger cracks were observed in the YSZ coating and the bonded coat as shown in arrow-3. Here the pores and cracks increasing with this powder particles boundary between this nanorange inside this nano-sized YSZ coated process may support remove this stressed power produced throughout the thermal shocking.

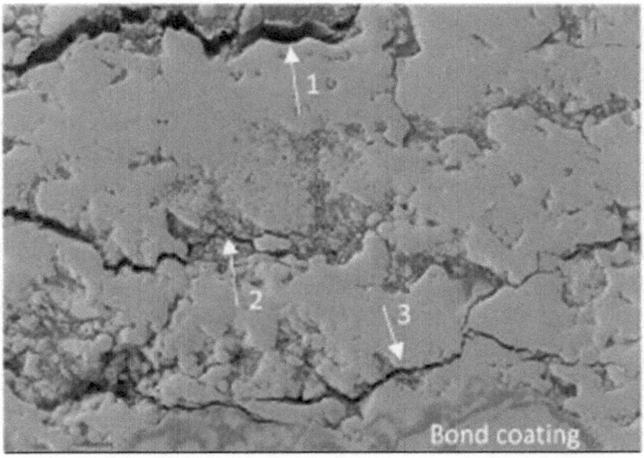

FIGURE 9.6 Cross-Section of the Thermal Cycling Test Sample with 60% Nanoscale [12].

9.3.6 Sintering Effects and Creep Behavior

The main interests in the application of nanostructured thermal spray coatings at high temperatures are their durability in connection to sintering-related impacts. Many researchers have observed that the sintering effects may harden nanostructured regions and be the main causing premature failure in TBCs [27]. The agglomerates used to make these coatings showed that the only nanostructured YSZ grains by size range vary from 15 to 130 nm. After heating for 48 h at 1000 °C, each unique YSZ nano-sized grains changed into a partially melted agglomerated stretched size of the order of 300 nm [28]. Here that was marked in this specific nano-sized YSZ powder grains approximately 250 nm in this surface coating process. While everyone those circumstances that were seen some little porosity system displayed within that nanostructure and led for the improved in the increased heating range. The creep value of that nanostructured YSZ coated process represents a larger one than that of the conventional process. The work energies vary from 165 to 192 kJ/mol and further stress exponents range from 2.2 to 1.3 for nanostructured and traditional one, respectively. This principal creep system provides an increase for creep value for the nanostructured YSZ known to be grain edges slides. This increase in creep value for that nanostructured YSZ happens to extended rest when stressed to higher heat, that is a required perspective. Though the increased rest to elevated heat temperatures can start for improvement for the stress when cooled, it can prompt early breakdown for the coated surface. In the opposite sides, while earlier explained, nano-sized coated process lead that shows greater toughness value if the comparison over traditional coated process, that could exceed this stress impact throughout the cooling process [28]. This article represents the necessary creep behavior could be affected by contamination in the metal's surface throughout. These variations under creep behavior in nano-sized and traditional YSZ coated process can have affected through that level of coated surface pureness.

9.4 OTHER PROPERTIES OF THE NANOCOATING

9.4.1 *Deposited Efficiency*

Various researchers have found that the deposited effectiveness rates for nano-sized agglomerated grains were greater as compared to the traditional coated surface. It was noted as that for four distinct plasma energy stages, deposition efficiency rates of nanostructured YSZ (diameter −80/+20 μm) were two times greater than those for conventional (diameter −100/+30 μm) [29]. As the similar energy, although three distinct spray gaps the deposition efficiency for this nanostructured YSZ coating was about 1.2 rates greater. Li et al. mentioned that optimal deposition efficiency for nano-sized grains (diameter nearly −60/+10 μm) was 1.4 times greater than optimal deposition efficiency of traditional coated grain (diameter nearly -60/+6 μm) [30]. Ctibor et al. mentioned that traditional TiO_2 powder grains that power consumed during thermal spray did weigh 0.6 kW/kg, on the other hand, the agglomerated nano-sized TiO_2 feedstock weighed 0.4 kW/kg [31]. Comparing the deposition efficiency values of nanostructures (approximately size −62/+14 μm) and traditional coated grains (approximately size 53/+24 μm) Al_2O_3-13 wt.% TiO_2 powders, the deposition efficiency rates of the nano-sized metals were 1.5 times greater than the traditional spray process. Individual likely description of that greater deposition efficiency amounts for nano-sized grains that depended at this large surface field for this nano-sized agglomerated grains. The larger surface region of the surface-coated process could support this consumption for the large quantities of heat energy. These grains' dwell period increased during the jet spray, and helped this molten grain boundary to hold on to the outside surface layer throughout the thermal spray process. This further assisted for improving this adhesion and cohesion for the depositing grains to the base metal during this surface coating process.

9.4.2 *Homogeneity*

Ctibor et al. lately investigated that mechanical characteristics for the nano-sized and traditional TiO_2 thermal spray-coated process embedded through water-stabilized plasma by the depth-sensing nanoindentation method [32]. This technique is one of the highly valuable techniques used to examine the mechanical characteristics for the metals. The quality of the spray jet in the coated structure formed through the method generally is decided by a significant amount of the surface coat imperfections, non-homogeneousness, and high variations in their coating characteristics. Ctibor et al. mentioned the application for the nano-sized feedstock system that decreased the possibility for larger defects inside the coating and helps to create a smoother surface quality. Notwithstanding this, there were evidence where the average rates for the hardness including modulus of elasticity for the nano-sized TiO_2 and traditional coated process were quite similar, and this nano-sized coated process showed more durability and strength. These measurements can support to describe these excellent mechanical characteristics for the nanostructured TiO_2 surface coated process that were examined by different authors [33]. Recent developments in the designing of deposition of thermal barrier coatings have been elaborated by the authors in another publication [34].

9.5 CONCLUSION

In this study, below mentioned results could be credited to the TBCs produced through nano-sized agglomerated grain powders. The spray-drying and sintering individual methods are used for manufactured, nanostructured ceramic agglomerated feedstock powders. These agglomerates are microscopic and usually porous in nature. The bimodal nanostructure produced through powder grains were completely in a melted and partially melted condition inside the jet spray during the surface coating process. These partially melted grains remained under observation so as to develop everywhere on the coated nanostructures, adding to this coated/base-metal interface. This nanozone can prepare denser microstructure in nature and provide higher mechanical strength for surface coating. On the other hand, the highly dense nanozones possibly happen when some melted portion of the partially melted powder grains completely infiltrate inside the capillary tube for that agglomerated throughout the spraying process. The arrangement of nanozone plays a crucial part to maintain the surface quality and mechanical properties that depend upon the main factors density and porosity that regulated through this mechanism. Many authors have calculated the thermal diffusivity for the nano YSZ and traditional coated process done at temperature of 1200 °C. When this experiment has been performed at a higher temperature, lower thermal diffusivity was found throughout for the nano-sized YSZ coating. The thermal shock tests have been conducted on nanostructured and conventional coatings and the service life, durability, and strength of the coated layer have been evaluated. This experiment has shown the results of nanostructured and traditional coating process in the thermal shock resistance test to analyze the resistance efficiency for the durability of the coating. The greater temperature leads to an improvement in the diameter and physical shape for the powder grains that has been founded inside the nanostructures. This nanostructure porosity can be promoted through nanozones for higher temperature stability of the coating. The creep analyses showed that a greater creep value for nanostructured YSZ coatings should appear within this increased rest during stress to higher temperatures, that gives useful aspect. Nevertheless, the thermal shock experiments described within this article relevant for this period exhibit effective outcomes to the nanostructured coated surface. There are higher deposition efficiency levels of the nanostructured agglomerated ceramic powders as compared to the conventional. This large deposition efficiency represented the large outside coating area of the nano-sized grains, which supports greater quantities of heat consumed for the coating process.

REFERENCES

1. Chen, W. R., Wu, X., Marple, B. R. and Patnaik, P. C. (2005) "Oxidation and crack nucleation/growth in an air-plasma-sprayed thermal barrier coating with NiCrAlY bond coat", *Surface & Coatings Technology*, 197, pp. 109.
2. Padture, N. P., Gell, M. and Jordan, E. H. (2002) "Thermal barrier coatings for gas-turbine engine applications", *Science*, 296, pp. 280–284.
3. Tian, Y. S., Chen, C. Z., Wang, D. Y. and Ji, Q. (2005) "Recent developments in zirconia thermal barrier coatings", *Surface & Coatings Technology*, 12, pp. 369–378.

4. Koch, C. C. (2002) *Nanostructured Materials—Processing, Properties and Applications.* Noyes Publications, William Andrew Publishing, Norwich, NY, USA.
5. Lu, Y. L. and Liaw, P. K. (2001) "The mechanical properties of nanostructured materials", *Journal of the Minerals Metals & Materials Society*, 53 (3), pp. 31–35.
6. Iijima, S. (1991) "Helical microtubules of graphitic carbon", *Nature*, 354, pp. 56–58.
7. Khor, K. A. and Yu, L. G. (2015) "Global research trends in thermal sprayed coatings technology analyzed with bibliometrics tools", *Journal of Thermal Spray Technology*, 24(8), pp. 1346e1354.
8. Zhao, Y. and Gao, Y. (2015) "Deposition of nanostructured YSZ coating from spray-dried particles with no heat treatment", *Applied Surface Science*, 346, pp. 406–414.
9. Lima, R. S. and Marple, B. R. (2005) "Superior performance of high- velocity oxyfuel-sprayed nanostructured TiO_2 in comparison to air plasma-sprayed conventional Al_2O_3-$13TiO_2$", *Journal of Thermal Spray Technology*, 14(3), pp. 397–404.
10. Turunen, E., Varis, T., Gustafsson, T. E., Keskinen, J., Falt, T. and Hannula, S.-P. (2006) "Parameter optimization of HVOF sprayed nanostructured alumina and alumina-nickel composite coatings", *Surface Coatings Technology*, 200, pp. 4987–4994.
11. Lin X., Zeng, Y., Zhou, X. and Ding, C. (2003) "Microstructure of alumina-3wt.% titania coatings by plasma spraying with nanostructured powders", *Materials Science and Engineering A*, 357, pp. 228–234.
12. Yang, D., Gao*, Y., Liu, H. and Sun, C. (2017) "Thermal shock resistance of bimodal structured thermal barrier coatings by atmospheric plasma spraying using nanostructured partially stabilized zirconia", *Surface & Coatings Technology*, 315, pp. 9–16.
13. Zhou, F., Deng, C., Wang, Y., Liu, M., Wang, L., Wang, Y. and Zhang, X. (2019) "Characterisation of multi-scale synergistic toughened nanostructured YSZ thermal barrier coatings: From feedstocks to coatings", *Journal of the European Ceramic Society*, 40, pp. 1443–1452.
14. Tao, S., Liang, B., Ding, C., Lao, H. and Code, C. (2005) "Wear characteristics of plasma-sprayed nanostructured Yttria partially stabilized zirconia coatings", *Journal of Thermal Spray Technology*, 14(4), pp. 518–523.
15. Lima, R. S. and Marple, B. R. (2000) "From APS to HVOF spraying of conventional and nanostructured titania feedstock powders: A study on the enhancement of the mechanical properties", *Surface & Coatings Technology*, 200, pp. 3428–3437.
16. Wang, J., Sun, J., Zhang, H., Dong, S., Jiang, J., Deng, L., Zhou, X. and Cao, X. (2018) "Effect of spraying power on microstructure and property of nanostructured YSZ thermal barrier coatings", *Journal of Alloys and Compounds*, 730, pp. 471–482.
17. Zhang, J., Yin, Y., Jing, L. and Hong, Z. (2003) "Fabrication and properties of $Fe_3AleAl_2O_3$ graded coatings", *Journal of Materials Processing Technology*, 134, pp. 206–209.
18. Huang, W., Zhao, Y., Fan, X., Meng, X., Wang, Y., Cai, X., Cao, X. and Wang, Z. (2013) "Effect of bond coats on thermal shock resistance of thermal barrier coatings deposited onto polymer matrix composites via air plasma spray process", *Journal of Thermal Spray Technology*, 22, pp. 918–925.
19. Bansal, P., Padture, N. P. and Vasiliev, A. (2003) "Improved interfacial mechanical properties of Al_2O_3-13wt.% TiO_2 plasma-sprayed coatings derived from nanocrystalline powders", *Acta Materialia*, 51, pp. 2959–2970.
20. Chen, H., Zhang, Y. and Ding, C. (2002) "Tribological properties of nanostructured zirconia coatings deposited by plasma spraying", *Wear*, 253, pp. 885–893.
21. Liu, X., Zhang, B. and Deng, Z. (2002) "Grinding nanostructured ceramic coatings: Surface observation and material removal mechanisms", *International Journal of Machine Tools and Manufacture*, 42, pp. 1665–1676.
22. Gell, M., Jordan, E. H., Sohn, Y. H., Goberman, D., Shaw, L. and Xiao, T. D. (2001) "Development and implementation of plasma sprayed nanostructured ceramic coatings", *Surface & Coatings Technology*, 146–147, pp. 48–54.

23. Chen, H., Zhou, X. and Ding, C. (2003) "Investigation of the thermomechanical properties of a plasma-sprayed nanostructured zirconia coating", *Journal of the European Ceramic Society*, 23, pp. 1449–1455.
24. Taylor, T. A. (1992) "Thermal properties and microstructure of two thermal barrier coatings", *Surface & Coatings Technology*, 54/55, pp. 53–57.
25. Taylor, R. E., Wang, X. and Xu, X. (1999) "Thermophysical properties of thermal barrier coatings", *Surface & Coatings Technology*, 120–121, pp. 89–95.
26. Lima, R. S. and Marple, B. R. (2008) "Nanostructured YSZ thermal barrier coatings engineered to counteract sintering effects", *Materials Science and Engineering A*, 485 (1–2), pp. 182–193.
27. Wang, N., Zhou, C., Gong, S. and Xu, H. (2007) "Heat treatment of nanostructured thermal barrier coatings", *Ceramics International*, 33, pp.1075–1081.
28. Soltani, R., Garcia, E., Coyle, T. W., Mostaghimi, J., Lima, R. S., Marple, B. R. and Moreau, C. (2006) "Thermo-mechanical behavior of nanostructured plasma sprayed zirconia coatings", *Journal of Thermal Spray Technology*, 15, pp. 675–662.
29. Chen, H., Lee, S. W., Du, H., Ding, C. X. and Choi, C. H. (2004) "Influence of feedstock and spraying parameters on the depositing efficiency and microhardness of plasma-sprayed zirconia coatings", *Materials Letters*, 58, pp. 1241–1245.
30. Li, J. F., Liao, H., Wang, X. Y., Normand, B., Ji, V., Ding, C. X. and Coddet, C. (2004) "Improvement in wear resistance of plasma-sprayed Yttria stabilized zirconia coating using nanostructured powder", *Tribology International*, 37, pp. 77–84.
31. Ctibor, P., Neufuss, K., Dubsky, J., Kolman, B., Rohan, P. and Chraska, P. (2006) "Spraying of agglomerated TiO2 nanopowder by water-stabilized plasma", *PDF file in Proceedings of the International Thermal Spray Conference 2006*, B. R. Marple, M. M. Hyland, Y.-C. Lau, R. S. Lima and J. Voyer(eds.), ASM International, Materials Park, OH.
32. Ctibor, P., Bohac, P., Stranyanek, M. and Ctvrtlik, R. (2006) "Structured and mechanical properties of plasma sprayed coatings of titania and alumina", *Journal of the European Ceramic Society*, 26, pp. 3509–3514.
33. Kim, G. E., Walker, J., Jr. and Williams, J. B., Jr., Nanostructured Titania Coated Titanium, US Patent 6,835,449 B2, Dec 28, 2004.
34. Mehta, A., Vasudev, H. and Singh, S. (2020) "Materials today: Proceedings Recent developments in the designing of deposition of thermal barrier coatings – A review", *Materials Today: Proceedings*, 26, pp. 1336-1342, doi: 10.1016/j.matpr.2020.02.271.

10 Selection of Glass Substrates to be used as Electrodes in Dye-Sensitized Solar Cells

Shivani Arora Abrol, Cherry Bhargava, and Rajeev Sharma

10.1 INTRODUCTION AND AVAILABILITY OF DIFFERENT GLASS SUBSTRATE MATERIALS

Recent solar studies have attracted DSSCs studies because of their low production cost, high power conversion efficiencies and easy fabrications when compared to a normal silicon solar cell. There are many factors that influence the above parameters, mainly its efficiency. One such parameter is nature of the transparent substrate of the glass substrate and its resistivity. Mainly, two transparent and conductive oxides also called as TCO are used for forming the substrate of DSSC. These are indium doped tin oxide, named as (ITO) and another being fluorine doped tin oxide, names as (FTO). There is a huge diversity of cell configuration and therefore the material used for it also diversifies. This makes it very difficult for an appropriate selection of a TCO material for the glass substrate of DSSC as it offers a decisive influence on the performance.

The most prominently used TCO material for thin-film solar-cell manufacturing is F-doped tin oxide, FTO. Apart from this, indium-doped tin oxide (ITO) and antimony-doped tin oxide (ATO) have also come up as promising substitutes [1]. FTO is used extensively due to its high heat-resistant properties (normally up to 600 °C) as compared to ITO, which is less heat resistant, although it is thermally more stable [2]. The structural image of a dye-sensitized solar cell is shown in Figure 10.1.

10.1.1 Importance of the TiO_2 Layer and the Counter Electrode

A deposition of thick layer (10–20 nm) on TCO changes its transmittance properties and the roughness of the surface [1]. Also, there are limitations to both substrates, i.e. ITO & FTO, for a range of infrared light radiations. Hence, it becomes crucial to

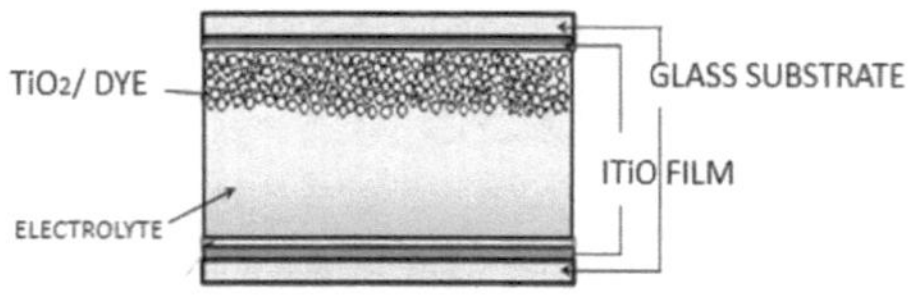

FIGURE 10.1 Structural Image of a DSSC

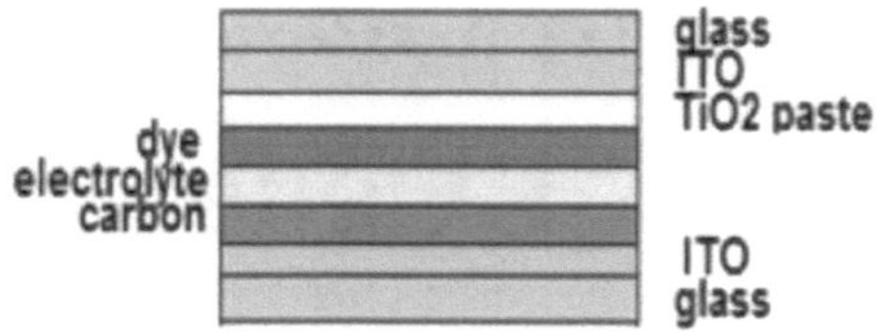

FIGURE 10.2 Overlapped TCO Structure with TiO2 paste

improve the photovoltaic efficiency of the DSSC, which is obtained by introducing a layer of a dye-sensitized TiO_2 in contact with the electrolyte. Figure 10.1 shows the structural image of such a DSSC. The introduction of the TiO_2 coating endows high photoelectric properties to the cell. The overlapping structure of TCO with the TiO_2 layer is shown in Figure 10.2.

The performance of a DSSC depends on the molecules liberated from the dye and semiconductor electrodes, as a sensitizer. Basically, three processes occur in a DSSC simultaneously. Firstly, the dye gets absorbed at the TiO2 layer of the electrode, which further interacts with the sunlight and liberates an electron from the lower orbit of the atomic structure to the excited state [3–4]. During this process, photons from the source of light (sun) penetrate into the cell and the process of photoexcitation takes place because the cell itself gets excited with the dye electrons. Secondly, the chemical diffusion of electrons from dye to TiO_2 layer into the ITO conductive layer takes place. To complete the circuit, the electron is returned to the cell dye and brings it in a normalized state with the use of the electrolyte. The DSSC is called a sandwiched cell because two conducting glasses overlap the layers of dye and electrolytes, as shown in Figure 10.2 [5]. Hence, the anode electrode is coated by the TiO_2 layer, which is sensitized by the dye and the second TCO counter electrode is coated by the carbon or graphite coating to enhance electrolytic interaction. Figure 10.3 shows how the titanium

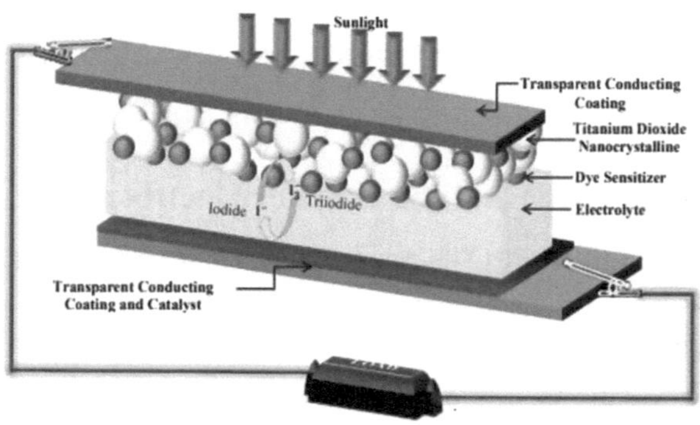

FIGURE 10.3 Titanium Diox ide Nanocrystalline Structure Sandwiched between the TCO Layers

dioxide nanocrystalline structure is sandwiched between the different layers between the electrodes of DSSC.

The various photovoltaic characteristics of the three coated substrates can be seen in the Table 10.1 below [3]. It can be clearly seen that with a high current density of 10.96 mA/cm^2, FTO exhibits the best conducting properties.

With the deposition of the TiO2 layer on ITO/FTO glass substrates, the ideality factor reduces, which indicates that the properties of the junction of a DSSC are improved–which was the problem of the presence of a shunt resistance at the junction. This happens due to the fact that the contact properties between the electrodes (TiO_2 coated ITO/FTO) and dye improve. The IPCE (Increased Photon to Current Conversion Efficiency) factor also increases due to an improved transmittance caused by TiO_2 layer insertion [2].

An appropriate texture of the glass substrate surface is achieved by a TCO layer having high optical transmission, good electrical conductivity and the beneficial property of light scattering, i.e. high infrared reflectivity [6]. An advantage of using TCO is that controlling the chemical in film deposition becomes easy, due to which it is used in many applications like liquid crystal displays, LEDs, etc. Their electroluminescent properties also make them useful in determination of glucose level in solutions, in the field of biology [7].

10.2 FEATURES OF VARIOUS TCO-COATED GLASS SUBSTRATES

Various TCOs have different properties like transparency, ability of light scattering etc., which are mainly determined by their structures. The different structures affect the electrical properties of a solar cell vastly as they determine the interfacing area of the glass substrate with other layers of the cell [8,9]. Features such as transmittance – which is higher for ITO in visible light than a FTO glass of the same thickness – and reflectance – which is higher for FTO as compared to ITO for the infrared zone – become important for determining the efficiency of a DSSC [7].

TABLE 10.1
Photovoltaic Characteristics using FTO, ITO and ITiO Substrates on Electrodes

Parameters	FTO	ITO	ITiO
Vsc (V)	0.78	0.63	0.75
Isc (mA)	3.06	2.59	2.94
Jsc Ma/cm^2)	10.96	8.23	10.85
Fill Factor	0.53	0.37	0.47
Efficiency (%)	6.47	2.73	5.64
Vmax	0.66	0.61	0.64
Area (cm^2)	0.25	0.25	0.2

The selected TCO should have the following features:

i. Neutral colour: A neutral-coloured glass inhibits the reflector colours, which leads to increased light transmittances and minimum haze for optimal clear visibility.
ii. Electrically conductive nature: The TCO should have good electrical conductivity. Due to this feature, a good heated and thermal control is obtained. Further, the transmittance of electromagnetic radiations and electrostatic dissipation is reduced.
iii. *Diverse nature*: The substrate should be available in a variety of glass thicknesses and resistivities of surface area for increased flexibility.
iv. *Unlimited shelf life*: Substances like pyrolytic surfaces provide durability in terms of least rubs and scrapes and, hence, are preferred. Also, with time, the surface should not get oxidised or change its colour.
v. *Ease of fabrication*: The durability of the glass in terms of handling, its ability to bear cutting stresses & lamination, heat strengthening, etc. are the few characteristics needed for easy fabrication of the substrate.

10.3 ITO-COATED GLASS SUBSTRATE

For effective and optimal conductivity, a cell would need conductive glass slides. Indium Tin Oxide-coated glass comes under the category of TCO-conductive glass. These are manufactured by spreading carefully (under vacuum-enclosed conditions at a constant temperature of 300 °C) a Tin Oxide layer that is thin and uniform on one side. This makes the glass transparent and highly conductive with very low resistance. The conventional thickness of an ITO is in the range 1.1 to 0.5 mm. The other side of the glass remains insulated.

The main area of application of ITO is the field of research and laboratories for bulk applications. These conductive glass substrates are used in the development of organic solar cells based on dye sensitization.

10.3.1 *FTO-coated Glass Substrate*

FTO-coated glass substrates mostly come in square or rectangular shapes but can be cut in a circular shape as well. Their standard thickness is approximately 25 nm. An FTO can effectively work in high temperature ranges, upto 350 °C. These glass substrates are chemically inert, relatively stable for all weather conditions, have high physical abrasion tolerance, are mechanically hard, have high temperature resistance and are less expensive as compared to ITO. FTO glass substrates have an advantage over ITO as they do not require indium to be diffused into n-type TiO_2 more often. They also exhibit a wide range of thermal and heating glass performances and upsurge the transmittance of light, thus optimizing electrical conductivity.

FTO is an electrically conductive glass and is ideally used for applications such as optoelectronics, thin-film photovoltaics, touch screens, RFI, energy-saving windows and other electro-optical and insulating applications.

10.4 COMPARISON OF ITO- AND FTO-COATED GLASS SUBSTRATES

ITO & FTO glass substrates can be studied on the basis of various attributes. A few of them are enlisted in Table 10.2 below.

To summarize, FTO glass substrates have the following advantages over ITO glass substrates:

- FTO is more transparent
- FTO is more stable against heating and environment abrasions
- ITO films have a transmittance of over 80% while FTO films exhibit a transmittance of about 75% in the visible region
- FTO has lager conductivity
- Indium can diffuse to the adjacent layers of ITO, altering their characteristics

TABLE 10.2
Comparison of ITO & FTO Glass Substrates

S.No.	Attribute	ITO coated glass	FTO coated glass
1.	*Response to visible light*	Layer shows medium transparency in visible light	Surface layer is better transparent to visible light
2.	*Temperature range*	ITO-coated glass can be used maximum at 350°C	FTO glass coating works well on higher temperature 600°C
3.	*Usability*	Glass slides usability is suitable for inverted work	Rarely used for inverted work
4.	*Reflectance*	Lower reflectance in infrared zone	Higher reflectance in infrared zone
5.	*Size*	Average grain size of ITO is 257 nm (SEM Result)	Average grain size of FTO is 190 nm (SEM Result)
6.	*Response with temperature rise*	Resistance of ITO glass substrate increases with temperature	Resistivity of FTO coated glass substrate is constant up to 600°C
7.	*Thermal stability*	Has a lower thermal stability	Has an excellent thermal stability
8.	*Conductivity*	Has moderate conductivity	Has good conductivity
9.	*Construction*	There is a passivation layer on the glass surface, then ITO coated on the passivation layer.	FTO directly coated on glass surface
10.	*Physical abrasion tolerance*	ITO coating is moderately tolerable for physical abrasion	FTO layer is high tolerance to physical abrasion
11.	*Structure*	Has a cubic structure in nature	Consist tetragonal structure
12.	*Cost*	ITO glass is quite expensive	FTO-coated glass is cheaper as compared to ITO glass.

- ITO has a sheet resistance of 18Ω/cm^2 in contrast to FTO's sheet resistance of 8.5/cm^2
- FTO is less expensive

10.5 CONCLUSION

As discussed, the efficiency and stable nature of organic dye-based DSSCs improve upon using FTO-coated glass substrates as electrodes. The coating of the TiO_2 layer further improves the interference characteristics between the layers and hence leads to better transfer of charge.

On the other hand, the sheet resistivity of the ITO glass substrate deteriorates upon heating above the temperature of 400° C [10].

Also, the IPCE, fill factor, photocurrent densities and open-circuit voltages for the cell came out to be high when FTO was used as a glass substrate in them compared to ITO [10].

It was also seen that the FTO glass substrate was thermally more stable and gave better performance at temperatures as high as 600° C.

REFERENCES

1. Y. Beomjin and K. Kyungkon et al. (2010) "Enhanced charge collection efficiency by thin TiO2 film deposition on FTO coated ITO conductive oxide in dye sensitized solar cells", *Journal of Material Chemistry*, p. 4392 Accepted March 9, 2010, first published on April 23rd, doi: 10.1039/b926145a.www.rsc.org/materials
2. S. Cornelia and G. Constantin (2010) "Comparison of dye-sensitized solar cells performance based on transparent conductive ITO & FTO", *Thin Solid Films*, 519, p. 596, doi: 10.1016/j.tsf.2010.07.002.
3. B. Woon-Hyuk and C. Mijung (2010) "Use of fluorine doped tin oxide instead of indium tin oxide in highly efficient air fabricated inverted polymer solar cells", *Applied Physics Letters*, 96, pp. 13506-2, doi: 10.1063/1.3374406.http://apl.aip.org/.
4. C. Woo-Jin, K. Dong-Joo, et al. (2012) "Characterization of Transparent Conductive ITO, ITiO and FTO films for application in photoelectrochemical cells", *Journal of Nanoscience and Nanotechnology*, 12, pp. 3394–3397, doi: 10.1166/jnn.2012.5571.
5. L. Latifa Hanum, A. Tri, et al. (2018) "Electrical, optical and structural properties of FTO thin films fabricated by spray ultrasonic nebulizer technique from SnCl4 precursor", *AIP Conference Proceedings of the International Seminar on Metallurgy and Materials*, pp. 02001–02008, doi: 10.1063/1.5038281.
6. J. Mikkel, N. Kion and C. Kerbs Federik (2008) "Stability/ Degradation of polymer solar cells", *Solar Energy Materials And Solar Cells*, 92, p. 686, doi: 10.1016/j.solmatr.2008.01.005.
7. M. Ait Aouaj, R. Diaz, et al. (2009) "Comparative Study Of ITO And FTO Thin Films Grown By Spray Pyrolysis", *Material Research Bulletin*, 44, p. 1459, doi: 10.1016/j.materresbull.2009.02.019.
8. M. Joachim, et al (2003) "Role Of The Glass/ TCO Substrate In The Thin Film Silicon Solar Cell," in *3rdworld conference on PhotoVoltaic Energy Conversion*, Osaka, Japan, May 11–18, 5P-D4-3, pp. 1839–1842.
9. A. Shanian and O. Savadogo (2005) "TOPSIS multiple criteria decision support analysis for

material selection of metallic bipolar plates for polymer electrolyte fuel cell", *Journal of Power Sources*, 159, p. 1095, doi: 10.1016/j.jpowsour.2005.12.092.www.sciencedirect.com

10. M. Mazalan, M. Mohd Noh, et al (2013) "Development of dye-sensitized solar cell (DSSC) using patterned Indium Tin Oxide (ITO) Glass., *3rdIEEE conference on Clean Energy & Technology (CEAT)*, 5P-D4-3, pp. 187–191, 978-1-4799-3238-2/13/$31.00.
11. K. Doon-Joo, M. Byung-Ho, et al (2011) "Comparision of transparent conductive indium tin oxide, titanium- doped indium oxide and fluorine doped tin oxide films for dye sensitised solar cell applications", *Journal of Electrical Engineering & Technology*, 6, (5), pp. 684–687,10.5370/JEET.2011.6.5.684.

11 Advanced Materials for Biomedical Nanotechnology

Dr. Mousmee Sharma and Dr. Parteek Prasher

11.1 INTRODUCTION

Nanotechnology provides profitable solutions for managing the clinical difficulties associated with biomedicine [1]. The advanced nanomaterials evade complex biomedical phenomenon including drug efflux and prompt a targeted delivery of the molecular medicine while supplementing molecular imaging and biomedical diagnosis [2]. Characteristic physicochemical properties of nanomaterials such as surface plasmon resonance, photothermal effect, and magnetothermal effect revolutionized theranostics by promoting the bioimaging of morbid cells and annihilation of cancer cells [3]. The nanomaterials such as nanotubes and functionalized nanoparticles assist targeted drug delivery to the deliberated site with high precision (Patra et al.). Further, the conjugation of the nanoscale systems with the biomacromolecules provides applications as gene transfection in molecular medicine. The noble metal nanoparticles with representative biocidal and oligodynamic effect present a robust candidature for the development of next generation antibiotics against drug-resistant and susceptible strains [4]. Similarly, the functionalized magnetic metal nanoparticles serve as image contrast agents in magnetic resonance imaging (MRI) and computed tomography [5]. The physiological toxicity of the metal nanoparticles limits their biological applications; however, their surface fabrication with desired molecules poises harmful effects on living systems, in addition to providing supplementary functionalities for further conjugation [6]. Nevertheless, a complex metabolic profile of metal nanoparticles, ability to generate oxidative stress, and extraction from body restrict extensive applications. Recent developments identified biodegradable, nontoxic nanosystems including polymersomes, and liposomes with diverse applications in biomedicine [7]. This chapter focuses on the progress of advanced nanomaterials in biomedical sciences, current perspectives, and future challenges.

11.2 ADVANCED NANOMATERIALS FOR DRUG DELIVERY

The success of representative drug-delivery paradigm depends on target specificity of the carrier systems, potency to cross the blood–brain barrier, considerable biotolerance, and biodegradation in systemic circulation after releasing the cargo drug molecules [8]. Moreover, the drugs are susceptible to lose their bioactivity and are prone to degradation in the presence of enzymes and changes in physiological pH or temperature. These factors decide the therapeutic efficacy, pharmacokinetics, cellular uptake, distribution and metabolism of the drug, and its subsequent clearance from the body [9]. From functionalized metal nanoparticles to carbon nanotubes and biodegradable liposomes and polymersomes, the nanotechnology has traversed a long journey for the development of advanced materials for an optimum drug delivery at the deliberated sites [10,11]. The advanced nanomaterials prolong the drug release at the target sites to achieve the desired beneficial effects with high physiological tolerance to the surrounding tissues. The nanomaterials present excellent results in delivering the oral and injectable drugs, in addition to improving the drug delivery via ocular, nasal, transdermal, and pulmonary routes [12]. The application of polymersomes for RNA transfection in molecular medicine ensures its delivery to the target cell's nucleus while providing protection against the cellular proteases and cytoplasmic degradation [13]. However, the utility of biomaterials in drug delivery faces persistent challenges such as the success of sustained release biomaterials varies from patient to patient, and that it requires repeated doses to achieve optimum therapeutic effect [14]. Similarly, it is difficult to appraise the metabolism and physiological clearance of metal-based nanosystems thereby raising critical concerns regarding their toxicity [15]. Apparently, the crossing of blood–brain barrier presents another major hurdle in the success of drug-delivering biomaterials thereby necessitating the development of rationally engineered theranostics nanosystems to counter this challenge [16].

11.2.1 *Carbon Nanotubes*

Carbon nanotubes are the new generation, advanced nanomaterials with interesting biomedical properties owing to having a hollow structure with a large surface area and considerable hydrophobicity well suitable for the delivery of drug molecules and biomolecules [17]. Characteristic optoelectronic and photothermal properties further extend the application of carbon nanotubes in photodynamic therapy and photoacoustic imaging [18]. Further, the excellent conducting properties of carbon nanotubes promote their application in the development of enzyme biosensors, cancer biosensors, and gene biosensors [19]. The surface functionalization of carbon nanotubes improves their dispersion in cellular environment and provides functional groups for selectively conjugating to desired biomacromolecules and ligands for precisely targeting the morbid sites [20]. Surface functionalization also supports their cellular entry via endocytosis and membrane adsorption followed by stimuli responsive intracellular release of the cargo molecules [21]. Importantly, the positioning of functionalized nanotubes perpendicular to the cell membranes prompts their uptake and internalization without effecting the cellular viability [22]. The subcutaneous and abdominal administration of carbon nanotubes leads to their absorption through the lymphatic canal, with a small portion remaining in the local tissues [20]. The persistence of anticancer-drug-loaded carbon nanotubes in lymph nodes minimizes the chances of tumor recurrence by lymphatic metastasis due to the annihilation of the metastatic cancer cells [10,23]. The administration of drug-carrying carbon nanotubes in blood directly through veins distributes them in vital organs including liver, heart, spleen, and kidneys, and their clearance from systemic circulation depends on the nature of surface functionality [20]. Reportedly, the presence of polyethylene glycol functionalization improves the blood half-life of carbon nanotubes due to the lowering of carrier immunogenicity hence averting their phagocytosis by the reticuloendothelial system [24].

Li et al. [25] developed pH-responsive, magnetic-targeted drug-delivery vehicle composed of carbon nanotube–hydroxyapatite composite loaded with magnetic nanoparticles for carrying the anticancer drug doxorubicin. The composite system demonstrated high drug-loading capacity, and the pH response restrained the drug release in optimum physiological conditions, but in peculiar cellular environment hence minimizing the undesired side effects. In addition, the ferromagnetic property of the carrier system enabled the drug transport to the target site under magnetic fields. Pistone et al. [26] reported pH- and temperature-responsive polymer-gated multiwalled carbon nanotubes for doxorubicin delivery. The fabrication with biocompatible polylactide enables the nanosystem to form hydrogen bond with poly (ethylene glycol) (PEG), leading to the entrapment of the cargo drug molecule within the polymeric chains. The in-vitro investigation of the drug-release properties and antiproliferative effect of the carrier system on human cancer cell lines suggested the direct dependence of the drug release on the degree of functionalization of carbon nanotube material. Seyfoori et al. [27] reported pH-responsive smart anticancer drug-delivery vector system based on carbon nanotube-based hybrid nanogels for delivering doxorubicin. The vector system exhibited superior drug-loading capacity with low responsiveness to pH in acidic medium, which improved on coating with magnetic nanoparticles. Farvadi et al. [28] reported an improved delivery of doxorubicin by using poly-ionic complex of single-walled carbon nanotubes and PEG-grafted-hyperbranched polyethyleneimine. The nanosystem demonstrated a pH-responsive release of doxorubicin in acidic pH with a burst release of the drug at pH 7.4 in the absence of polyethyleneimine graft. Interestingly, the presence of polyethyleneimine graft improved the drug-loading efficiency of the vector nanosystem and prompted the control release of the drug under same conditions. Yan et al. [29] reported an effective delivery of doxorubicin via single-walled carbon-nanotubes functionalized with asparagine-glycine-arginine (NGR) peptide. Further loading of the functionalized carbon nanotube with MRI contrast agent facilitated the tumor diagnosis in physiological environment. The hybrid nanosystem efficiently accumulated and entered the tumor cells in animal models due to the presence of peptide appendage, which facilitated drug internalization to demonstrate the optimum antitumor chemotherapeutic effect and tumor diagnosis due to the loading of contrast agent. Uttekar et al. [30] demonstrated a precise delivery of doxorubicin via folic acid anchored, acid-functionalized single-walled carbon nanotubes, which graft to the cargo drug via π–π stacking interactions. The nanosystem presented a superior drug-entrapment efficiency, high stability in the biological environment, and minimal toxicity. Notably, the nanosystem exhibited 84% drug-entrapment efficiency and an optimum drug release mainly at acidic pH. Yang et al. [31] reported novel, pH-responsive drug-delivery system comprising multiwalled carbon nanotubes with larger inner diameter. The nanosystem demonstrated high loading efficiency for cisplatin and doxorubicin where the former encapsulates inside the inner cavity of nanotubes and the latter anchors to the outer surface. Pourjavadi et al. 2016 developed dendritic multiwalled carbon nanotubes containing thermoresponsive shells for loading anticancer drugs. Interestingly, the dehydration of polymeric shell at body temperature promoted the release of encapsulated drug via diffusion-controlled mechanism. The anchoring of PAMAM on the surface of carbon nanotubes improved the drug-loading efficiency into the dendrimer cavity, and its further grafting with poly(N-isopropyl amide) afforded thermal sensitivity for a controlled release. The studies validated the potential applications of the nanosystem in treating hyperthermia and targeted tumor therapy. Notably, the drug-release efficiency of carbon nanotubes depends on length and incubation time, where the small-sized carbon nanotubes display superior efficiency after 48 hours of incubation, compared to the large-sized counterparts [32].

11.2.2 *Polymersomes*

Polymersomes comprise amphiphilic copolymer vesicles enclosing aqueous cavity for accommodating the cargo drug molecules via passive and active loading approaches [33]. The former strategy incorporates the solubilization of hydrophobic payload in a suitable solvent, whereas the latter comprises the drug loading onto the polymersome based on salt and pH gradient. The incorporation of appropriate moieties on the surface of polymersome including monoclonal antibodies, aptamer, peptides, and small organic molecules improves their biodistribution by selective cellular uptake and reduced toxicity toward the healthy tissues [34]. Importantly, the engineering of stimuli-responsive polymersomes promotes controlled drug release and improved bioavailability at the target site. The stimuli include magnetic field, pH, temperature, redox potential, and light that prompt the drug release by smart polymersomes [35,36]. As such, the presence of acidic pH in the tumor microenvironment, extracellular matrix of tumor cells, inflammatory cells, and cellular components including lysosomes and endosomes act as favorable sites for the release of drugs by pH-sensitive polymersomes [36,37]. However, a slow response to the pH stimulus results in a slower drug release, which apparently results in the induction of drug resistance in the cells [38,39]. Similarly, the bioreducible polymersomes containing disulfide functionalities display sensitivity to redox changes in the tumor microenvironment caused by Glutathione (GSH) and cysteine and homocysteine balance [40]. Specifically, the tumor site possesses extracellular oxidative environments and the intracellular reductive environments that support the drug delivery by redox-responsive polymersomes. The disulfide functionality reportedly improves the release of cargo drug molecules in reducing environment; however, the presence of reducing agents in systemic circulation premature drug leakage occurs hence effecting the drug-delivering efficacy of the redox-sensitive polymersome [41].

Zhang et al. [42] reported photothermal-responsive nanosized polymersomes as anticancer drug-delivery vehicles for both hydrophobic and hydrophilic drugs. The nanovehicles comprised porous silicon nanoparticles conjugated with gold nanoparticles encapsulated into biocompatible, amphiphilic diblock copolymer-based polymersomes. The nanosystem presented superior drug-loading efficiency, high cellular-compatibility, and lower cytotoxicity toward healthy cells. Scherer et al. [43] reported nanosized polymersomes based on pentafluorophenyl ester as drug-delivery vehicles. Techniques such as cryo transmission electron microscopy (cryoTEM) and light scattering validate the vesicle formation, which efficiently encapsulated hydrophilic cargo molecules including small interfering ribonucleic acid (siRNA). Importantly, the nanovehicles demonstrated aggregation in human blood serum and minimal toxicity in vitro. Zhou et al. [44] developed light-sensitive, block amphiphilic polymersomes as drug-delivery vehicle for doxorubicin hydrochloride. The presence of quaternary ammonium functionality affords hydrophilicity to the polymersome and promotes electrostatic adsorption with folic acid, hence enabling the selective targeting of cancer cells via over-expression of folate receptor. The exposure to light resulted in a photocleavage of o-nitrobenzyl functionality, leading to a disintegration of polymersome due to the transformation of its structure from cationic amphiphilic to hydrophilic zwitter ionic state, hence facilitating the drug release. Tang et al. [45] developed ROS-sensitive, laser-triggered, self-immolative smart polymersomes for cancer therapy. The encapsulation of zinc phthalocyanine in polymersome bilayers prevented the water insolubility and aggregation and improved the biocompatibility. The nanosystem afforded efficient loading of both hydrophilic and hydrophobic drugs. Kulkarni et al. [46] identified mitochondria-targeted fluorescent polymersomes for an effective drug delivery to the cancer cells. The presence of triphenylphosphonium moiety favored mitochondrial localization, and the dansyl groups exhibited fluorescence emission. In addition, the presence of PEG polymer ensured improved half-life in systemic circulation and suitability for the targeted delivery of drugs to cancer cells. Kozlovskaya et al. [47] reported thermal-responsive polymersomes for mitigating cardiotoxicity induced by doxorubicin, caused by an irreversible damage of the cardiac muscles and dysregulation of immune system. The polymersomes displayed exceptional drug-loading capacity toward doxorubicin, with a high encapsulation efficiency due to spontaneous drug loading from its aqueous solution at the room temperature. The histological analysis for the polymersome-encapsulated doxorubicin did not indicate toxicity signatures, while they appeared in the case of liposome carrier. Zhang et al. [48] presented bright fluorescent polymersomes with aggregation-induced emission for an in-vivo investigation of drug delivery and distribution. The polymeric membranes underwent self-assembly in water by nanoprecipitation with dioxane, or tetrahydrofuran cosolvent, resulting in the closure of amphiphilic block copolymers bilayer lamellae to give polymersomes with thickness 10–15 nm. The self-assembly prompted fluorescence emission in the polymersomes useful for the monitoring of transport and distribution of drugs and bioconjugates in the living cells. Chao et al. [49] reported biodegradable polymersomes for the delivery of doxorubicin. Methoxy poly(ethylene glycol)-b-poly(epsilon-caprolactone) (mPEG-b-PCL) copolymer served as the precursor for the synthesis of polymersomes with hydrophobic membrane of thickness 10 nm and nano-scale particle size of 60 nm. These polymersomes elevated the cytotoxicity and intracellular accumulation of doxorubicin in the target MCF-7/ADR cells, while significantly improving the bioavailability and circulation time in vivo. Cellari et al. [50] reported drug-triggered self-assembly of triblock copolymers into polymersomes, which assisted the synergistic co-delivery of paclitaxel and platinum drugs. Interestingly, the polymersome system displayed high drug-loading content for the cargo drugs and provided stability against enzymatic degradation.

11.3 ADVANCED NANOMATERIALS IN THERANOSTICS

The unique physicochemical characteristics of nanomaterials endow multidimensional properties including cell imaging, drug delivery, and cancer therapy, collectively referred as theranostics with advanced properties compared to representative approaches [12]. The nanomaterials such as quantum dots and magnetic nanomaterials serve as excellent resource for the development of theranostics with multifunctional properties [51]. The prominent application of quantum dots and magnetic nanoparticles includes monitoring of the intra/ extracellular events, drug metabolism, pharmacokinetics, and toxicity profile of the cargo drug molecules via fluorescence, photothermal imaging, and magnetic imaging in response to changes in the biological environment [52]. The tumor cells demonstrate abnormal physicochemical environment with uncharacteristic pH, temperature, and metabolism as compared to the healthy cells, which serves as the stimuli for functioning of rationally designed theranostics [53]. Further conjugation of quantum dots and magnetic nanoparticles with biomolecules and functional head groups provides the privilege of intracellular drug delivery via covalent/non-covalent conjugation [54]. Importantly, the quantum dots display extraordinary resistance toward photobleaching, demonstrate high fluorescence stability compared to the organic fluorophores and fluorescent proteins, and possess broad excitation spectra and size-tunable emission spectra [55]. These properties ensure long-term monitoring of intramolecular and intermolecular interactions in live cells and tissues. Similarly, the superparamagnetism in theranostic metal nanoparticles serve as image contrast improvement agents in MRI and tomography while assisting the in-vivo magnetic tracking of the loaded drug, or therapeutic agent. The theranostic nanoparticles display extensive biological applications, however a poor clearance rate from systemic circulation poses a significant challenge in clinical success. [5].

11.3.1 *Quantum Dots*

Drug delivery by nanoparticles promotes reduced toxicity, improved bioavailability, better half-life in systemic circulation, and controlled release. However, the clinical success of nanodrug-delivery vehicles necessitates the appraisal of the physiological fate of nanoformulations in vivo including their distribution, degradation, and clearance. Quantum dots present high efficacy for addressing these exigencies by offering the real-time monitoring of nanovehicles and drug release at both cellular and systemic levels. Quantum dots referred as nanoscale semiconductor materials present characteristic, tunable opto-electronic properties including bright, intense fluorescence for delivering interesting applications. In addition, the quantum dots offer superior photochemical stability, high quantum yield, and size-maneuverable light emission. As a semiconductor absorbs a photon, and the electron is promoted to the conduction band hence creating a hole in the valence band. Coulomb attraction keeps the electron and the hole together due to which the electron orbits the hole at a fixed average distance. When the conduction electrons move back to the valence band, they emit light whose color depends on the energy difference between the conduction band and valence band. For smaller nanoparticles, the high energy difference between the bands results in a deeper blue color; however, for large-sized nanoparticles, the lower energy difference between the two bands results in red color. The contemporary theranostic platform requires materials capable of simultaneous biosensing, bioimaging, and therapy at the deliberated site for which the quantum dots present a robust candidature. The quantum dots function as the principal nanocarrier of cargo therapeutic molecule, in addition to functioning as fluorescent labels in composite nanomaterials. Importantly, the quantum dots present lower toxicity, physiological benevolence, and broad excitation spectra that further validate their application in the representative nano-theranostics.

Cai et al. [56] reported pH-responsive zinc oxide quantum dots for an intracellular controlled release of doxorubicin to lung cancer cells. The presence of dicarboxyl-terminated PEG affords stability to the quantum dot in physiological fluids, whereas the conjugation with hyaluronic acid prompts specific binding to the overexpressed glycoprotein CD44 in cancer cells. Notably, the pH-responsive ZnO quantum dots after cellular uptake furnished Zn^{+2} ions in acidic endosomes and lysosomes, hence triggering the dissociation of metal–drug complex thereby causing a controlled drug release. Yao et al. [57] reported graphene quantum dots capped magnetic mesoporous silica nanoparticles for controlled drug release of doxorubicin and synergistic attenuation of cancer cells. The nanosystem displayed pH-responsive release of the cargo drug in acidic pH and generated hyperthermia for a selective annihilation of cancer cells. However, the nanosystem displayed lower therapeutic efficacy compared to the free doxorubicin mainly because of the partial internalization of the nanosystem carrying the cargo drug thereby resulting in a lower drug concentration in the target cells. Similarly, the conjugation of mesoporous silica nanoparticles with graphene quantum dots before endocytosis for mitigating toxicity of the nanosystem also alters its drug release characteristics. Dong et al. [58] developed arginine-glycine-aspartic-acid-conjugated graphene quantum dots for targeted drug delivery of doxorubicin and to provide fluorescence imaging properties for tracking and monitoring of the delivered drug. Notably, the nanosystem demonstrated pH-responsive release of the cargo drug with negligible toxicity to the healthy cells. The utilization of the nanocarrier for drug delivery improved the efficacy of doxorubicin without the requirement of dose increase. Notably, the nanosystem displayed effective nuclei penetration post 16 hours of incubation hence suggesting an efficient nuclear delivery of the cargo drug with improved the cytotoxicity toward U251 glioma cells. Huan et al. [59] developed nucleolus targeting fluorescent quantum dots. The quantum dots possess good water dispersibility, superior photostability, and high compatibility toward biological systems. The coupling of the quantum dots with a photosensitizer led to a remarkable enhancement of phototherapeutic efficiency for rapidly targeting tumors via intravenous administration of the nanosensor. Dong et al. [58] developed fluorescent PEGylated quantum dots by refluxing graphitic carbon nitride (g-C_3N_4) in acidic medium, followed by its hydrothermal treatment with a surface passivation agent such as diamine-tethered oligomeric poly(ethylene glycol). The drug release by quantum dots occurred in response to pH changes in the morbid cells, with minimal toxicity due to PEGylation. Notably, the high photoluminescence of fluorescent quantum dots promotes the visualization of drug delivery without the employment of external dyes. Justin et al. (2016) reported photoluminescent and superparamagnetic, reduced graphene oxide–iron oxide quantum dots for applications in drug delivery and photothermal therapy. The quantum dots possessed negligible residual magnetization and displayed low cytotoxicity to the health cells at lower concentration. The drug loading on the surface of quantum dots occurred at ration 0.31:1, and the loaded drug achieved a stable but complete release from the carrier quantum dots in a time duration over 8 hours. Khodadadei et al. [60] developed fluorescent nitrogen-doped graphene quantum dots via pyrolysis of citric acid as a carbon source and urea as a source of nitrogen. The loading of anticancer drug methotrexate on graphene quantum dots via π–π stacking interactions resulted in a highly efficient drug-delivery system. In addition, the layered structure of the quantum dots offered a larger surface area for an effective intercalation of the cargo drug between the layers. Notably, the free drug rapidly diffused in the target cells causing a high toxicity to the healthy cells, but its delivery via quantum dots resulted in a controlled release with cytotoxicity directed toward the target cancer cells. Hence, the quantum dots serve as excellent materials for drug delivery and monitoring of drug behavior.

11.3.2 *Magnetic Nanoparticles*

The functionalized magnetic nanoparticles present biosensing applications for biomedical diagnostics, hyperthermia, MRI, and controlled drug delivery. The nanoparticles with magnetic behavior form a vital component in anticancer theranostics due to their potency to track the chemotherapeutic movement through the body, while improving the drug efficacy and minimizing side effects. Notably, the appropriately engineered magnetic nanoparticles display improved plasma pharmacokinetics with superior tumor selectivity and provide supplementary functionalities for internalization into target cells. Importantly, the nature of magnetic nanoparticle's surface and nanoparticle hydrodynamic size determine their pharmacokinetics with the reticuloendothelial system responsible for their clearance from systemic circulation and plasma half-life. Interestingly, the magnetic nanoparticles generate heat in the presence of a variable magnetic field due to magnetic hysteresis loss referred as magnetic hyperthermia, which presents application in the non-invasive thermal ablation of cancer cells. This technique delivers promising results, but the local overheating may cause damage to the normal tissues. Another significant challenge for the application of magnetic nanoparticles is the necessity of improved magnetic field gradients. The magnetic capturing of magnetic nanoparticles customarily occurs at small distances from the magnet source, hence suggesting their application mainly for the treatment of superficial tumors. In addition, it is desirable to have an improved focus of the flux gradient toward the target cells for a better therapeutic effect. Similarly, the heterogeneity of tumor vasculature and fenestration size results in the heterogeneous accumulation of magnetic nanoparticles in tumor site. However, the utilization of externally applied forces such as focused ultrasound reportedly enhances the penetration of magnetic nanoparticles in tumors and promotes their homogeneous delivery to the tumors.

Amirshaghaghi et al. [61] reported dual mode theragnostic applications of superparamagnetic iron oxide nanoparticle (SPION) nanoclusters for imaging and photodynamic therapy. The presence of chlorin e6 coating enables the solubilization of hydrophobic SPION as highly stabilized, water-soluble nanoclusters without the application of external amphiphiles or carriers. The nanoclusters effectively localize in tumor cells via improved permeability and retention, while being detectable by magnetic resonance (MR) and optical imaging techniques. Sabareeswaran et al. [62] studied the effect of surface-engineered SPIONs on mast cell infiltration for theranostic applications. The surface modification of SPIONs demonstrated a significant improvement in biocompatibility and lowered the levels of antioxidants such as GSH and superoxide dimustase (SOD) due to an elevated recruitment of mast cells in vital organs. Notably, the generation of oxidative stress with progressive intracellular degradation of SPIONs adversely affects the cellular activity and impacts the recruitment of mast cells in vital organs in vivo. Luo et al. [63] reported the theranostic application of graphene oxide engineered with ultrasmall SPIONs. The nanosystem displayed pH-sensitive, potential chemotherapeutic applications for T_1-weighted magnetic resonance (T_1-MR) imaging. The nanosystem reportedly accumulated in the spleen and liver after 4 hours of administration, followed by a successful clearance from the body without altering the cell morphology in vital organs. Thomas et al. [64] reported gene delivery applications and MR contrast agent property of SPIONs loaded on poly(L-lysine)/hyaluronic acid micelles. The nanosystem efficiently transferred foreign DNA molecule, assisted by the poly(L-lysine) appendage functioning as DNA-carrier. The nanosystem displayed an average particle size of 200 nm, with spherical morphology. The nanosystem displayed lower toxicity to the NIH3T3 (murine fibroblast cells) and demonstrated highly efficient DNA transfected into CT-26 cell line. Huang et al. [68] reported folic-acid-conjugated SPIONs for target-specific drug delivery in cancer theranostics. The monodispersed SPIONs coated with PEG and PEI polymers are further conjugated to folic acid via EDC/NHS coupling to obtain the desired nanosystem for an effective delivery of doxorubicin. The nanosystem displayed hydrodynamic diameter in the range 23–67 nm and displayed marked colloidal stability in PBS solution. The nanosystem displayed high r_2 relaxivity, and accumulated in the tumor cells, which provided diagnostic applications by Magnetic Resonance Imaging. Shang et al. [66] reported polymeric nanoparticles loaded with SPIONs and doxorubicin for an efficient drug delivery and MRI detection properties. The nanosystem exhibited marked water solubility and colloidal stability, with highly potent targeting of tumor cells. Notably, the nanosystem displayed superior T_2 contrast in MRI technique, suggesting its potential in biosensing applications. Salunkhe et al. [67] reported the application of SPIONs for MRI-guided magneto-chemotherapy in cancer theranostics. The high magnetic moment iron oxide nanoparticles displayed average diameter of 12 nm and high magnetization value of 92 emu/g. The nanosystem demonstrated MRI-guided magneto-chemotherapy on breast cancer cells (MCF-7) with significant 96% killing of cancer cells in 30 min of the application of magneto-chemotherapy. Mauro et al. [68] reported polyaminoacid nanogels embedded with SPIONs for the treatment of tumor microenvironment and for the annihilation of breast cancer cells. The nanomedicine comprised SPION core and hydrophilic cross-linked shell affording the encapsulation of hydrophilic and hydrophobic molecules. Reportedly, the doxorubicin anchored to the hydrophobic SPIONs surface and collagenase-2 interacted with the hydrophilic shell via hydrogen bonds. Interestingly, the local degradation of extracellular matrix and its remodeling in solid tumors by proteolytic compound such as collagenase-2 potentially enhance the penetration of nanomedicine in tumor cells. This also promotes the sustained release of the cargo drug in tumor cells hence enabling a synergistic anticancer effect on the highly invasive breast tumors.

REFERENCES

1. Kaushik, A. (2019) "Biomedical nanotechnology related grand challenges and perspectives", *Frontiers in Nanotechnology*, 1, pp. 1–4.
2. Nune, S. K., Gunda, P., Thallapally, P. K., Lin, Y. Y., Forrest, M. L., Berkland, C. J. (2009) "Nanoparticles for biomedical imaging", *Expert Opinion On Drug Delivery*, 6, pp. 1175–1194.
3. Vines, J. B., Yoon, J. H., Ryu, N. E., Lim, D. J., Park, H. (2019) "Gold nanoparticles for photothermal cancer therapy", *Frontiers in Chemistry*, 7, Article 167.
4. Prasher, P., Singh, M., Mudila, H. (2018) "Silver nanoparticles as antimicrobial therapeutics: Current perspectives and future challenges", *3 Biotech,* 8, 411.
5. Jeong, Y., Hwang, H. S., Na. K. (2018) "Theranostics and contrast agents for magnetic resonance imaging", *Biomaterials Research*, 22, 20.
6. Zhang, X. Q., Xu, X., Bertrand, N., Pridgen, E., Swami, A., Farokhzad, O. C. (2012) "Interactions of nanomaterials and biological systems: Implications to personalized nanomedicine", *Advanced Drug Delivery Reviews,* 64, pp. 1363–1384.
7. Chowdhury, A., Kunjiappan, S., Panneerselvam, T., Somasundaram, B., Bhattacharjee, C. (2017) "Nanotechnology and nanocarrier-based approaches on treatment of degenerative diseases", *International Nano Letters*, 7, pp. 91–122.
8. Dean, S. N., Turner, K. B., Medintz, I. L., Walper, S. A. (2017) "Targeting and delivery of therapeutic enzymes", *Therapeutic Delivery*, 8, pp. 577–595.
9. Balamuralidhara, V., Pramodkumar, T. M., Srujana, N., Venkatesh, M. P., Vishal Gupta, N., Krishna, K. L., Gangadharappa, H. V. (2011) "pH sensitive drug delivery systems: A review", *American Journal of Drug Discovery and Development*, 1, pp. 24–48.
10. Rastogi, V., Yadav, P., Bhattacharya, S. S., Mishra, A. K., Verma, N., Verma, A., Pandit, J. K. (2014) "Carbon nanotubes: An emerging drug carrier for targeting cancer cells", *Journal of Drug Delivery*, 2014, Article 670815.
11. Mabrouk, M., Rajendran, R., Soliman, I. E., Ashour, M. M., Beherei, H. H., Tohamy, K. M., Thomas, S., Kalarikkal, N., Arthanareeswaran, G., Das, D. B. (2019) "Nanoparticle-and nanoporous-membrane-mediated delivery of therapeutics", *Pharmaceutics,* 11, Article 294.

12. Patra, J. K., Das, G., Fraceto, L. F., Campos, E. V. R., Rodriguez-Torres, M., Rodriguez-Torres, M. P., Acosta-Torres, L. S., Diaz-Torres, L. A., Grillo, R., Swamy, M. K., Sharma, S., Habtemariam, S., Shin, H. S. (2018) "Nano based drug delivery systems: Recent developments and future prospects", *Journal of Nanobiotechnology*, 16, Article 71.
13. Patel, A., Patel, M., Yang, X., Mitra, A. K. (2014) "Recent advances in protein and peptide drug delivery: A special emphasis on polymeric nanoparticles", *Protein & Peptide Letters,* 1, pp. 1102–1120.
14. Kowalski, P. S., Bhattacharya, C., Afewerki, S., Langer, R. S. (2018) "Smart biomaterials: Recent advances and future directions", *ACS Biomaterials Science & Engineering*, 4, 3809–3817.
15. Gupta, R., Xie, H. (2018) "Nanoparticles in daily life: Applications, toxicity and regulations", *Journal of Environmental Pathology, Toxicology and Oncology*, 37, pp. 209–230.
16. Tang, W., Fan, W., Lau, J., Deng, L., Shena, Z., Chen, X. (2019) "Emerging blood–brain-barrier-crossing nanotechnology for brain cancer theranostics", *Chemical Society Reviews,* 48, pp. 2967–3014.
17. Maiti, D., Tong, X., Mou, X., Yang, K. (2018) "Carbon-based nanomaterials for biomedical applications: A recent study", *Frontiers in Pharmacology*, 9, 1401.
18. Li, W., Wang, X., Wang, J., Guo, Y., Lu, S. Y., Li, C. M., Kang, Y., Wang, Z. G., Ran, H. T., Cao, Y., Liu, H. (2018) "Enhanced photoacoustic and photothermal effect of functionalized polypyrrole nanoparticles for near-infrared theranostic treatment of tumor", *Biomacromolecules,* 20, pp. 401–411.
19. Sireesha, M., Jagadeesh Babu, V., Kranthi Kiran, A. S., Ramakrishna, S. (2018) "A review on carbon nanotubes in biosensor devices and their applications in medicine", *Nanocomposites*, 4, pp. 36–57.
20. Zhang, W., Zhang, Z., Zhang, Y. (2011) "The application of carbon nanotubes in target drug delivery systems for cancer therapies", *Nanoscale Research Letters*, 6, 555.
21. Sigismund, S., Confalonieri, S., Ciliberto, A., Polo, S., Scita, G., Fiore P. P. (2012) "Endocytosis and signaling: Cell logistics shape the eukaryotic cell plan", *Physiological Reviews*, 92, pp. 273–366.
22. Elhissi, A. M. A., Ahmed, W., Hassan, I., Dhanak, V. R., Emanuele, A. (2012) "Carbon nanotubes in cancer therapy and drug delivery", *Journal of Drug Delivery*, 2012, Article 837327.
23. Ji, J., Liu, M., Meng, Y., Liu, R., Yan, Y., Dong, J., Guo, Z., Ye, C. (2016) "Experimental study of magnetic multi-walled carbon nanotube-doxorubicin conjugate in a lymph node metastatic model of breast cancer", *Medical Science Monitor*, 7, pp. 2363–2673.
24. Suk, J. S., Xu, Q., Kim, N., Hanes, J., Ensign, L. M. (2016) "PEGylation as a strategy for improving nanoparticle-based drug and gene delivery", *Advanced Drug Delivery Reviews*, 99, pp. 28–51.
25. Li, H., Sun, X., Li, Y., Li, B., Liang, C., Wang, H. (2019) "Preparation and properties of carbon nanotube (Fe)/hydroxyapatite composite as magnetic targeted drug delivery carrier", *Materials Science and Engineering C*, 97, pp. 222–229.
26. Pistone, A., Iannazzo, D., Ansari, S., Milone, C., Salamo, M., Galvagno, S., Cirmi, S., Navarra, M. (2016) "Tunable doxorubicin release from polymer-gated multiwalled carbon nanotubes", *International Journal of Pharmaceutics*, 515, pp. 30–36.
27. Seyfoori, M., Sarfarazijami, S., Ebrahimi, S. A. S. (2019) "pH-responsive carbon nanotube-based hybrid nanogels as the smart anticancer drug carrier", *Artificial Cells, Nanomedicine, and Biotechnology*, 47, pp. 1437–1443.
28. Farvadi, F., Tamaddon, A. M., Sobhani, Z., Abolm aali, S. S. (2017) "Polyionic complex of single-walled carbon nanotubes and PEG-grafted-hyperbranched polyethyleneimine (PEG-PEI-SWNT) for an improved doxorubicin loading and delivery: Development and

in vitro characterization", *Artificial Cells, Nanomedicine, and Biotechnology*, 45, pp. 855–863.
29. Yan, C., Chen, C., Hou, L., Zhang, H., Che, Y., Qi, Y., Zhang, X., Cheng, J., Zhang, Z. (2017) "Single-walled carbon nanotube-loaded doxorubicin and Gd-DTPA for targeted drug delivery and magnetic resonance imaging", *Journal of Drug Targeting*, 25, pp. 163–171.
30. Uttekar, P. S., Lakade, S. H., Beldar, B. K., Harde, M. T. (2019) "Facile synthesis of multi-walled carbon nanotube via folic acid grafted nanoparticle for precise delivery of doxorubicin", *IET Nanobiotechnology*, 13, pp. 688–696.
31. Yang, T., Wu, Z., Wang, P., Mu, T., Qin, H., Zhu, Z., Wang, J., Sui, L. (2017) "A large-inner-diameter multi-walled carbon nanotube-based dual-drug delivery system with pH-sensitive release properties", *Journal of Materials Science: Materials in Medicine*, 28, p. 110.
32. Sciortino, N., Fedeli, S., Paoli, P., Brandi, A., Chiarugi, P., Severi, M., Cicchi, S. (2017) "Multiwalled carbon nanotubes for drug delivery: Efficiency related to length and incubation time", *International Journal of Pharmaceutics*, 521, pp. 69–72.
33. Messager, L., Gaitzsch, J., Chierico, L., Battaglia, G. (2014) "Novel aspects of encapsulation and delivery using polymersomes", *Current Opinion in Pharmacology*, 18, pp. 104–111.
34. Anajafi, T., Mallik, S. (2015) "Polymersome-based drug-delivery strategies for cancer therapeutics", *Therapeutic Delivery*, 6, pp. 521–534.
35. Saravana, K. K., Hu, X., Ali, D. M., Wang, M. H. (2019) "Emerging strategies in stimuli-responsive nanocarriers as the drug delivery system for enhanced cancer therapy", *Current Pharmaceutical Design*, 25, pp. 2609–2625.
36. Wang, Y., Shim, M. S., Levinson, N. S., Sung, H. W., Xia, Y. (2014) "Stimuli-responsive materials for controlled release of theranostic agents", *Advanced Functional Materials*, 24, pp. 4206–4220.
37. Alsehli, M. (2020) "Polymeric nanocarriers as stimuli-responsive systems for targeted tumor (cancer) therapy: Recent advances in drug delivery", *Saudi Pharmaceutical Journal*, 28, pp. 255–265.
38. Wong, P. T., Choi, S. K. (2015) "Mechanisms of drug release in nanotherapeutic delivery systems", *Chemical Reviews*, 115, pp. 3388–3432.
39. Housman, G., Byler, S., Heerboth, S., Lapinska, K., Longacre, M., Snyder, N., Sarkar, S. (2014) "Drug resistance in cancer: An overview", *Cancers (Basel)*, 6, pp. 1769–1792.
40. Nehate, C., Nayal, A., Koul, V. (2019). "Redox responsive polymersomes for enhanced doxorubicin delivery", *ACS Biomaterials Science and Engineering*, 5, pp. 70–80.
41. Guo, X., Cheng, Y., Zhao, X. (2018) "Advances in redox-responsive drug delivery systems of tumor microenvironment", *Journal of Nanobiotechnology*, 16, 74.
42. Zhang, H., Cui, W., Qu, X., Wu, H., Qu, L., Zhang, X., Makila, E., Salonen, J., Zhu, Y., Yang, Z., Chen, D., Santos, H. A., Hai, M., Weitz, D. A. (2019) "Photothermal-responsive nanosized hybrid polymersome as versatile therapeutics codelivery nanovehicle for effective tumor suppression", *Proceedings of the National Academy of Sciences*, 116, pp. 7744–7749.
43. Scherer, M., Fischer, K., Depoix, F., Thiermann, R., Mohr, K., Zentel, R. (2016) "Pentafluorophenyl ester-based polymersomes as nanosized drug-delivery vehicles", *Macromolecular Rapid Communications*, 37, pp. 60–66.
44. Zhou, Y., Chen, R., Yang, H., Bao, C., Fan, J., Wang, C., Lin, Q., Zhu, L. (2020) "Light-responsive polymersomes with a charge-switch for targeted drug delivery", *Journal of Materials Chemistry B*, 8, pp. 727–735.
45. Tang, Q., Hu, P., Peng, H., Zhang, N., Zheng, Q., He, Y. (2020) "Near-infrared laser-triggered, self-immolative smart polymersomes for in vivo cancer therapy", *International Journal of Nanomedicine*, 15, pp. 137–149.
46. Kulkarni, P. S., Haldar, M. K., Confeld, M. I., Langaas, C. J., Yang, X., Qian, S. Y., Mallik, S. (2016) "Mitochondria-targeted fluorescent polymersomes for drug delivery to cancer cells", *Polymer Chemistry*, 7, pp. 4151–4154.

47. Kozlovskaya, V., Liu, F., Yang, Y., Ingle, K., Qian, S., Halade, G. V., Urban, V. S., Kharlampieva, E. (2019) "Temperature-responsive polymersomes of poly(3-methyl-N-vinylcaprolactam)-block-poly(N-vinylpyrrolidone) to decrease doxorubicin-induced cardiotoxicity", *Biomacromolecules*, 20, pp. 3989–4000.
48. Zhang, N., Chen, H., Fan, Y., Zhou, L., Trepout, S., Guo, J., Li, M.-H. (2018) "Fluorescent polymersomes with aggregation-induced emission", *ACS Nano*, 12, pp. 4025–4035.
49. Chao, Y., Liang, Y., Fang, G., He, H., Yao, Q., Xu, H., Chen, Y., Tang, X. (2017) "Biodegradable polymersomes as nanocarriers for doxorubicin hydrochloride: Enhanced cytotoxicity in MCF-7/ADR cells and prolonged blood circulation", *Pharmaceutical Research*, 34, pp. 610–618.
50. Cellari, M., Wong, S., Lu, H., Wright, J. A., de Souza, P., Stenzel, M. H. (2017) "Drug induced self-assembly of triblock copolymers into polymersomes for the synergistic dual-drug delivery of platinum drugs and paclitaxel", *Polymer Chemistry*, 8, pp. 6289–6299.
51. Matea, C. T., Mocan, T., Tabaran, F., Pop, T., Mosteanu, O., Puia, C., Iancu, C., Mocan, L. (2017) "Quantum dots in imaging, drug delivery and sensor applications", *International Journal of Nanomedicine*, 12, pp. 5421–5431.
52. Probst, C. E., Zrazhevskiy, P., Bagalkot, V., Gao, X. (2013) "Quantum dots as a platform for nanoparticle drug delivery vehicle design", *Advanced Drug Delivery Reviews*, 65, pp. 703–718.
53. Gubala, V., Johnston, L. J., Krug, H. F., Moore, C. J., Ober. C. K., Schwenk, M., Vert, M. (2018) "Engineered nanomaterials and human health: Part 2. Applications and nanotoxicology (IUPAC Technical Report)", *Pure and Applied Chemistry*, 90, pp. 1325–1356.
54. Banerjee, A., Pons, T., Lequeux, N., Dubertret, B. (2016) "Quantum dots–DNA bioconjugates: Synthesis to applications", *Interface Focus*, 6, Article 20160064.
55. Kairdolf, B. A., Smith, A. M., Stokes, T. H., Wang, M. D., Young, A. N., Nie, S. (2013) "Semiconductor quantum dots for bioimaging and biodiagnostic applications", *Annual Review of Analytical Chemistry*, 6, pp. 143–162.
56. Cai, X., Luo, Y., Zhang, W., Du, D., Lin, Y. (2016) "pH-sensitive ZnO quantum dots–doxorubicin nanoparticles for lung cancer targeted drug delivery", *ACS Applied Materials & Interfaces*, 34, pp. 22442–22450.
57. Yao, X., Niu, X., Ma, K., Huang, P., Grothe, J., Kaskel, S., Zhu, Y. (2017) "Graphene quantum dots-capped magnetic mesoporous silica nanoparticles as a multifunctional platform for controlled drug delivery, magnetic hyperthermia, and photothermal therapy", *Small,* 13, p.1602225.
58. Dong, J., Wang, K., Sun, L., Sun, B., Yang, M., Chen, H., Wang, Y., Sun, J., Dong, L. (2018) "Application of graphene quantum dots for simultaneous fluorescence imaging and tumor-targeted drug delivery", *Sensors and Actuators B: Chemical*, 256, pp. 616–623.
59. Huan X.-W., Bao, Y.-W., Wu, F. G. (2018) "Fluorescent carbon quantum dots with intrinsic nucleolus-targeting capability for nucleolus imaging and enhanced cytosolic and nuclear drug delivery", *ACS Applied Materials & Interfaces*, 10, pp. 10664–10677.
60. Khodadadei, F., Safarian, S., Ghanbari, N. (2017) "Methotrexate-loaded nitrogen-doped graphene quantum dots nanocarriers as an efficient anticancer drug delivery system", *Materials Science and Engineering: C*, 79, pp. 280–285.
61. Amirshaghaghi, A., Yan, L., et al. (2019) "Chlorin e6-coated superparamagnetic iron oxide nanoparticle (SPION) nanoclusters as a theranostic agent for dual-mode imaging and photodynamic therapy", *Scientific Reports*, 9, 2613.
62. Sabareeswaran, A., Ansar, E. B., Varma, P. R., Varma, H., Mohanan. P. V., Kumary, T. V. (2016) "Effect of surface-modified superparamagnetic iron oxide nanoparticles (SPIONS) on mast cell infiltration: An acute in vivo study", *Nanomedicine: Nanotechnology, Biology and Medicine*, 12, pp. 1523–1533.

63. Luo, Y., Tang, Y., Chen, Q., Zhou, X., Wang, N., Ma, M., Cheng, Y., Chen, H. (2019) "Engineering graphene oxide with ultrasmall SPIONs and smart drug release for cancer theranostics", *Chemical Communications*, 55, pp. 1963–1966.
64. Thomas, R. G., Muthiah, M., Moon, M., Park, I.-K., Jeong, Y. Y. (2017) "SPION loaded poly(L-lysine)/hyaluronic acid micelles as MR contrast agent and gene delivery vehicle for cancer theranostics", *Macromolecular Research*, 25, pp. 446–451.
65. Huang, Y., Mao, K., Zhang, B., Zhao, Y. (2017) "Superparamagnetic iron oxide nanoparticles conjugated with folic acid for dual target-specific drug delivery and MRI in cancer theranostics", *Materials Science and Engineering: C Journal*, 70, pp. 763–771.
66. Shang, L., Wang, Q.-Y., Chen, K.-L., Qu, J., Zhou, Q.-H., Luo, J.-B., Lin, J. (2017) "SPIONs/DOX loaded polymer nanoparticles for MRI detection and efficient cell targeting drug delivery", *RSC Advances*, 7, pp. 47715–47725.
67. Salunkhe, A., Khot, V., Patil, S. I., Tofail, S. A. M., Bauer, J., Thorat, N. D. (2020) "MRI guided magneto-chemotherapy with high-magnetic-moment iron oxide nanoparticles for cancer theranostics", *ACS Applied Bio Materials*, 3, pp. 2305–2313. doi: 10.1021/acsabm.0c00077.
68. Mauro, N., Scialabba, C., Puleio, R., Varvara, P., Licciardi, M., Cavallaro, G., Giammona, G. (2019) "SPIONs embedded in polyamino acid nanogels to synergistically treat tumor microenvironment and breast cancer cells", *International Journal of Pharmaceutics*, 555, pp. 207–219.
69. Dong, J., Zhao, Y., Chen, H., Liu, L., Zhang, W., Sun, B., Yang, M., Wang, Y., Dong, L. (2018) "Fabrication of PEGylated graphitic carbon nitride quantum dots as traceable, pH-sensitive drug delivery systems", *New Journal of Chemistry*, 42, pp. 14263–14270.
70. Justin, R., Tao, K. et al. (2016) "Photoluminescent and superparamagnetic reduced graphene oxide–iron oxide quantum dots for dual-modality imaging, drug delivery and photothermal therapy", *Carbon*, 97, pp. 54–70.
71. Pourjavadi, A., Tehrani, Z. M., Shirvani, T., Doulabi, M., Bumajdad, A., (2016) "Dendritic multi-walled carbon nanotube with thermoresponsive shells: A good carrier for anticancer drugs", *Journal of Industrial and Engineering Chemistry*, 35, pp. 332–340.
72. Salunkhe, Ashwini, Khot, Vishwajeet, Patil, S. I., Tofail, Syed A.M., Bauer, Joanna, & Thorat, Nanasaheb D. (2020). MRI Guided Magneto-chemotherapy with High-Magnetic-Moment Iron Oxide Nanoparticles for Cancer Theranostics. *ACS Applied Bio Materials*, 3, pp.2305–231310.1021/acsabm.0c00077.

12 Graphene Oxide as Drug Carriers

Problems and Solutions

Deepika Sharma, Rajesh Kumar, Mangesh Pradeep Kulkarni, Chandan Bhogendra Jha, Sheetu, Rashi Mathur, Gurvinder Singh, Pardeep Kumar Sharma, and Ankit Sharma

12.1 INTRODUCTION

12.1.1 DRUG CARRIER

A drug carrier can be defined as any substance or underlying layer that is used in the advancement of drug delivery, which aids in increasing the selectivity, proficiency and/or safety of drug administration. These are predominantly used for controlled release of a drug into systemic circulation. With the aid of these carriers, the frequency of drug administration and its hostile properties are reduced. Even the physicochemical properties of a drug can be masked, which has led to increase in the permeability of drugs across the biological membrane and increased the rate and extent of absorption. Additionally, the drug molecules captured inside the drug carrier system (DCS) could be sheltered from enzymatic deprivation also. Multiple drug molecules can be entrapped within a single unit of the drug carrier system, thus ensuring the administration of a great concentration of drug per receptor using a single targeting group can be achieved [1,2]. A carrier must be decomposable, non-immunogenic, and stable in blood [3].

One of the most naturally occurring elements in our ecosystem is carbon. Carbon is much more preferred over inorganic materials, as it is biologically friendly. Advancements in nanotechnology and nano-sciences have led to a step forward towards new drug-delivery systems [4]. Graphene has become an eye-catching element in research owing to its prodigious applications. Graphene is a mono-layer of graphite, which is biologically safe to use [5–7]. Graphene has mechanical, electrical, thermal properties and ease of functionalization [8]. Its two-dimensional structure, exhibiting high crystal quality, is applicable for biomedical research, whereas the one-dimensional structure is found to be cytotoxic [5]. Graphene is

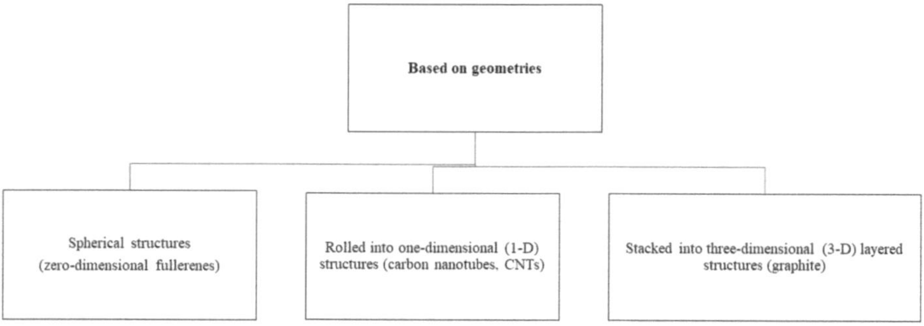

FIGURE 12.1 Different Structures Based on Geometries.

titled as the world's strongest, thinnest and stiffest material [9]. Graphene is an elementary structure for other graphitic materials. Other members of graphene depend upon the geometrical arrangement. These can also be wrapped into different structures, as shown in Figure 12.1.

Graphene oxide (GO) is produced by exfoliation of graphite layers [10]. Mass production of GO is carried out by chemical modification of graphite oxide. Chemical functionalization of reactive O_2 groups, present in graphene oxide, has led to a number of applications. The reactive groups in GO have been exfoliated in various solvents to form a uniform colloidal suspension [11]. The reaction is classified into two steps [12]:

1. Reduction: removal of oxygen from GO
2. Chemical functionalization: other chemical functionalities are added to graphene oxide

A nonolayer sheet of graphene oxide forms a stable suspension because of the water-loving oxygen group attached [13]. The oxygen molecules present on the GO surface allow the water molecules to intercalate in the interlayers of GO [14]. Tremendous colloidal stability is a result of the carboxyl groups present in GO [15].

Different types of bonding interactions are possible: these can be hydrogen bonding, π- π stacking, hydrophobic and electrostatic interactions. These bondings react to stimuli released by chemical substances, temperature, electric fields, ultraviolet or visible lights, pH, etc. [16–18]. Electronic properties, solubility and interfacial interactivity can be improved by covalently grafting polymer on graphene sheets [19].

12.1.2 Origin of Graphene Oxide

In 1859, a British chemist, B.C. Brodie, was experimenting on flakes of graphite. He prepared a slurry of graphite in the presence of fuming HNO_3 and added potash of chlorate (also called as potassium chlorate). At the end of reaction, he determined that the composition of resultant material was hydrogen, oxygen, and carbon, which resulted in an upturn in the mass of graphite flakes. On further oxidation, the oxygen content was increased with four oxidation cycles, resulting in maximum oxygen. The composition of C:H:O was found to be 61.04: 1.85: 37.11, respectively. He termed it as graphic acid because this was easily dispersed in water but not in lower pH (acidic media). Upon further heating this at 220°C, the composition of C:H:O further changed to 80.13: 0.58: 19.29. After many trials of studies, he revealed the molecular weight to be 33 [20].

After several years, L. Staudenmaier improved Brodie's reaction by adding potash chlorate along with sulphuric acid (H_2SO_4). This changed Brodie's multiple step reaction to a single-vessel reaction. Oxidation extent was also increased [21]. After 60 years, two scientists Hummers and Offeman tried another way of oxidation. They treated graphite with a pre-prepared mixture of potassium permanganate and conc. H_2SO_4. The outcome of this was the same level of oxidation taking place in the reaction [22].

GO formed in the reactions depends upon:

- Oxidants used,
- Source of graphite, and
- Reaction conditions.

Examples of oxidants:

- Nitric acid: highly reactive towards aromatic carbon and carbon nanotubes. Lactones, ketones and carboxyls are formed at the end of reaction [23,24]
- Potassium permanganate: in situ source of dioxygen, acts as a highly responsive species. It is also used for explosive purpose [25]
- Sulphuric acid [25]

12.1.3 Advantages of GO

- Low cost
- Ease of modification
- A greater surface area with two outer surfaces accessible for drug binding and the absence of toxic metal particles
- Greater drug loading ratio

The loading ratio of graphene nanomaterials (GNMs) could reach even up to 200%, which is considerably much greater as compared to other nanoparticles [26,27].

GO overrules the crystalline nanoparticles carbon nanotubes (CNTs) in drug delivery, showing lower toxicity and greater biocompatibility [28].

12.1.4 Structure of GO

Atoms of graphene are arrayed in a honeycomb-like pattern (Figure 12.2). This amphiphilic sheet contains a water-hating basal plane and water-loving edges [29].

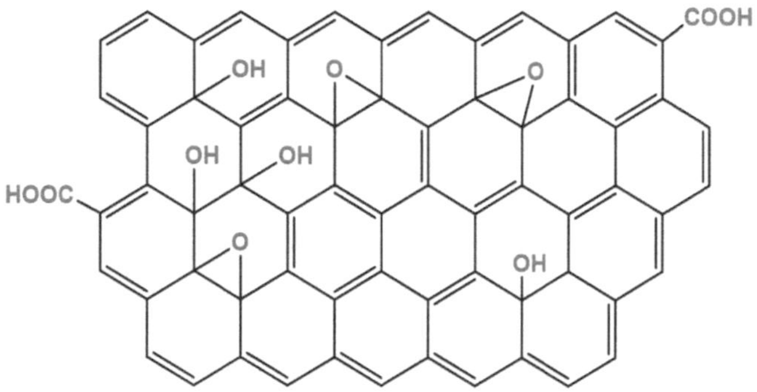

FIGURE 12.2 Chemical Structure of Graphene oxide.

GO usually occurs as a single layer or as sheets for a maximum of 10 layers. The thickness of a mono layer is 1–1.4 nm [30], so this makes graphene oxide flexible and thus, allows it to be folded into a gauge-like shape during the cellular uptake process [31] or in the biological medium [29]. GO can be characterized as a light-brown suspension. It is also a precursor of graphene [10]. Reduced graphene oxide (rGO) is synthesized by chemical or thermal reduction of GO. Strong or mild reducing agents can be used for it, e.g. sodium hydroxide and hydrazine [32]. After the reduction of GO, the water dispersibility of GO is reduced because the oxygen present also undergoes reduction [33]. This rGO can be used as a nano drug-carrier because drug loading is done by π-π and hydrophobic interactions [34].

12.1.5 Properties of GO

GO has several properties which attract its use in biomedical science:

12.1.5.1 Larger Surface Area

There are two planes and edges available for the attachment of biomolecules at GO. Approximately 2600 m^2/g surface is available, which is much larger than other nanomaterials [35,36]. GO has higher drug loading capacity owing to the availability of a greater surface area [37,38]. Drug loading of 235 wt% has been reported, which is much larger than that of liposomes [39] and polymeric micelles [40,41].

12.1.5.2 Distinctive Surface Properties

Graphene is hydrophobic in nature, which results in irreversible agglomeration [42] and protein adsorption [43], whereas graphene oxide is amphiphilic in nature and anchors a site for functionalization [44] along with this pH-dependent negative surface charge, which results in colloidal stability [45].

12.1.5.3 pH-sensitive Zeta Potential

At pH 3–12, stable GO suspensions were prepared, whereas the best stability was observed at pH 7 or 8 [46]. This dynamic property can be used to formulate a controlled release drug-delivery system. Drug release in an acidic environment was observed to be more as compared to neutral pH. This property can be used to design anti-cancer drug delivery systems [41].

12.1.5.4 Good Water Dispersibility

GO exhibits good water dispersibility as compared to CNTs [47]. When GO is dispersed in water, ionization of carboxylic acid and hydroxyl groups takes place, developing a negative charge, which is enough to cause an electrostatic repulsion, resulting in a stable dispersion [45].

12.1.5.5 Unique Intrinsic Optical Properties

GO exhibits properties comprising optical absorptions (for photothermal therapy) [48,49] and near-infrared photoluminescence (570 nm) (for live cell imaging) [50,51]. Conjugation of foreign moieties, such as fluorescence moieties, is not required by GO for direct tracking of the intracellular location of nano-GO (NGO) because of its photoluminescence nature [50].

12.1.6 Limitation of GO

Besides all the advantages, GO also possess a few limitations, and overcoming them may result in a drug carrier with a greater potential [52]. The limitations of GO include:

12.1.6.1 Aggregation in Biological Solution

Salts like sodium chloride, calcium chloride, etc., destabilize GO because of their ionic strength [53,54]. Proteins present biologically also destabilize GO by non-specific binding. Both the phenomena lead to the shielding of the electric double layer of GO [55].

12.1.6.2 Non-uniformity in Size

A wide distribution of size of GO can be noticed, which might be a result of chemical impurities and may lead to the non-biocompatibility of GO sheets [31].

12.1.7 Biocompatibility

Biocompatibility studies are needed to be carried out to check the compatibility of carrier in the biological medium. These studies are divided into two types, as explained below.

12.1.7.1 In vitro Biocompatibility

In vitro models are used for tests that involve phagocytes, non-phagocytic cells (endothelial and tumor cells) and red blood cells (RBCs) [52].

Hemocompatibility

It is important to conduct toxicity studies for I.V. injections because RBCs are the primary site of interaction. Hemocompatibility study was started in the year 2011 for GO [56]. After a 3 h incubation period for nano-sized GO (350 nm) and micro-sized (3 μm) graphene sheets, it was detected that nano-sized GO induced a severe hemolytic effect (70% hemolysis at 25 μg/mL) whereas micro-sized graphene sheets exhibited 10% hemolysis at 100 μg/mL. This was due to the strong electrostatic interactions between the negatively charged GO surface and the lipid bilayer of the red blood cell membrane [54]. On the other hand, in micro-sized (3 μm) graphene sheets, good hemocompatibility was noticed due to the less aggregated area of graphene oxide available for red blood cells to interact. Surface coating can also improve the hemocompatibility of GO. Examples for surface coating are heparin and chitosan [54,57]. Surface coating reduces the contact between GO and red blood cells. The hemolysis of cell caused by GO can also be minimized by adding 1% tween 80 surfactant, which can significantly reduce the interaction between graphene oxide and blood cells [52,58].

Inflammation Responses

GO nanocarriers are highly prone to being removed out by macrophages prior to reaching the desired spot. This can be overcome by sustaining the particle size approximately 150 nm and coating with hydrophilic material that results in declining the opsonin-protein interaction [52].

Cytotoxicity

In mammalian cells, GO cytotoxicity was tested and it was observed that micro-sized graphene oxide resulted in higher cytotoxicity as compared to nano-sized graphene oxide. It was due to the quicker sedimentation rate and formation of compact graphene oxide aggregates on the top of the adherent cells in the wells, thus preventing the accessibility of nutrients for the progress of cells [52,54,56].

Nano-sized GO, as a carrier, has been preferred over micro-sized GO due to lower toxic potential, weaker inflammation response, and better uptake in cells [52].

12.1.7.2 *In vivo* Biocompatibility

In vivo toxicity

Jeong et al. observed that when microinjection of NGO (99 nm) was delivered to zebrafish, it resulted in apoptosis and morphological defects. On the other hand, when GO-PEG (301.3 ± 87.2 nm) was delivered, it expressively diminished the toxic effects [59]. The same extent of angiogenesis was observed in both but the mechanism is still unknown. GO-PEG proved to be an effective drug carrier since it was observed in mice that GO-PEG loaded with drug effectively destroyed tumour cells and there was no reoccurrence of tumour for the next 40 days [60]. Along with this, around two-fold increase in life span was observed as compared to the mice treated with free drug [61].

Pathological Changes

At a dose of 0.2–0.5 mg/mouse, both the particle sizes (micro as well as nano-GO) accumulated in lungs, spleen and liver [56]. The retention time in lungs was up to one month [62]. The accumulation of GO led to pulmonary edema, granuloma formation and dose-dependent inflammatory cell infiltration [63]. The accumulation of GO can be reduced by coating. For example, dextran was coated on GO which led to no noticeable toxicity in spleen [64]. The accumulation threat can also be reduced by adding 1% tween 80 in a prepared formulation of GO. No pathological changes were detected in liver, blood cells, spleen and testes while using GO/tween [58].

Inflammation Response

Yue an co-workers [31] reported for the inflammation response. They administered micro-GO (2 µm) and nano-GO (350 nm) through the neck region by subcutaneous route in mice and observed that micro-GO caused much severe inflammation as compared to nano-GO. Micro-GO resulted in tissue impairment, and also foreign body response [63]. Inflammation response could be overcome by PEGylated GO [65].

Clearance

Clearance pathway of GO is dependent upon the size of nanoparticles and not upon the coating used. Micro sized GO were eliminated by liver through secretion into the biliary tract [62] whereas nano-GO (size lesser than 10 nm) were eliminated through the renal route [56]. GO-PEG (5 nm) were cleared by hepatobiliary pathway because of the size greater than that for renal filtration [66]. GO-Dextran (GO-DEX) particles were cleared by two different pathways because of their wide distribution [52,64].

- Renal pathway: In urine, small GO-DEX were excreted
- Fecal pathway: Larger GO-DEX were excreted in fecal matter

12.2 FUNCTIONALIZATION OF GO

The functionalization of graphene using polymer and inorganic materials can be achieved through covalent and non-covalent modification (Table 12.1). Modifications involve hydrogen bonding, π- π interactions and hydrophobic interactions. Polymers can be attached or encapsulated by functionalization of graphene derivatives. Few examples of natural polymers are hyaluronic acid and chitosan, and that of synthetic polymer are polyethylene glycol polyethyleneimine (PEI) and Pluronic F127 (PF127).

Functionalization of graphene using markers e.g. SPIONs (super paramagnetic iron oxide nanoparticles) [77], gold nanoparticles [78] and silver nanoparticles [79] may help in site specific targeting of drug molecules as well as multifunctioning and synergistic effects.

12.3 GRAPHENE AND GO AS A DRUG CARRIER

- **Gene delivery**: Graphene oxide sheets were modified by polyethyleneimine (PEI), and genes were loaded. Plasmid DNA was loaded by covalent

TABLE 12.1
List of a Few Materials Used For Surface Modification

Material	Type	Advantage	Outcome	Reference
PEI	Synthetic polymer	• Non-viral vector • Used for gene delivery	• Enhanced chemotherapy efficacy of drug	[67]
PEG	Synthetic polymer	• FDA approved • Soluble in both water and organic solvent • Nontoxic and highly biocompatible	• Improved solubility and stability	[68]
PF127	Synthetic polymer	• Non- toxic • Biocompatible • Thermosensitivity	• Improved water dispersibility • Improved stability • High drug loading	[37,69]
Hyaluronic acid (HA)	Natural polysaccharides	• Non-immunogenic • Non-toxic • Biocompatible • Biodegradable	• Reduced cytotoxicity • High drug loading • Receptor mediated drug targeting	[70,71]
Chitosan	Natural polysaccharide	• Biodegradable • Non-toxic • Biocompatible	• Controlled release of water-hating drugs • Improved stability	[72,73]

		• pH sensitive		
SPIONs	Inorganic material	• pH sensitive • Targeted site of action	• Multifunctional drug delivery system • Dual targeting	[74]
Dextran	Polysaccharide	• Natural reducing agent • Biocompatible	• Small reductions in cell viability were observed at very high concentration of GO-DEX	[75]
Gelatin	Natural and nontoxic polymer	• Biocompatible • Economic	• Reduced toxicity of gelatin-conjugated graphene	[76]

conjugation. Genes were delivered to cells, with aid of complexation through the electrostatic interactions [80]. Arrangement of PEI on GO was linear [81] and also branched [82]. When compared this with simple complex of plasmid with PEI, it was witnessed that high gene transfection efficiency and low cytotoxicity were witnessed in GO conjugated with PEI and loaded with plasmid DNA [83].

- **Cancer treatment**: Functionalization of nano-graphene oxide (NGO) with six arm polyethylene glycol resulted in higher cellular uptake and higher therapeutic efficiency when applied over cancer cell lines [51,84]. NGO derivatives have high absorption of near IR, which is the basis for application of GO in phototherapy. Nano Graphene oxide derivatives caused induction of oxidative stress, depolarization of mitochondria, apoptotic and necrotic cell death as a result of caspase activation [85]. GO conjugated with chemotherapy drugs (Doxorubicin (DOX) and cisplatin) could progress the slaying of MCF-7 cells that were resistant to DOX and cisplatin [86].

Chemo-phototherapy can also be a new road to treat cancer. Nano graphene oxide was functionalized with polyvinyl pyrrolidine (PVP). NGO-PVP was conjugated with folic acid (FA) via covalent amide bonds. The prepared FA-NGO-PVP was loaded with anticancer drug doxorubicin. In vitro experiments were performed which resulted in targeted drug delivery with high therapeutic efficacy [87].

- **pH responsive drug delivery**: Small molecule drugs which have pH sensitive drug release profile, can be delivered using GO as a carrier. Graphene oxide functionalization was done with poly(2-(diethylamino) ethyl methacrylate) (PDEA) covalently by surface initiated *in situ* atom transfer radical polymerization. Camptothecin (CPT), a hydrophobic anti-cancer drug was loaded to GO-PDEA. When the drug loaded GO-PDEA was studied for its release, it was observed that CPT was released at lower pH (acidic environment) and no release at basic or neutral media was observed. As cancer cells are having acidic environment, drugs can be directly targeted to the site without harming other healthy cells [88].
- **Antimicrobial activity**: Silver functionalized graphene oxide had synergistic action [89]. GO is a promising material for antibacterial activity. GO works by physical and chemical interaction with the bacterial cell [90]. Primary target of GO is cell membrane, this could be verified by seeing morphological changes in cell membrane, leakage of RNA and intracellular electrolytes, uptake of membrane-impermeable dyes, and changes in the trans membrane potential [91,92]. Sharp edges of GO penetrate physically and disrupt the integrity. Oxidative nature of GO results in lipid peroxidation, ultimately damaging the bacterial cells [93].

12.3.1 Factors affecting GO success [4]

- Assembling a carrier with a prime loading capacity
- Grade of safety and biocompatibility, a necessity for biomedical application

- Strategical system that is able to discharge drugs in a controlled way at a targeted site (tumor) for fruitful healing

A simpler approach for targeting the drug is to directly restrain it onto the modified GO surface.

12.3.2 Release of drug from GO

Biological application depends upon the discharge of drug. The controlled release of drugs further depends upon their structural and physical characterizations. For example, drug release from GO for large molecular drug is different from that of smaller drug molecules. Drug affinity towards GO sheets is different with different drugs (Table 12.2), for example ibuprofen has greater affinity towards GO sheets as compared to 5-Fluorouracil (5-FU. This is due to the hydrophobic nature of ibuprofenm which results in stronger π-π interactions whereas hydrophilic nature of 5-FU results in resonance of benzenoid, which leads to weaker π-π interactions comparatively [11]. The list of patents on GO-based theragnostic agents is summarized Table 12.3.

12.4 CONCLUSION AND FUTURE PERSPECTIVES

Graphene oxide, owing to its remarkable chemical and structural characteristics, has been increasingly used as a drug-delivery carrier over the past few years, since it has been proved to be superior over other similar delivery systems. They can be designed into complex multifunctional drug delivery systems incorporated with combination therapy, which is difficult with other nanomaterials. The work done so far is a witness to the significant progress that has been made and led to the application of these biomaterials in the biomedical field. The results of initial pre-clinical studies have been satisfactory; however, some challenges are still to be overcome to establish their clinical potential. Particle size control is one of the major challenges that need to be overcome to get reproducibility of particle dimensions. Though most of the available literature reveals otherwise, biocompatibility and thus toxicity are still the other significant limitations that need to be addressed. There is a need to conduct more *in vivo* toxicity studies with animal models to overcome the safety concerns. The future is going to desperately demand performing extensive studies using animal models as well as cell lines to establish the actual potential of graphene and graphene oxide nanomaterials. The advancements achieved in the form of nanomedicine open the gateway towards their applications in more areas with proven clinical potential. Graphene-based nanoplatforms, thus, can be anticipated as the material of choice for future nanomedicines.

TABLE 12.2
Graphene Oxide and Drug Interactions

GO composite	Drug	Outcome of the study	References
Graphene oxide-functionalized ovalbumin-polymethyl methacrylate	Doxorubicin	Drug was fruitfully loaded on Protein-polymeric carriers and controlled release was attained	[94]
O-nanoplatelets (GONPs)	Cisplatin	In addition to their role as drug carrier, GO-NPs were also able to potentiate the anticancer effect of CP in A549 cells significantly	[95]
Polyvinylpyrrolidone (PVP)-functionalized graphene oxide (GO-PVP)	Quercetin and Gefitinib	Stronger impact of Cocktailed drug system, significantly more toxic toward PA-1 cells compared to the toxicity toward IOSE-364 cells	[96]
Graphene oxide flakes	Curcumin	Activity against Methicillin-resistant *Staphylococcus aureus* (MRSA)	[97]
TiO_2@ZO-GO hybrid nanocomposites	Curcumin	Due to anionic charge present on GO sheet pH dependent drug release was seen whereas drug release from TiO_2@ZO-GO was higher at neutral pH as compared to acidic pH	[98]
Dopamine (DA) conjugated graphene oxide	Methotrexate	Drug delivery was raised towards DA receptor positive human breast adenocarcinoma cell line	[99]
Sodium alginate functionalized GO	5-FU	Inhibited the tumor growth and liver metastasis as well as prolonged the survival time of mice	[100]
Nano graphene oxide	Gallic acid	Sustained release and inhibitory effect to cancer cell growth without affecting normal cell growth	[101]
Graphene oxide nanosheet functionalization with methoxy polyethylene glycol (mPEG)	Pirfenidone	Higher dug release was noticed in acidic environment hence, this can be effective therapy	[102]

		for acidic inflammatory lesions after severe SAH.	
Cysteine polymethacrylic acid cross-linked nano graphene oxide polyethylene glycol carrier ($CPMAA_2$-GON-PEG)	DOX	Six-fold faster release rate was observed at acidic pH	[103]
Nano graphene oxide disulfide linked polyethylene glycol (NGO-SS-PE)	DOX	NGO-SS-PEG showed a higher efficacy than NGO-PEG for antitumor therapy compared with NGO-PEG	[104]
NGO was coated with dual type of polymers i.e. polyethylene glycol (PEG) and 2,3-dimethylmaleic anhydride (DA)	DOX	Cellular uptake was increased in tumor environment pH and the release of DOX was accelerated in acidic environment inside the cell lysosomes, enhanced cell slaying for drug-resistant cancer cells under the tumor micro environmental pH in comparison with free DOX. Synergistic action could be noticed by combining chemo and photo therapy	[105]
Nano-sized GO-PEG	Paclitaxel (PTX)	Able to quickly enter A546 and MCF-7 cells and it was evidenced that broad range of PTX showed cytotoxicity for A546 and MCF-7 cells	[10]
GO	DOX	pH dependent release. Best for curing tumor	[28]
Polyethyleneimine poly(sodium 4-styrenesulfonate) graphene oxide (PPGO)	Adriamycin (ADR), miR-21	PPG significantly enhanced the accumulation of ADR in MCF-7/ADR-resistant cells exhibiting much higher cytotoxicity than free ADR	[106]
Superparamagnetic GO	Doxorubicin	Active and passive targeting	[107]
Polyacrylic acid graphene oxide (PAA-GO)	BCNU	Thermal stability was increased of the drug and considerably prolonged the half-life of bound BCNU from 19 to 43 hours	[108]

(*Continued*)

TABLE 12.2 (Continued)

GO composite	Drug	Outcome of the study	References
Graphene/Fe_3O_4	DOX	Drugs released via dual targeting i.e. magnetic or electrical stimulation	[109]
Graphene oxide-polysebacic anhydride	Levofloxacin	Longer and controlled drug release	[110]
Graphene oxide	Gentamycin sulfate	Efficient loading of drug and having synergistic antibacterial activity	[111]
Folic acid graphene oxide (FA-GO)	DOX and CPT	Co-delivery of both drugs had a synergistic effect and higher cytotoxicity than GO loaded with either DOX or CPT alone	[86]
Polyvinyl alcohol graphene oxide (GO/PVA)	VB-12	pH-responsive polymer. Best for curing cancer	[112]

TABLE 12.3
List of Patents on GO-based Theragnostic Agents

Patents

Patent No.	Title	Publication date	Reference
US20180193261	Method for preparing hydrogel containing reduced graphene oxide	07/12/2018	[113]
9675714	Graphene based theranostics for tumor targeted drug/gene delivery and imaging	06/13/2017	[114]
US20160089443	Protein-graphene nanocomposite drug carrier	03/31/2016	[115]
US20150283239	Graphene derivative-based composition for drug delivery and preparation method thereof	10/08/2015	[116]

REFERENCES

1. Jătariu, A. N., Popa, M. and Peptu, C. A. (2010). "Different particulate systems—bypass the biological barriers?" *Journal of Drug Targeting,*18, pp. 243–253.
2. Kabanov, A. and Batrakova, E. (2004). "New technologies for drug delivery across the blood brain barrier", *Current Pharmaceutical Design*, 10, pp. 1355–1363.
3. Küçüktürkmen, B. and Bozkır, A. (2019). *A new approach for drug targeting to the central nervous system: Lipid nanoparticles, Nanoarchitectonics in Biomedicine.* Elsevier, pp. 335–369.

4. Liu, J., Cui, L. and Losic, D. (2013). "Graphene and graphene oxide as new nanocarriers for drug delivery applications", *Acta Biomaterialia*, 9, pp. 9243–9257.
5. Geim, A. K. and Novoselov, K. S. (2010). *The rise of graphene, Nanoscience and Technology: A Collection of Reviews from Nature Journals*. World Scientific, pp. 11–19.
6. Novoselov, K.S., Geim, A.K., Morozov, S.V., Jiang, D., Zhang, Y., Dubonos, S.V., Grigorieva, I.V. and Firsov, A.A. (2004). "Electric field effect in atomically thin carbon films", *Science*, 306, pp. 666–669.
7. Suk, J. W., Piner, R. D., An, J. and Ruoff, R. S. (2010). "Mechanical properties of monolayer graphene oxide", *ACS Nano*, 4, pp. 6557–6564.
8. An, J., Gou, Y., Yang, C., Hu, F. and Wang, C. (2013). "Synthesis of a biocompatible gelatin functionalized graphene nanosheets and its application for drug delivery", *Materials Science and Engineering: C*, 33, pp. 2827–2837.
9. Georgakilas, V., Otyepka, M., Bourlinos, A. B., Chandra, V., Kim, N., Kemp, K. C., Hobza, P., Zboril, R. and Kim, K.S. (2012). "Functionalization of graphene: covalent and non-covalent approaches, derivatives and applications", *Chemical Reviews*, 112, pp. 6156–6214.
10. Xu, Z., Wang, S., Li, Y., Wang, M., Shi, P. and Huang, X. (2014). "Covalent functionalization of graphene oxide with biocompatible poly (ethylene glycol) for delivery of paclitaxel", *ACS Applied Materials & Interfaces*, 6, pp. 17268–17276.
11. Rana, V. K., Choi, M. C., Kong, J. Y., Kim, G. Y., Kim, M. J., Kim, S. H., Mishra, S., Singh, R. P. and Ha, C. S. (2011). "Synthesis and drug-delivery behavior of chitosan-functionalized graphene oxide hybrid nanosheets", *Macromolecular Materials and Engineering*, 296, pp. 131–140.
12. Dreyer, D. R., Park, S., Bielawski, C. W. and Ruoff, R. S. (2010). "The chemistry of graphene oxide", *Chemical Society Reviews*, 39, pp. 228–240.
13. Lerf, A., He, H., Forster, M. and Klinowski, J. (1998). "Structure of graphite oxide revisited", *Journal of Physical Chemistry B*, 102, pp. 4477–4482.
14. Stankovich, S., Dikin, D. A., Piner, R. D., Kohlhaas, K. A., Kleinhammes, A., Jia, Y., Wu, Y., Nguyen, S. T. and Ruoff, R. S. (2007). "Synthesis of graphene-based nanosheets via chemical reduction of exfoliated graphite oxide", *Carbon*, 45, pp. 1558–1565.
15. Rourke, J. P., Pandey, P. A., Moore, J. J., Bates, M., Kinloch, I. A., Young, R. J. and Wilson, N. R. (2011). "The real graphene oxide revealed: stripping the oxidative debris from the graphene-like sheets", *Angewandte Chemie International Edition*, 50, pp. 3173–3177.
16. Chunder, A., Liu, J. and Zhai, L. (2010). "Reduced graphene oxide/poly (3-hexylthiophene) supramolecular composites", *Macromolecular Rapid Communications*, 31, pp. 380–384.
17. Lee, S. H., Dreyer, D. R., An, J., Velamakanni, A., Piner, R. D., Park, S., Zhu, Y., Kim, S. O., Bielawski, C. W. and Ruoff, R. S. (2010). "Polymer brushes via controlled, surface-initiated atom transfer radical polymerization (ATRP) from graphene oxide", *Macromolecular Rapid Communications*, 31, pp. 281–288.
18. Zhu, Y., Stoller, M. D., Cai, W., Velamakanni, A., Piner, R. D., Chen, D. and Ruoff, R. S. (2010). "Exfoliation of graphite oxide in propylene carbonate and thermal reduction of the resulting graphene oxide platelets", *ACS Nano*, 4, pp. 1227–1233.
19. Veca, L. M., Lu, F., Meziani, M. J., Cao, L., Zhang, P., Qi, G., Qu, L., Shrestha, M. and Sun, Y.-P. (2009). "Polymer functionalization and solubilization of carbon nanosheets", *Chemical Communications*, pp. 2565–2567.
20. Brodie, B. C. (1859). *XIII. On the atomic weight of graphite*. Philosophical Transactions of the Royal Society of London, pp. 249–259.
21. Staudenmaier, L. (1898). "Verfahren zur darstellung der graphitsäure", *Berichte der deutschen chemischen Gesellschaft*, 31, pp. 1481–1487.
22. Hummers Jr, W. S. and Offeman, R. E. (1958). "Preparation of graphitic oxide", *Journal of the American Chemical Society*, 80, pp. 1339–1339.

23. Lakshminarayanan, P. V., Toghiani, H. and Pittman Jr, C. U. (2004). "Nitric acid oxidation of vapor grown carbon nanofibers", *Carbon*, 42, pp. 2433–2442.
24. Zhang, N., Wang, L.Y., Liu, H. and Cai, Q.K. (2008). "Nitric acid oxidation on carbon dispersion and suspension stability. Surface and Interface Analysis: An International Journal devoted to the development and application of techniques for the analysis of surfaces", *Interfaces and Thin Films*, 40, pp. 1190–1194.
25. Cotton, F. A., Wilkinson, G., Murillo, C. A., Bochmann, M. and Grimes, R. (1988). *Advanced inorganic chemistry*. Wiley New York.
26. Davis, M. E., Chen, Z. and Shin, D. M. (2010). "Nanoparticle therapeutics: an emerging treatment modality for cancer", *Nanoscience And Technology: A Collection of Reviews from Nature Journals*. World Scientific, pp. 239–250.
27. Zhang, Y., Ali, S. F., Dervishi, E., Xu, Y., Li, Z., Casciano, D. and Biris, A. S. (2010b). "Cytotoxicity effects of graphene and single-wall carbon nanotubes in neural phaeochromocytoma-derived PC12 cells", *ACS Nano*, 4, pp. 3181–3186.
28. Mendes, R. G., Bachmatiuk, A., Büchner, B., Cuniberti, G. and Rümmeli, M. H. (2013). "Carbon nanostructures as multi-functional drug delivery platforms", *Journal of Materials Chemistry B*, 1, pp. 401–428.
29. Mu, Q., Su, G., Li, L., Gilbertson, B.O., Yu, L. H., Zhang, Q., Sun, Y.-P. and Yan, B. (2012). "Size-dependent cell uptake of protein-coated graphene oxide nanosheets", *ACS Applied Materials & Interfaces*, 4, pp. 2259–2266.
30. Paredes, J., Villar-Rodil, S., Martínez-Alonso, A. and Tascon, J. (2008). "Graphene oxide dispersions in organic solvents", *Langmuir*, 24, pp. 10560–10564.
31. Yue, H., Wei, W., Yue, Z., Wang, B., Luo, N., Gao, Y., Ma, D., Ma, G. and Su, Z. (2012). "The role of the lateral dimension of graphene oxide in the regulation of cellular responses", *Biomaterials*, 33, pp. 4013–4021.
32. Tkachev, S., Buslaeva, E.Y., Naumkin, A., Kotova, S., Laure, I. and Gubin, S. (2012). "Reduced graphene oxide", *Inorganic Materials*, 48, pp. 796–802.
33. Shao, Y., Wang, J., Wu, H., Liu, J., Aksay, I. A. and Lin, Y. (2010). "Graphene based electrochemical sensors and biosensors: a review", *Electroanalysis: An International Journal Devoted to Fundamental and Practical Aspects of Electroanalysis*, 22, pp. 1027–1036.
34. Muthoosamy, K., G Bai, R. and Manickam, S. (2014). "Graphene and graphene oxide as a docking station for modern drug delivery system", *Current Drug Delivery*, 11, pp. 701–718.
35. Hakimi, M. and Alimard, P. (2012). "Graphene: synthesis and applications in biotechnology-a review".
36. Yang, R., Tang, Z., Yan, J., Kang, H., Kim, Y., Zhu, Z. and Tan, W. (2008a) "Noncovalent assembly of carbon nanotubes and single-stranded DNA: an effective sensing platform for probing biomolecular interactions", *Analytical Chemistry*, 80, pp. 7408–7413.
37. Hu, H., Yu, J., Li, Y., Zhao, J. and Dong, H. (2012). "Engineering of a novel pluronic F127/graphene nanohybrid for pH responsive drug delivery", *Journal of Biomedical Materials Research Part A*, 100, pp. 141–148.
38. Zhang, R., Hummelgård, M., Lv, G. and Olin, H. (2011a). "Real time monitoring of the drug release of rhodamine B on graphene oxide", *Carbon*, 49, pp. 1126–1132.
39. Sun, W., Zhang, N., Li, A., Zou, W. and Xu, W. (2008a). "Preparation and evaluation of N3-O-toluyl-fluorouracil-loaded liposomes", *International journal of Pharmaceutics*, 353, pp. 243–250.
40. Kim, S., Shi, Y., Kim, J. Y., Park, K. and Cheng, J.-X. (2010). "Overcoming the barriers in micellar drug delivery: loading efficiency, *in vivo* stability, and micelle–cell interaction", *Expert Opinion On Drug Delivery* 7, pp. 49–62.

41. Yang, X., Zhang, X., Liu, Z., Ma, Y., Huang, Y. and Chen, Y. (2008b). "High-efficiency loading and controlled release of doxorubicin hydrochloride on graphene oxide", *Journal of Physical Chemistry C*, 112, pp. 17554–17558.
42. Kuila, T., Bose, S., Mishra, A. K., Khanra, P., Kim, N. H. and Lee, J. H. (2012). "Chemical functionalization of graphene and its applications", *Progress in Materials Science*, 57, pp. 1061–1105.
43. Sanchez, V. C., Jachak, A., Hurt, R. H. and Kane, A. B. (2011). "Biological interactions of graphene-family nanomaterials: an interdisciplinary review", *Chemical Research in Toxicology*, 25, pp. 15–34.
44. Xie, G., Cheng, J., Li, Y., Xi, P., Chen, F., Liu, H., Hou, F., Shi, Y., Huang, L. and Xu, Z. (2012). "Fluorescent graphene oxide composites synthesis and its biocompatibility study", *Journal of Materials Chemistry*, 22, pp. 9308–9314.
45. Li, D., Müller, M. B., Gilje, S., Kaner, R. B. and Wallace, G. G. (2008). "Processable aqueous dispersions of graphene nanosheets", *Nature Nanotechnology*, 3, pp. 101.
46. Chen, J.-T., Fu, Y.-J., An, Q.-F., Lo, S.-C., Huang, S.-H., Hung, W.-S., Hu, C.-C., Lee, K.-R. and Lai, J.-Y. (2013). "Tuning nanostructure of graphene oxide/polyelectrolyte LbL assemblies by controlling pH of GO suspension to fabricate transparent and super gas barrier films" *Nanoscale*, 5, pp. 9081–9088.
47. Bussy, C., Ali-Boucetta, H. and Kostarelos, K. (2012). "Safety considerations for graphene: lessons learnt from carbon nanotubes", *Accounts of Chemical Research*, 46, pp. 692–701.
48. Vila, M., Portolés, M., Marques, P., Feito, M., Matesanz, M., Ramírez-Santillán, C., Gonçalves, G., Cruz, S., Nieto, A. and Vallet-Regi, M. (2012). "Cell uptake survey of pegylated nanographene oxide", *Nanotechnology*, 23, pp. 465103.
49. Wate, P. S., Banerjee, S.S., Jalota-Badhwar, A., Mascarenhas, R. R., Zope, K. R., Khandare, J. and Misra, R.D.K. (2012). "Cellular imaging using biocompatible dendrimer-functionalized graphene oxide-based fluorescent probe anchored with magnetic nanoparticles", *Nanotechnology*, 23, pp. 415101.
50. Mao, H. Y., Laurent, S., Chen, W., Akhavan, O., Imani, M., Ashkarran, A. A. and Mahmoudi, M. (2013). "Graphene: promises, facts, opportunities, and challenges in nanomedicine", *Chemical Reviews*, 113, pp. 3407–3424.
51. Sun, X., Liu, Z., Welsher, K., Robinson, J. T., Goodwin, A., Zaric, S. and Dai, H. (2008b). "Nano-graphene oxide for cellular imaging and drug delivery", *Nano Research*, 1, pp. 203–212.
52. Kiew, S. F., Kiew, L. V., Lee, H. B., Imae, T. and Chung, L.Y. (2016). "Assessing biocompatibility of graphene oxide-based nanocarriers: a review", *Journal of Controlled Release*, 226, pp. 217–228.
53. Chowdhury, I., Duch, M. C., Mansukhani, N. D., Hersam, M. C. and Bouchard, D. (2014). "Deposition and release of graphene oxide nanomaterials using a quartz crystal microbalance", *Environmental Science & Technology*, 48, pp. 961–969.
54. Liao, K.-H., Lin, Y.-S., Macosko, C. W. and Haynes, C. L. (2011). "Cytotoxicity of graphene oxide and graphene in human erythrocytes and skin fibroblasts", *ACS Applied Materials & Interfaces*, 3, pp. 2607–2615.
55. Pan, Y., Sahoo, N. G. and Li, L. (2012). "The application of graphene oxide in drug delivery", *Expert Opinion on Drug Delivery*, 9, pp. 1365–1376.
56. Zhang, X., Yin, J., Peng, C., Hu, W., Zhu, Z., Li, W., Fan, C. and Huang, Q. (2011d). "Distribution and biocompatibility studies of graphene oxide in mice after intravenous administration", *Carbon*, 49, pp. 986–995.
57. Cheng, C., Nie, S., Li, S., Peng, H., Yang, H., Ma, L., Sun, S. and Zhao, C. (2013). "Biopolymer functionalized reduced graphene oxide with enhanced biocompatibility via mussel inspired coatings/anchors", *Journal of Materials Chemistry B*, 1, pp. 265–275.

58. Qu, G., Wang, X., Liu, Q., Liu, R., Yin, N., Ma, J., Chen, L., He, J., Liu, S. and Jiang, G. (2013). "The ex vivo and *in vivo* biological performances of graphene oxide and the impact of surfactant on graphene oxide's biocompatibility", *Journal of Environmental Sciences*, 25, pp. 873–881.
59. Jeong, J., Cho, H.-J., Choi, M., Lee, W. S., Chung, B. H. and Lee, J.-S. (2015). "*In vivo* toxicity assessment of angiogenesis and the live distribution of nano-graphene oxide and its PEGylated derivatives using the developing zebrafish embryo", *Carbon*, 93, pp. 431–440.
60. Zhang, W., Guo, Z., Huang, D., Liu, Z., Guo, X. and Zhong, H. (2011c). "Synergistic effect of chemo-photothermal therapy using PEGylated graphene oxide", *Biomaterials*, 32, pp. 8555–8561.
61. Rong, P., Yang, K., Srivastan, A., Kiesewetter, D. O., Yue, X., Wang, F., Nie, L., Bhirde, A., Wang, Z. and Liu, Z. (2014). "Photosensitizer loaded nano-graphene for multimodality imaging guided tumor photodynamic therapy", *Theranostics*, 4, pp. 229.
62. Ruiz, O. N., Fernando, K.S., Wang, B., Brown, N. A., Luo, P. G., McNamara, N. D., Vangsness, M., Sun, Y.-P. and Bunker, C.E. (2011). "Graphene oxide: a nonspecific enhancer of cellular growth", *ACS Nano*, 5, pp. 8100–8107.
63. Sydlik, S. A., Jhunjhunwala, S., Webber, M. J., Anderson, D. G. and Langer, R. (2015). "*In vivo* compatibility of graphene oxide with differing oxidation states", *ACS Nano*, 9, pp. 3866–3874.
64. Zhang, S., Yang, K., Feng, L. and Liu, Z. (2011b). "In vitro and *in vivo* behaviors of dextran functionalized graphene", *Carbon*, 49, pp. 4040–4049.
65. Yang, K., Gong, H., Shi, X., Wan, J., Zhang, Y. and Liu, Z. (2013). "*In vivo* biodistribution and toxicology of functionalized nano-graphene oxide in mice after oral and intraperitoneal administration", *Biomaterials*, 34, pp. 2787–2795.
66. Hong, H., Yang, K., Zhang, Y., Engle, J. W., Feng, L., Yang, Y., Nayak, T. R., Goel, S., Bean, J. and Theuer, C. P. (2012). "*In vivo* targeting and imaging of tumor vasculature with radiolabeled, antibody-conjugated nanographene", *ACS Nano*, 6, pp. 2361–2370.
67. Shi, J., Zhang, H., Wang, L., Li, L., Wang, H., Wang, Z., Li, Z., Chen, C., Hou, L. and Zhang, C. (2013). "PEI-derivatized fullerene drug delivery using folate as a homing device targeting to tumor", *Biomaterials*, 34, pp. 251–261.
68. Kolate, A., Baradia, D., Patil, S., Vhora, I., Kore, G. and Misra, A. (2014). "PEG—a versatile conjugating ligand for drugs and drug delivery systems", *Journal of Controlled Release*, 192, pp. 67–81.
69. Huang, S.-J., Hsu, Z.-R. and Wang, L.-F. (2014). "Synthesis and characterization of pluronic-block-poly (N, N-dimethylamino-2-ethyl methacrylate) pentablock copolymers for drug/gene co-delivery systems", *RSC Advances*, 4, pp. 31552–31563.
70. Luo, Y., Cai, X., Li, H., Lin, Y. and Du, D. (2016). "Hyaluronic acid-modified multifunctional Q-graphene for targeted killing of drug-resistant lung cancer cells", *ACS Applied Materials & Interfaces*, 8, pp. 4048–4055.
71. Wu, H., Shi, H., Wang, Y., Jia, X., Tang, C., Zhang, J. and Yang, S. (2014). "Hyaluronic acid conjugated graphene oxide for targeted drug delivery", *Carbon*, 69, pp. 379–389.
72. Wen, H., Yin, C., Du, A., Deng, L., He, Y. and He, L. (2015). "Folate conjugated PEG–chitosan/graphene oxide nanocomplexes as potential carriers for pH-triggered drug release", *Journal of Controlled Release*, 213. pp. e44–e45.
73. Zamora-Mora, V., Fernández-Gutiérrez, M., González-Gómez, Á., Sanz, B., San Roman, J., Goya, G. F., Hernández, R. and Mijangos, C. (2017). "Chitosan nanoparticles for combined drug delivery and magnetic hyperthermia: From preparation to in vitro studies", *Carbohydrate Polymers*, 157, pp. 361–370.
74. Shagholani, H., Ghoreishi, S. M. and Mousazadeh, M. (2015). "Improvement of interaction between PVA and chitosan via magnetite nanoparticles for drug delivery application", *International Journal of Biological Macromolecules*, 78, pp. 130–136.

75. Gautam, S. (2017). "Graphene oxide: a potential drug carrier for cancer therapy", *Research and Reviews: A Journal of Pharmaceutical Science*, 8, pp. 21–31.
76. Santoro, M., Tatara, A. M. and Mikos, A. G. (2014). "Gelatin carriers for drug and cell delivery in tissue engineering", *Journal of Controlled Release*, 190, pp. 210–218.
77. Shen, J.-M., Gao, F.-Y., Guan, L.-P., Su, W., Yang, Y.-J., Li, Q.-R. and Jin, Z.-C. (2014). "Graphene oxide–Fe 3 O 4 nanocomposite for combination of dual-drug chemotherapy with photothermal therapy", *RSC Advances*, 4, pp. 18473–18484.
78. Gao, S., Zhang, L., Wang, G., Yang, K., Chen, M., Tian, R., Ma, Q. and Zhu, L. (2016). "Hybrid graphene/Au activatable theranostic agent for multimodalities imaging guided enhanced photothermal therapy", *Biomaterials*, 79, pp. 36–45.
79. Tang, J., Chen, Q., Xu, L., Zhang, S., Feng, L., Cheng, L., Xu, H., Liu, Z. and Peng, R. (2013). "Graphene oxide–silver nanocomposite as a highly effective antibacterial agent with species-specific mechanisms", *ACS Applied Materials & Interfaces*, 5, pp. 3867–3874.
80. Feng, L., Zhang, S. and Liu, Z. (2011). "Graphene based gene transfection", *Nanoscale*, 3, pp. 1252–1257.
81. Chen, B., Liu, M., Zhang, L., Huang, J., Yao, J. and Zhang, Z. (2011). "Polyethylenimine-functionalized graphene oxide as an efficient gene delivery vector", *Journal of Materials Chemistry*, 21, pp. 7736–7741.
82. Kim, H., Namgung, R., Singha, K., Oh, I.-K. and Kim, W. J. (2011). "Graphene oxide–polyethylenimine nanoconstruct as a gene delivery vector and bioimaging tool", *Bioconjugate Chemistry*, 22, pp. 2558–2567.
83. Chung, C., Kim, Y.-K., Shin, D., Ryoo, S.-R., Hong, B. H. and Min, D.-H. (2013). "Biomedical applications of graphene and graphene oxide", *Accounts of Chemical Research*, 46, pp. 2211–2224.
84. Liu, Z., Robinson, J.T., Sun, X. and Dai, H. (2008). "PEGylated nanographene oxide for delivery of water-insoluble cancer drugs", *Journal of the American Chemical Society*, 130, pp. 10876–10877.
85. Markovic, Z. M., Harhaji-Trajkovic, L. M., Todorovic-Markovic, B. M., Kepić, D.P., Arsikin, K.M., Jovanović, S.P., Pantovic, A.C., Dramićanin, M.D. and Trajkovic, V.S. (2011). "In vitro comparison of the photothermal anticancer activity of graphene nanoparticles and carbon nanotubes", *Biomaterials*, 32, pp. 1121–1129.
86. Zhang, L., Xia, J., Zhao, Q., Liu, L. and Zhang, Z. (2010a). "Functional graphene oxide as a nanocarrier for controlled loading and targeted delivery of mixed anticancer drugs", *Small*, 6, pp. 537–544.
87. Qin, X., Guo, Z., Liu, Z., Zhang, W., Wan, M. and Yang, B. (2013). "Folic acid-conjugated graphene oxide for cancer targeted chemo-photothermal therapy", *Journal of Photochemistry and Photobiology B: Biology*, 120, pp. 156–162.
88. Kavitha, T., Abdi, S.I.H. and Park, S.-Y. (2013). "pH-sensitive nanocargo based on smart polymer functionalized graphene oxide for site-specific drug delivery", *Physical Chemistry Chemical Physics*, 15, pp. 5176–5185.
89. De Faria, A. F., Perreault, F.o., Shaulsky, E., Arias Chavez, L. H. and Elimelech, M. (2015). "Antimicrobial electrospun biopolymer nanofiber mats functionalized with graphene oxide–silver nanocomposites", *ACS Applied Materials & Interfaces*, 7, pp. 12751–12759.
90. Perreault, F., De Faria, A. F., Nejati, S. and Elimelech, M. (2015b). "Antimicrobial properties of graphene oxide nanosheets: why size matters", *ACS Nano*, 9, pp. 7226–7236.
91. Chen, J., Peng, H., Wang, X., Shao, F., Yuan, Z. and Han, H. (2014). "Graphene oxide exhibits broad-spectrum antimicrobial activity against bacterial phytopathogens and fungal conidia by intertwining and membrane perturbation", *Nanoscale*, 6, pp. 1879–1889.

92. Perreault, F., De Faria, A. F. and Elimelech, M. (2015a). "Environmental applications of graphene-based nanomaterials", *Chemical Society Reviews*, 44, pp. 5861–5896.
93. Gurunathan, S., Han, J. W., Dayem, A. A., Eppakayala, V. and Kim, J.-H. (2012). "Oxidative stress-mediated antibacterial activity of graphene oxide and reduced graphene oxide in Pseudomonas aeruginosa", *International Journal of Nanomedicine*, 7, pp. 5901.
94. Prabakaran, S., Jeyaraj, M., Nagaraj, A., Sadasivuni, K. K. and Rajan, M. (2019). *Polymethyl methacrylate–ovalbumin@ graphene oxide drug carrier system for high antiproliferative cancer drug delivery*. Applied Nanoscience, pp. 1–14.
95. Rosli, N.F., Fojtů, M., Fisher, A.C. and Pumera, M. (2019). "Graphene oxide nanoplatelets potentiate anticancer effect of cisplatin in human lung cancer cells", *Langmuir*, 35, pp. 3176–3182.
96. Tiwari, H., Karki, N., Pal, M., Basak, S., Verma, R. K., Bal, R., Kandpal, N.D., Bisht, G. and Sahoo, N. G. (2019). "Functionalized graphene oxide as a nanocarrier for dual drug delivery applications: The synergistic effect of quercetin and gefitinib against ovarian cancer cells", *Colloids and Surfaces B: Biointerfaces*, 178, pp. 452–459.
97. Bugli, F., Cacaci, M., Palmieri, V., Di Santo, R., Torelli, R., Ciasca, G., Di Vito, M., Vitali, A., Conti, C. and Sanguinetti, M. (2018). "Curcumin-loaded graphene oxide flakes as an effective antibacterial system against methicillin-resistant Staphylococcus aureus", *Interface Focus*, 8, pp. 20170059.
98. Zamani, M., Rostami, M., Aghajanzadeh, M., Manjili, H.K., Rostamizadeh, K. and Danafar, H. (2018). "Mesoporous titanium dioxide@ zinc oxide–graphene oxide nanocarriers for colon-specific drug delivery", *Journal of Materials Science*, 53, pp. 1634–1645.
99. Masoudipour, E., Kashanian, S. and Maleki, N. (2017). "A targeted drug delivery system based on dopamine functionalized nano graphene oxide", *Chemical Physics Letters*, 668, pp. 56–63.
100. Zhang, B., Yan, Y., Shen, Q., Ma, D., Huang, L., Cai, X. and Tan, S. (2017 "A colon targeted drug delivery system based on alginate modificated graphene oxide for colorectal liver metastasis", *Materials Science and Engineering: C*, 79, pp. 185–190.
101. Dorniani, D., Saifullah, B., Barahuie, F., Arulselvan, P., Hussein, M. Z. B., Fakurazi, S. and Twyman, L. J. (2016). "Graphene oxide-gallic acid nanodelivery system for cancer therapy", *Nanoscale Research Letters*, 11, pp. 491.
102. Yang, L., Wang, F., Han, H., Yang, L., Zhang, G. and Fan, Z. (2015). "Functionalized graphene oxide as a drug carrier for loading pirfenidone in treatment of subarachnoid hemorrhage", *Colloids and Surfaces B: Biointerfaces,* 129, pp. 21–29.
103. Zhao, X., Yang, L., Li, X., Jia, X., Liu, L., Zeng, J., Guo, J. and Liu, P. (2015). "Functionalized graphene oxide nanoparticles for cancer cell-specific delivery of antitumor drug", *Bioconjugate Chemistry*, 26, pp. 128–136.
104. Xiong, H., Guo, Z., Zhang, W., Zhong, H., Liu, S. and Ji, Y. (2014). "Redox-responsive biodegradable PEGylated nanographene oxide for efficiently chemo-photothermal therapy: A comparative study with non-biodegradable PEGylated nanographene oxide", *Journal of Photochemistry and Photobiology B: Biology*, 138, pp. 191–201.
105. Feng, L., Li, K., Shi, X., Gao, M., Liu, J. and Liu, Z. (2014). "Smart pH-responsive nanocarriers based on nano-graphene oxide for combined chemo-and photothermal therapy overcoming drug resistance", *Advanced Healthcare Materials*, 3, pp. 1261–1271.
106. Zhi, F., Dong, H., Jia, X., Guo, W., Lu, H., Yang, Y., Ju, H., Zhang, X. and Hu, Y. (2013). "Functionalized graphene oxide mediated adriamycin delivery and miR-21 gene silencing to overcome tumor multidrug resistance in vitro", *PloS One*, 8, pp. e60034.

107. Wang, Z., Zhou, C., Xia, J., Via, B., Xia, Y., Zhang, F., Li, Y. and Xia, L. (2013). "Fabrication and characterization of a triple functionalization of graphene oxide with Fe3O4, folic acid and doxorubicin as dual-targeted drug nanocarrier", *Colloids and Surfaces B: Biointerfaces*, 106, pp. 60–65.
108. Lu, Y.-J., Yang, H.-W., Hung, S.-C., Huang, C.-Y., Li, S.-M., Ma, C.-C.M., Chen, P.-Y., Tsai, H.-C., Wei, K.-C. and Chen, J.-P. (2012). "Improving thermal stability and efficacy of BCNU in treating glioma cells using PAA-functionalized graphene oxide", *International Journal of Nanomedicine*, 7, pp. 1737.
109. Liu, H.-W., Hu, S.-H., Chen, Y.-W. and Chen, S.-Y. (2012). "Characterization and drug release behavior of highly responsive chip-like electrically modulated reduced graphene oxide–poly (vinyl alcohol) membranes", *Journal of Materials Chemistry*, 22, pp. 17311–17320.
110. Gao, J., Bao, F., Feng, L., Shen, K., Zhu, Q., Wang, D., Chen, T., Ma, R. and Yan, C. (2011). "Functionalized graphene oxide modified polysebacic anhydride as drug carrier for levofloxacin controlled release", *RSC Advances*, 1, pp. 1737–1744.
111. Pandey, H., Parashar, V., Parashar, R., Prakash, R., Ramteke, P.W. and Pandey, A.C. (2011). "Controlled drug release characteristics and enhanced antibacterial effect of graphene nanosheets containing gentamicin sulfate", *Nanoscale*, 3, pp. 4104–4108.
112. Bai, H., Li, C., Wang, X. and Shi, G. (2010). "A pH-sensitive graphene oxide composite hydrogel", *Chemical Communications*, 46, pp. 2376–2378.
113. Lee, J. Y. G., Kim, Seminand J. O., Hyerim (2018). *Method For Preparing Hydrogel Containing Reduced Graphene Oxide*. Gwangju Institute of Science and Technology (Gwangju, KR), United States.
114. Mohapatra, S. L. and Wang, Chunyan (2017). *Graphene based theranostics for tumor targeted drug/gene delivery and imaging*. University of South Florida (Tampa, FL, US), United States.
115. Hu, S.-h.T.C., Chen, San-yuan, Lai, Yen-ho, Chiang, Chih-sheng and Chiang, Min-yu (2016). *Protein-Graphene Nanocomposite Drug Carrier*. National Chiao Tung University (Hsinchu City, TW), United States.
116. Lee, H. S.-s. and Some, Surajit (2015). *Graphene Derivative-Based Composition For Drug Delivery and Preparation Method Thereof*. Research & Business Foundation Sungkyunkwan University (Suwon-si, KR), United States.

13 A Synoptic Overview on Ancient Alchemy Sudha Varg (Calcium-Containing Drugs)

An applied Nanomedicine

Saurabh Singh, Simranjeet Kaur, Dileep Singh Baghel, Nitika Anand, Sakshi Sabharwal, Vibhu Khanna, Arun Kumar, and Iqbaljit Kaur

13.1 INTRODUCTION

The National Institute of Health (USA) defines nanomedicine as "molecular-scale medical intervention for the purpose of prevention, diagnosis and treatment of disease" [1]. According to the European Science Foundation, "Nanomedicine is the science and technology of diagnosing, treating and preventing disease and traumatic injury, of relieving pain and of preserving and improving human health using molecular tools and molecular knowledge of the human body" [2]. But the unique definition given by the European Technology Platform on Nanomedicine is "Nanomedicine is the application of nanotechnology to health. It exploits the improved and often novel physical, chemical, and biological properties of materials at the nanometric scale" [3].

Bhasma is an exclusive Ayurvedic herbo-mineral-metallic compound with size in nano-dimensions. This is an ancient formulation described in "*Rasa Shastra,*" which helps prevent chronic diseases and rapid absorption better as compared to herbs [4]. The benefits of nanomedicines (*Bhasma*) are multifold. Safety-related investigations already described in the classical texts of Ayurveda and the latest AYUSH guidelines for safer manufacturing practices like 'Schedule T guidelines' and toxicological evaluation as per OECD guidelines take care of ecology and environment. Calcium is now a daily requirement for people. In Ayurveda, the *sudha varga* drug is co-related with calcium compounds in the modern era and they belong to the category of minerals. The nanomedicines (*Bhasma*) prepared from these drugs are highly beneficial for the treatment of several chronic diseases and also helpful to fulfil the daily calcium supplement needs in a safer way. The drugs of *sudha varga* have been classified in ancient texts of Ayurveda, and several scholars have given their own opinion to modify these classifications. The present chapter will insist on the adoption of natural resources of calcium, which are already available in the form of nanomedicines in our traditional system of medicines.

13.2 HISTORY OF INDIAN NANOMEDICINE

The Indian healthcare system expects the sale of nanomedicines to grow to a value of USD 1.6 Billion in the next 10 to 15 years [5]. It is predicted that India will be at the top 3rd position in the healthcare market in 2020 [6]. The Indian government grants research and development funds for nanomedicines with the goal to fulfil social needs (Figure 13.1). The Department of Science recognized a nano mission program in 2007 to encourage basic research. In India, some studies were done to distinguish nanotechnology and nanomedicine in healthcare. In 2006, Mr. Jain defined the status of research on nanomedicines in India by revealing all the research that has been done in various institutes all over the country [7]. While in 2014, Kumar and Desai gave the example of the projects initiated by the government of India to support nano-biotechnology and performed a "SWOT" analysis to find the strengths and weaknesses in this particular area [8–10]. Ali and Sinha in 2014 highlighted the library catalogue on nano-biotechnology, but no details were found [11]. They also investigated the utilization of nanotechnology in the Indian healthcare sector and made efforts to recognize the various stakeholders [12,13]. In 2011, Bhattacharya and Shilpa, in 2014, Anand, and in 2016 Shefali described a few nanotechnology-based formulations in medicine [14–16].

13.3 IMPORTANCE OF SUDHA VARGA BHASMA (NANOMEDICINES)

Bhasma helps preserve best alkalinity for optimal health, provides absorbed and usable calcium, intestines and liver, strengthens the bones and teeth, treats the nervous system, cures insomnia, removes unwanted matter from kidneys, depression, keeps rhythmic heart beating, arrhythmias and minerals balance, maintains the metabolism of iron in the body, breakdowns heavy metals and drug residues in the body, neutralizes harmful acids that lead to illness, achieves a healthy alkaline level by neutralizing acid, and protects the body from free radical damage [17].

Sudha varga dravyas can play a significant role in curing diseases like *grahni*, *amlapitta*, *parinamashool*, *swasa kasa* and *hridya roga*. These drugs are used as supplements of calcium and also in several processes of *rasa shastra* like- *parad bandhana* and *melan*. The drugs belonging to this *varga* have calcium in their composition. Calcium helps maintain the body structure, strengthens the bones, movement of muscles, secretion of GIT, cardiac physiology, etc.

13.4 ORIGIN AND CLASSIFICATION OF SUDHA VARGA

In *Charka Samhita* and *Sushruta Samhita, Sudha varga* is known as *Parthiva varga* and in *Rasa Ratnakara* and *Rasarnava,* it is known as *Shukla varga.* It has

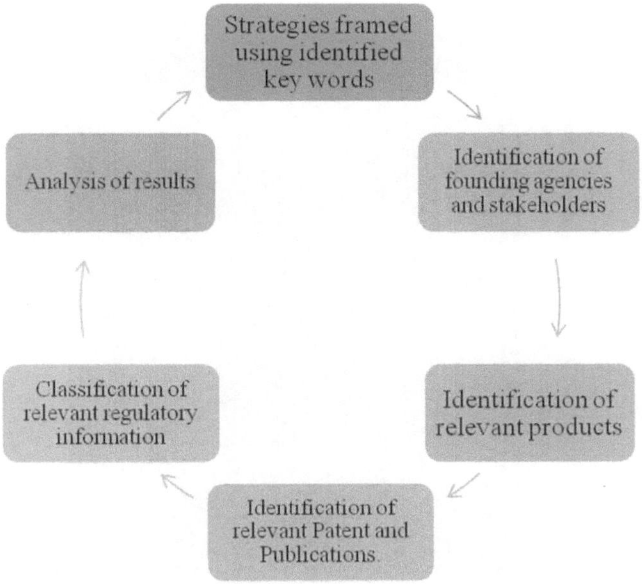

FIGURE 13.1 Approach Adopted for Mapping Nanomedicine Novelty in India.

only four drugs: *sudha*, *sankha*, *varhatika* and *kurmaprista*. *Rasamritam* includes these drugs under "*sudha vijnaneeyam*" based on the chemical composition and having *sudha*, *khatika*, *godanti*, *sankha*, *sambhuka(shudrankha)*, *muktasukti*, *kurmaparista*, *praval*, *mukta*, *mrigsringi*, *kukkutandtwak*, *swetanjan* and *hasti danta*. In the period of *samhitas,* a total of 8 drugs – *Asthi*, *mukta*, *praval*, *kukundatwak*, *shankh*, *sukti*, *varatika, and samudra phane* – were known as *sudha varga. Anandkanda* includes *sankha*, *sambuka(kshudrasankha)*, *muktasukti* – only three drugs – in its *sudha varga*. In the 20th century, *Rasatrangni* separated these drugs in different three groups: *Manasiladi Vignaniyan*, *Shankhadi Vignaniyan*, and *Ratanadi Vignaniyan. Ayurvediya Rasa Shastra S. mishra* described a greater number of drugs than other references, *sudha*, *khatika*, *godanti*, *sankha*, *sambhuka (kshudrasankha)*, *muktasukti*, *varhatika*, *kurmapristha*, *praval*, *mukta*, *kukutandatwak*, *ajasthi*, *badarashma*, and *vanshlochana* (Tabulated in Table 13.1). They are well known for their properties for the treatment of certain conditions like *Amalpitta*, *Grahni*, *Parinamashula*, *Swasa*, *Kasa*, *Haridra roga*, etc. It is also a rich source of food and calcium. All drugs in *sudha varga* are a compact form of calcium or its salts.

13.5 BHASMAS OF SUDHA VARG

A number of *bhasmas* like *shankha*, *sukti* etc., are available in market, which are used for various therapeutic purposes either individually or as active pharmaceutical ingredients in various *ayurvedic* formulations. These are tabulated in Table 13.2.

TABLE 13.1
Drugs of *Sudha Varga*

Sr. NO	Drug	Common Name	Origin	Images
1	*Sudha* [18]	Lime	Mineral	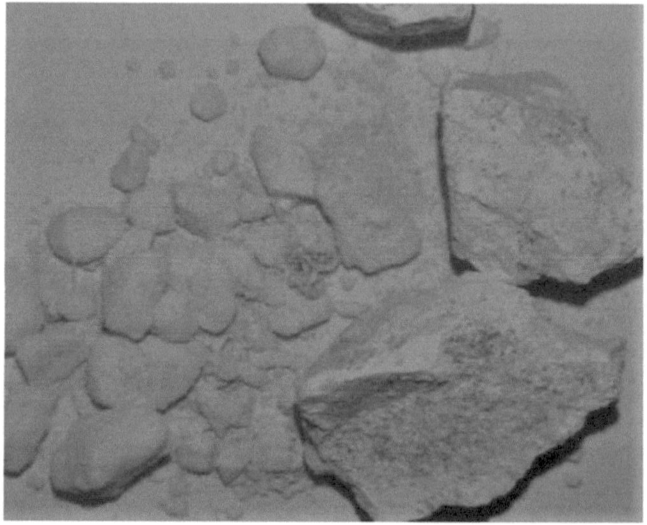 [18]

(*Continued*)

TABLE 13.1 (Continued)

Sr. NO	Drug	Common Name	Origin	Images
2	*Khatika*	Chalk	Mineral	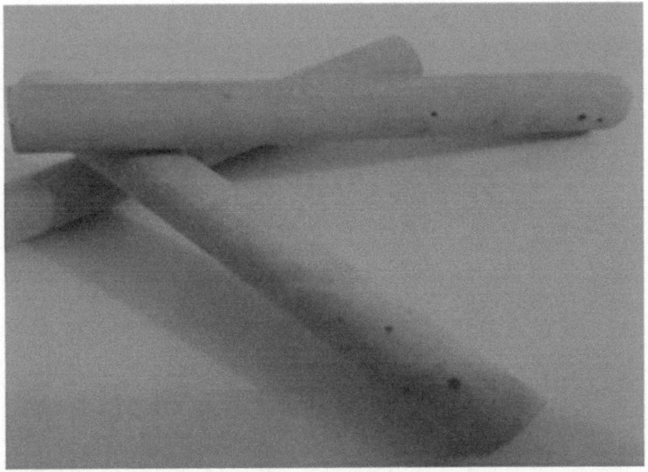 [19]
3	*Godanti*	Gypsum	Mineral	

(*Continued*)

TABLE 13.1 (Continued)

Sr. NO	Drug	Common Name	Origin	Images	
				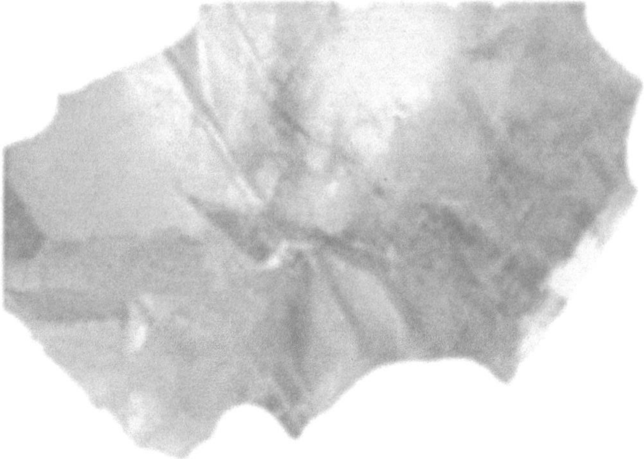	[20]

(Continued)

TABLE 13.1 (Continued)

Sr. NO	Drug	Common Name	Origin	Images
4	*Sankha*	Conch shell	Marine	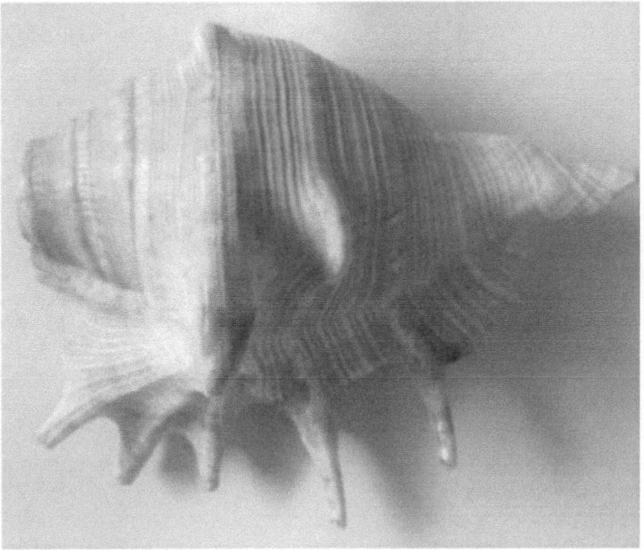 [21]

(*Continued*)

TABLE 13.1 (Continued)

Sr. NO	Drug	Common Name	Origin	Images	
5	*Shambuka*	Australian snail	Marine	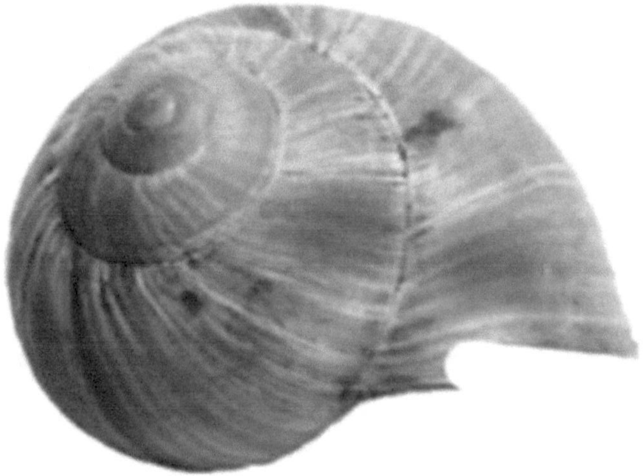	[22]

(Continued)

TABLE 13.1 (Continued)

Sr. NO	Drug	Common Name	Origin	Images
6	*Mukta sukti*	Pearl oyster shell	Marine	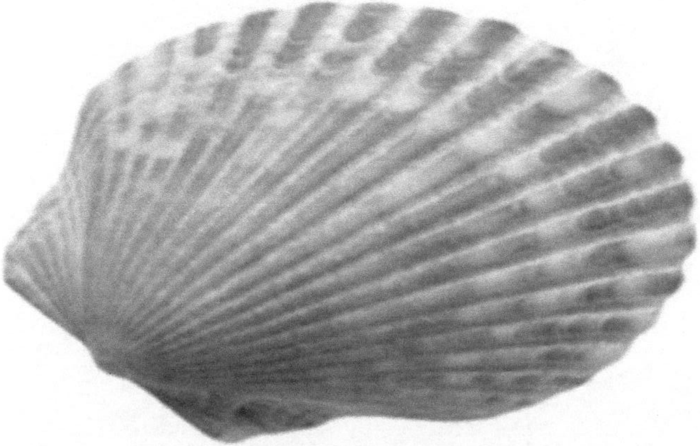 [23]

(Continued)

TABLE 13.1 (Continued)

Sr. NO	Drug	Common Name	Origin	Images	
7	*Kaparda*	Cowries shell	Marine	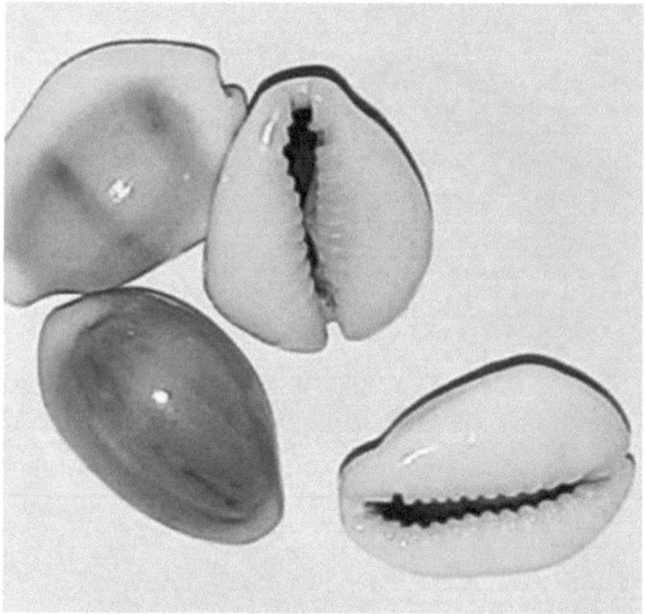	[24]

(Continued)

TABLE 13.1 (Continued)

Sr. NO	Drug	Common Name	Origin	Images	
8	*Kurmaprista*	Turtle shell	Marine	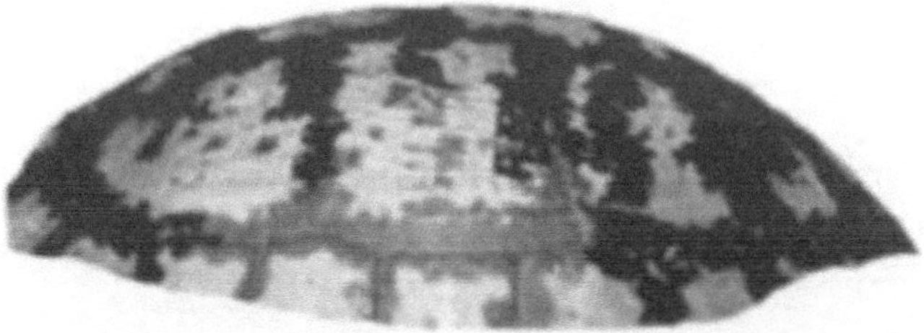	[25]
9	*Samundraphena*	Cattle fish bone	Marine		[26]

(Continued)

TABLE 13.1 (Continued)

Sr. NO	Drug	Common Name	Origin	Images
10	*Pravala*	Coral	Marine	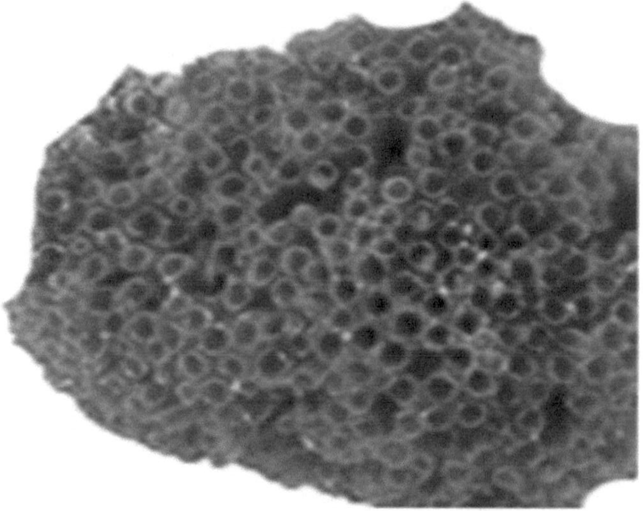 [27]

(Continued)

TABLE 13.1 (Continued)

Sr. NO	Drug	Common Name	Origin	Images
11	*Mukta*	Pearl	Marine	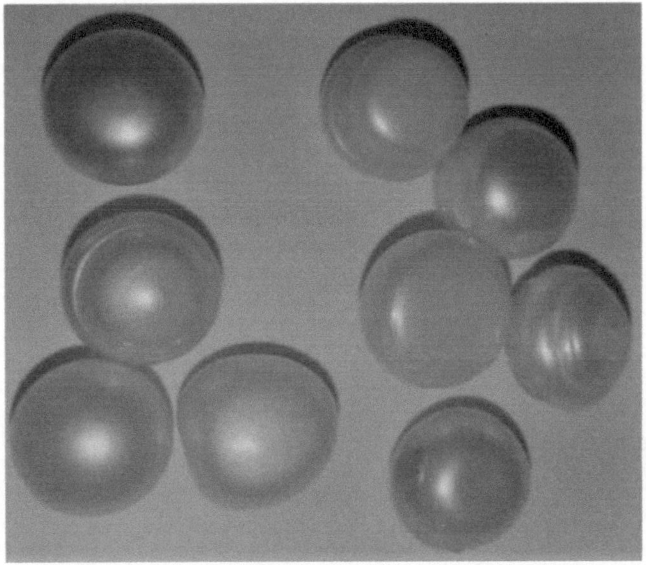 [28]

(*Continued*)

TABLE 13.1 (Continued)

Sr. NO	Drug	Common Name	Origin	Images	
12	*Mrigashringa*	Deer antlers	Animal	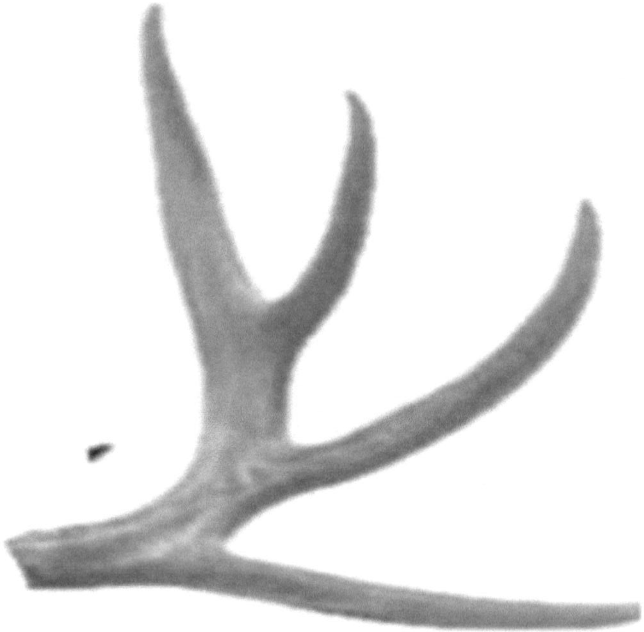	[29]

(Continued)

TABLE 13.1 (Continued)

Sr. NO	Drug	Common Name	Origin	Images	
13	*Kukkutanda twak*	Hen`s egg shell	Animal	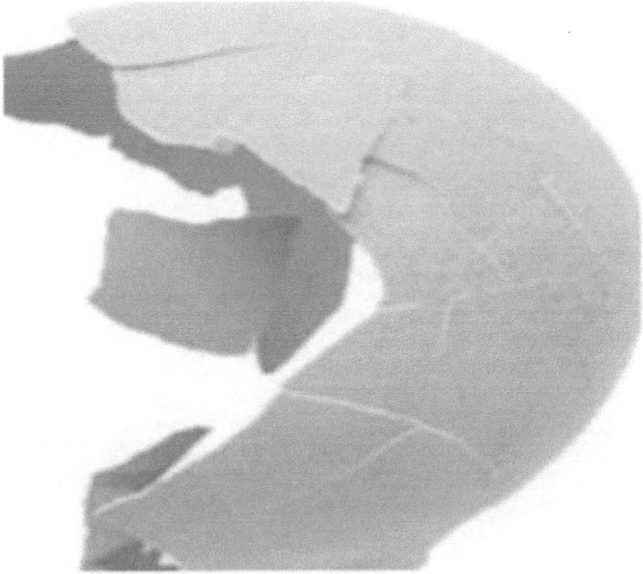	[30]

(*Continued*)

TABLE 13.1 (Continued)

Sr. NO	Drug	Common Name	Origin	Images
14	*Ajasthi*	Gout`s bone	Animal	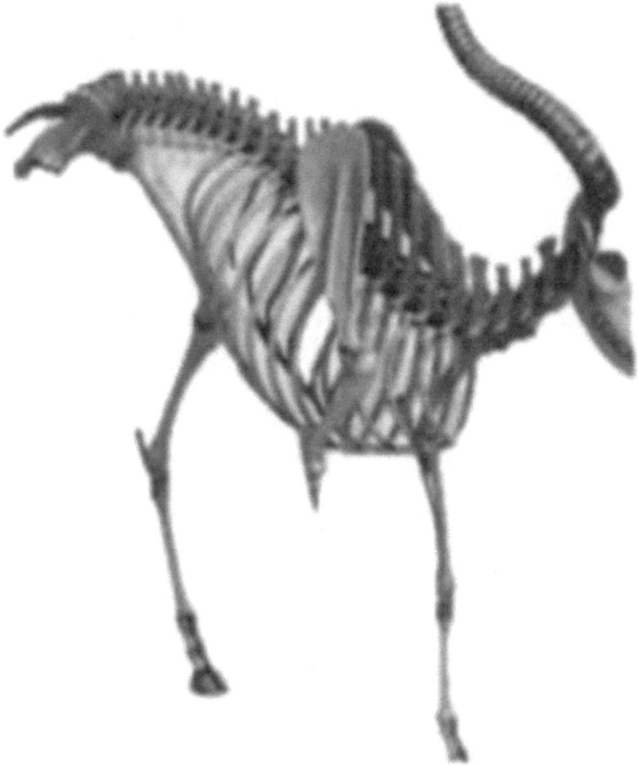 [31]

TABLE 13.2
Different Bhasmas Formulation of Sudha Varga

Sr. No	Important formulation	Compounds of formulation	Dose	USES	Side Effects:	Manufacture d by:	Reference
1	*Sudha bhasma*	-	-	-	-	-	-
2	*Khatika Bhasma*	-	-	-	-	-	-
3	*Godanti bhasma*	Purified Gypsum, aloe vera juice or lemon juice.	125 to 375 mg	Fever due to *Pitta* imbalance, *asthma*, anemia, chest injury, it improves strength and immunity.	Over- dosage may cause severe side effects including gastritis.	Divya Pharmacy, Shree Dhootapapes hwar Ltd.	*Rasa Tarangini* 11/241
4	*Sankha bhasma*	Purified Conch shell,	250–500 mg, 1–2 times	Coolant, complexion, gastritis, acidity, abdominal colic, malabsorption syndrome, dyspepsia, vomiting, nausea, acne, etc.	-	Divya Pharmacy, Dabur, Baidyanath	*Rasa Tarangini* 12/17 – 18
5	*Kshudrasankha (Shambhuka) bhasma*	-	-	-	-	-	-
6	*Mukta shukti Bhasma*	Purified Pearl Oyster,	125 – 250 mg, 1–2times	Gastritis, hyperacidity, cardiac diseases, urinary calculi,	Over-dosage may cause severe side effects.	Uma Ayurvedics pvt. Ltd. Dabur, Divya Pharmacy,	*Ayurveda prakasha* 2/327
7	*Varatika bhasma*						

(Continued)

TABLE 13.2 (Continued)

Sr. No	Important formulation	Compounds of formulation	Dose	USES	Side Effects:	Manufacture d by:	Reference
		Cowries, aloe vera juice, extracts,	125–250 mg,1–2 times	Digestive, *Asthma*, bronchitis, Tuberculosis, Chronic bronchial diseases.	Over- dosage may cause severe side effects, carefully used during, pregnancy, lactation	Divya Pharmacy, Baidyanath,.	*Ayurveda Prakasha* 3/100
8	*Kurmaprista Bhasma*	-	-	-	-	-	-
9	*Praval bhasma*	Coral, aloe vera juice extract/ *Shatavari* juice extract or *Jayanti* juice extract or cow milk,	250 mg, 1–2 times	Chronic respiratory diseases, bleeding disorders, Excessive sweating, improves digestive power,	Best avoided in pregnant and lactating mothers and chidren	Uma Ayurvedics pvt. Ltd. Dabur	*Rasatarangini* 23/129
10	*Mrigashringa bhasma*	Deer horn, Latex of *Arka*	250–500 mg,1–2 times	gastritis, *asthma*, bronchitis, cold, cough, heart burn etc.	-	Divya Pharmacy, Dabur, Baidyanath	*Rasa Tarangini* 12/105 – 107 .
11	*Kukkutanda twak bhasma*	Egg shell, Changeri.	125–500 mg	improve bone density, arthritis, osteoporosis, leucorrhea in women.	-	Baidyanath, Dabur	*Ayurveda Sara Sangraha*
12	*Ajasthi bhasma*	-	-	-	-	-	-
13	*Badarashma bhasma*	Lime Silicate, Radish juice	250–500 mg,1–2 times	Difficulty in urination and other urinary tract	-	Baidyanath, Divya Pharmacy	*Siddha Yoga Sangraha Ashmari*

(Continued)

TABLE 13.2 (Continued)

Sr. No	Important formulation	Compounds of formulation	Dose	USES	Side Effects:	Manufacture d by:	Reference
				disorders, external application in ring worm infection in children and urinary calculi			*Mutrakrichra Rogadhikara,* AFI Vol. 2, 14:4
14	*Vamshalochan a bhasma*	-	-	-	-	-	-
15	*Swetanjana Bhasma*	-	-	-	-	-	-
16	*Hastidanta Bhasma*	-	-	-	-	-	-

TABLE 13.3
Purification methods:

Sr. No.	Name	Synonyms	Appearance	Variety	Liquid media	Sodhana	Marana	Rf.
1	*Sudha*	*Curna, Curnaka, Sudha, Silaksara*	-	-	-	-	-	*Ayurve dya rasasha Stra*
2	*Sukti*	*Suktika, Muktasukti, Muktamata*	White color of *bhasma*	*Mukta sukti, Jala Sukti*	*Jayanti swarasa, nimbu swarasa, kamji*	*Swedana* by *dola yantra* for 3 hours	Give in presence of *ghritkumari swarasa* then *Gajaputa*	*R.T.* 12/65
3	*Sankha*	*Sankhaka, kambu, Samudraj,*	White color of *bhasma*	*Dakshanav arta, Vamavarta*	*Jambeera swarasa*	*Swedana* by *dola yantra* for 4 *prahara*	Give in presence of *kumari swarasa* then *gajaputa*	*R.T.* 12/6–7
4	*Badarasma*	-	-	-	*Kuluksth kwatha, kadalikanda*	*Nirvapa* 7 times	*Bhavana* of *mulaka swarasa* then	-
5	*Mriga Shringa*	*Ena sringa, mrga visanaka, harina sringa*	Black coloured *bhasma*, *shweta bhasm*, depend on procedure	-	*Arka dugdha*	-	*Maradana, Gajaputa*	*RT.* 12/ 105–107
6	*Khatika*	*Khatini, lekhani, Varnika*	-	*Khati Gourakhati*	Distilled water	Filtration	-	*R.T.*11/210
7	*Godhanti*	*Godantika, godanta,*	White color of *bhasma*	*Krishna rupa, Pinda kruti, Talakruti, Kourheyak, ruti,*	*Nimbu swarasa, dronapushpi swarasa*	*Swedana* by *dola yantra* 90 min	Give *sadharana puta*	*R.T.*12/103

(*Continued*)

TABLE 13.3 (Continued)

Sr. No.	Name	Synonyms	Appearance	Variety	Liquid media	Sodhana	Marana	Rf.
8	*Samudraphena*	*Phenaka, Abdhiphena, Dindira*	-	-	*Nimbu swarasa*	*Maradana* about 1 day	-	*R.T.*12/111–112
9	*Kukkutanda Twak*	*Sweta bhasma Sweranda bhasma*	White color of *bhasma*	-	Alkali media/ *nosad ra*	Macerated in liquid media 3–4 days then remove the outer cell of egg	*Maradana* with *Nimbu swarasa* then give *kukutputa*	-
10	*Kurmaprista*	-	-	-	-	Deep in distilled water about 12 hours then filter it	Give *gajaputa* presence of *ghritakumari swarasa.*	-

13.5.1 Shodhna and Marana (Purification and Calcination/Incineration)

In *rasashastra*, purification is an important tool of detoxification of metals, minerals and other classes of drugs. Purification is also important for *shdha varg* drugs. After purification, Marana is required for the preparation of *bhasma* (nanomedicines). Some examples with classical reference are tabulated in Table 13.3.

13.6 ANALYSIS OF BHASMA (SUDHA VARGA)

The entire confirmatory test should be done. To check if the process of *Bhasma* is completed or if more processess are required, various parameters have been defined in ancient texts (Tabulated in Table 13.4).

TABLE 13.4
Test (evaluation) of Bhasmas as per Ayurveda

Test	Characteristic	Procedure
Rekhapurnatwa	Fineness of *Bhasma* [35]	When the pinch of *Bhasma* is rubbed between thumb and index finger, *Bhasma* is inserted into lines and crevices of the fingers which is not easily removed by washing.
Apunarbha	No free metal present in *Bhasma* [35]	*Bhasma* is mixed with equal amount of *gunja*, *madhu*, *ghrita*, and borax and do *sandhibandhana*, and subjected to heat. After shelf cooling only *Bhasma* is found in the vessel.
Unam/Uttam	Lightness of *Bhasma* [35]	Little amount of *Bhasma* put on rice piece and rice piece is put over the water, if it is float over the surface, means *Bhasma* is ready.
Nirutha	No free metal present in *Bhasmaa* [35]	*Bhasm*a is mixed with a fixed weight of *rajat patra* and do *sandhibandhana*, and subjected to heat. After shelf cooling the weight of *rajat patra* is taken, if weight of *rajat patra* is increased, means *Bhasma* is not completely prepared.
Dantagre kachakachaabhav	Softness of *Bhasmaa* [35]	Little amount of *Bhasma* is putted between the teethes, *Bhasma* produced some sound or felt like rough, means it is not completely prepared.

(*Continued*)

TABLE 13.4 (Continued)

Test	Characteristic	Procedure
Nishchandrika	Lustreless [35]	*Bhasma* is observed under sunlight, if lustre is seen, means *Bhasma* is not prepared yet.
Sukshmatwam	Reduced particle size [35]	*Bhasma* should be like pollen grains of *ketakiraja*.
Dadhi Pariksha	Absence of free copper/ copper sulphate [35]	Little amount of *Bhasma* is pour on the surface of curd, if there is no discoloration observed, means *Bhasma* is ready [14].
Avami	Absence of free copper/ copper oxide/copper sulphate [35]	After administration of *Bhasma* no sensation of nausea is observed.
Niswadhutwa	Absence of free copper/ copper oxide/copper sulphate [35]	*Bhasma* should be tasteless.
Nirdhum	Fumeless *Bhasma* [35]	*Bhasma* should not produce fumes.

- **Modern analytical parameters for *Bhasma***
  Modern parameters are divided into four parts.
  a. Organoleptic evaluation
  b. Physical evaluation
  c. Chemical evaluation
  d. Instrumental evaluation

  - **Organoleptic Evaluation**
    In this, the colour, order, taste and touch of the *Bhasma* were noted (Tabulated in Table 13.5).
  - **Physical Evaluation**

TABLE 13.5
Parameters of Organoleptic Evaluation

Parameters	Characteristics
Colour	Colors for *Bhasmas* are specified according to the characteristics [34].
Odour	No odour is observed from well prepared *Bhasma* [34].
Taste	No taste is observed from well prepared *Bhasma* [34].
Touch	Soft and smooth touch is observed from well prepared *Bhasma* [34].

TABLE 13.6
Parameters of Physical evaluation

Parameters	Characteristics
Loss on drying	By this determination of amount of moisture content present in the sample when dried at 105°C [34].
Ash value	Helpful in the determining to illustrate the quality as well as purity of *Bhasma* [34].
Solubility	In this % of solubility of *Bhasma* is determined by dissolved in different solvents [34].
pH	Important parameter to check the acid neutralization capacity of Sudha varg (calcium) drugs
Extractive values	To check the solubility in various solvents

In physical evaluation some parameters are evaluated like loss on drying, ash value etc. (Tabulated in Table 13.6).

- **Chemical Evaluation**
  Chemical evaluation is further divided into two parts: Quantitative evaluation and Qualitative evaluation [32, 33].

- **Quantitative Evaluation**
  It is again further divided into three parts, as shown in Table 13.7.
- **Qualitative Evaluation**
  It includes NPST. Namburi-phased spot test is a technique to identify the purity and quality of Bhasma. In this test, Whatman paper number 1 is invariably impregnated in a suitable reagent and dried. The dried paper is tested with a drop of the solution of the substance under examination. As the reactant continues to react for a long time, the spot is studied at three different time intervals [34].

TABLE 13.7
Quantitative Evaluation of *Sudha Varga*

Parameters	Characteristics
Acid insoluble ash	It indicates the amount of inorganic content present in the sample [32,33].
Volumetric Analysis	This method is widely used in analysis. The measurement of volume of a solution of known concentration which is used to determine the concentration of the analyte [32,33,34].
Gravimetric Analysis	It helps to determine the atomic mass [32,33,35].

TABLE 13.8
Instruments Helpful in the Evaluation of *Sudha Varga Bhasma*

Instruments	Uses
X-ray diffraction (XRD)	Technique used to characterize the compound through crystalline phase
Scanning electron microscopy (SEM) and EDAX	Investigation of the morphologies and the elemental compositions of the *Bhasma* samples
Particle size distribution (PSD)	Determination of particle size
Fourier-transform infrared spectroscopy (FT-IR)	Record the FT-IR spectra and functional groups
Atomic absorption spectroscopy (AAS)	Use to detect the presence of metals

- **Instrumental Evaluation**
  Through instrumental analysis, qualitative, quantitative and as well as structural analysis can be done [36]. The techniques used are tabulated in Table 13.8.

13.7 PATENT AND PROPRIETARY AYURVEDIC MEDICINES

In the modern era, due to their high commercial value, lots of *Sudha varg* drugs are available in the form of patent and proprietary medicines, which are tabulated in Table 13.9. Besides, due to higher therapeutic values, scientists across

TABLE 13.9
Patent Proprietary Medicines of Sudha Varga

Sr. No.	Patent Product Name	Important Ingredients	Therapeutic effect	Dose
1.	"ACINILIN TAB (Koral)" [37]'	*"Shanka bhasma, Kapardika, Pravala bhasma, Apamarga kshar"*	"Hyper acidity, Peptic ulcer, Reflux oesophagitis, Dyspepsia, Gastric discomfort".	2 tablets thrice a day
2.	"AJICID CAP "(Ajmera) [37]	*"Jeera, Ajamoda, Pippali moola, Sajakshar, Gandhak vati,Shankh bhasma, Avipathikar choorna, Leela vilas ras."*	"Peptic ulcer, Gastritis, Flatulence"	1–2 capsules twice a day
3.		*"Abhrak bhasmam, Taamra bhasmam,*		

(*Continued*)

TABLE 13.9 (Continued)

Sr. No.	Patent Product Name	Important Ingredients	Therapeutic effect	Dose
	"AMLAPITTANTHAK YOG TAB" (Baidyanath) [37]	*Mandura bhasmam, Shank bhasmam etc."*	"Acidity, Loss of appetite, Indigestion, Vomiting, Nausea"	1–2 tablets twice a day
4.	"ANJAL TABLETS" (Ajmeera) [37]	*"Tribhuvankirtirasa, Sankhabhasma, Godanti bhasma, Spatika bhasma, Kavati bhasma, kaiphal etc."*	"Fever, Common cold, headache, Body pain etc."	1- 2 tablets twice a day
5.	"ANTI-MAL TAB" (Universal) [37]	*"Sudha thankan, Kuberakshar churna, Chirayata, Saptapamir, Kutaki, Hingul, Vatsanabh, Godanti bhasma etc"*	"Antipyretic and Analgesic"	1–2 tablets twice a day

the globe are working on calcium and related compounds and have applied for patents. Some of the important patent and proprietary medicines are tabulated in Table 13.10.

TABLE 13.10
Patents Related to Calcium and Similar Compounds

Sr. No	Title of Patent	Remarks	Patent no.
1.	Method and apparatus for on-site production of lime and sorbents for use in removal of gaseous pollutants [38]	Removal of gas phase pollutants by various methods which are provides by this invention.	US008999278B2, 07 April 2010
2.	Arsenic removal in conjunction with lime softening [39]	Lime is used to remove dissolved arsenic from an aqueous medium.	USOO68O298OB1, 12 Oct 2004
3.	Methods of manufacturing asphalt with lime pellets [40]	The invention provides asphalt cement manufactured with the use of lime pellets.	US007517401B2, 14 April 2009
4.	Process and system for producing commercial quality carbon dioxide from high solids lime mud [41]	Production of high quality carbon dioxide by this adaptation of this system and methods.	USOO8865101B2, 21 Oct 2014

(Continued)

TABLE 13.10 (Continued)

Sr. No	Title of Patent	Remarks	Patent no.
5.	Crude juice purification with reduced lime consumption [42]	Manufacturing of non sucrose substance and 2 apparatus for the purification of crude sugar beet juice with low lime consumption.	USOO9677144B2, 13 June 2017
6.	Method of preparing hydrated lime [43]	The invention is excellent sorbents for SO2 removal from gas streams.	US005223239A, 29 June 1993
7.	High capacity mobile lime slaker [44]	Method and apparatus for the formation of calcium hydroxide. This helps in continuous process, to make calcium hydroxide slurry from water and calcium oxide.	USOO6568842B1, 27 May 2003
8.	Continuous mixing and injection of lime-fly ash slurry [45]	Treatment of subsurface layer of the earth, to maintain the building strength and movement of subsurface water.	US4871283A, 03 Oct 1989
9.	Immobilization of lead and cadmium in solid residues from the combustion of refuse using lime and phosphate [46]	The purpose of this invention is to increase the immobilization of cadmium in solid residues and lead from combustion plants.	US4737356A, 12 April 1988
10.	Hydrated lime-fly ash-fine aggregate cement [47]	The hydrated lime fly ash-fine combined cements especially useful for protective coating, masonry mortar grouting compositions and soil stabilization.	US2564690A, 21 Aug 1951
11.	Layered nanoparticles [48]	The methods used to form a layered nano-particle, comprising providing a suspension. Firstly addition of core particles in a 1st liquid, and 2nd to the suspension, addition of reagent or precursor to the Suspension.	US009295654B2, 29 Mar 2016
12.			

(Continued)

TABLE 13.10 (Continued)

Sr. No	Title of Patent	Remarks	Patent no.
	Method of manufacturing skin care cream containing baked shell powder [49]	Preparation of cream which contain baked shell powder. It helps to cure inflammation of the skin. It is helpful for miliaria, athlete's foots, spots, freckles and exertanti-bacterial effects.	USOO8323699B2, 04 Dec 2012
13.	Method of Making Fermented Turtle Shell Powder Mixture [50]	The invention relates to a nutritional powder having a primary ingredient fermented Turtle shell powder that provides various health and medicinal benefits.	US 20150237904A1, 27 Aug 2015
14.	Chinese Herbal Oral Paste for Conditioning Blood Stasis Constitution and Processing Method therefor [51]	This invention is capable of achieving certain efficacy of strengthening physical health.	US 20190192603A1, 27 June 2019
15.	Traditional chinese pharmaceutical formulation for treatment of paradentosis & comma; process for preparation and use thereof [52]	Manufacturing of drug with the theoretical implementation to cure the symptoms, pathogens of periodontitis effectively.	US 20050170009A1, 04 Aug 2015
16.	Biomatrix hydrogels and methods of use thereof [53]	This invention helps in enhancing bone formation, regeneration of bones, cartilage formation.	US010342897B2, 09 July 2019
17.	Silicon oxycarbide, growth method of silicon oxycarbide layer, semiconductor device and manufacture method for semiconductor device [54]	The invention relates to manufacturing method of semiconductor device with different various suitable layers.	US008349722B2, 08 Jan 2013
18.	Surface-modified pearl pigment and process for producing the same [55]	In this leafing effect for the surface-modified in plane orientation is done.	USOO6858072B1, 22 Feb 2005
19.	Nano pearl cream [56]	The invention provides a cosmetic composition formed by intimately admixing the nano-meter sized ultra-fine pearl particles with Shielding and blocking ingredients.	US 2005022683OA1, 13 Oct 2005

(Continued)

TABLE 13.10 (Continued)

Sr. No	Title of Patent	Remarks	Patent no.
20.	Pearl polymer containing hollow pearls [57]	The invention relates to methods of manufacturing of pearl polymers, containing various homopolymers and copolymers.	US4208309A, 17 June 1980
21.	Stem cell lines from deer antlers, their application and culture methods [58]	Reconstruction of connective tissues, cartilage, bones, or lipid tissues in animals and humans with antlers of deer.	US008278096 B2, 02 Oct 2012
22.	Composition for making deer antler wine, method for making deer antler wine by using the composition, and deer antler wine made by the method [59]	The invention is to provide a ingredients for manufacturing of deer antler wine and the composition is used as a medium for fermentation to make the deer antler wine.	US 2012O164269A1, 28 June 2012
23.	Method of use of dicalcium phosphate as an antler scent [60]	The invention relates to dicalcium phosphate and, more particularly, to the use of dicalcium phosphate in aqueous solution for application to surfaces to create an antler scent of all species of deer on the Surfaces.	US 20120090557A1, 19 April 2012
24.	Deer antler extract for promoting angiogenesis [61]	Extraction of angiogenic extract from deer antlers and its composition. This is used to treat diseases, injuries and wounds in animals and humans.	USOO8067364B2, 29 Nov 2011
25.	Transcutaneous prosthesis [62]	This invention relates to transcutaneous prosthesis and includes a method of fitting a prosthesis having a transcutaneous component to a patient.	US 2014O107806A1, 17 April 2014
26.	Calcium Citrate-Malate as source of calcium to prevent bone diseases and increase bone strength in young animals and birds, especially young poultry, dogs, cats,	The invention relates to improvement of the health and development of bone in young animals and poul try. In addition, it enhances the eggshell quality of birds.	US 20140287088A1, 25 Sep 2014

(*Continued*)

TABLE 13.10 (Continued)

Sr. No	Title of Patent	Remarks	Patent no.
	swine, calves, and horses; and laying hens [63]	The addition of calcium citrate malate to feed of animals enhanced the bioavailability calcium for development.	
27.	Microinjection devices and methods of use [64]	This invention helps to manufacture devices of microinjection and describes the various methods to use.	USOO7339090B2, 04 Mar 2008
28.	Antibodies produced in the avian oviduct [65]	The invention relates to transgenic avians which produce antibodies in the egg white by introducing a nucleic acid sequence into the genome of an avian embryo wherein the nucleic acid sequence comprises a nucleotide sequence encoding an antibody and to the antibodies and to methods related thereto.	US 20100310552A1, 09 Dec 2010
29.	Joint Repair Using Mesenchymal Stem Cells [66]	By this invention repair of defected joints can be done. Which are defected with any injuries or by any diseases like osteoarthritis.	US 2013 0131804A1, 23 May 2013
30.	Fgf-2 variants having n-terminal deletions and increased receptor selectivity and uses thereof [67]	The invention relates to the design, manufacture and use of fibroblast growth factor (FGF) polypeptides having improved receptor specificity.	US 20180127475A1, 10 May 2018
31.	Bioactive complexes compositions and methods of use thereof [68]	By this invention, the bioavailability and efficacy are increased naturally. Because this composition is a complex of natural ingredients.	USOO7780873B2, 24 Aug 2010
32.	Compositions for regenerating tissue that has deteriorated, and methods for using such compositions [69]	The invention concerns the regeneration of tissues in a Subject that have degenerated as a result of a disease or disorder in the Subject.	USOO643271 OB1, 13 Aug 2002

(*Continued*)

TABLE 13.10 (Continued)

Sr. No	Title of Patent	Remarks	Patent no.
33.	Treatment methods using Dkk-1 antibodies [70]	The use of immunological fragments and antibodies by especially by using Dkk-1 polypeptides.	USOO81 0 1 184B2, 24 Jan 2012
34.	Platelet-derived growth factor compositions and methods for the treatment of osteochondral defects [71]	This invention relates to compositions and methods for treating an injury or a defect in a cartilage and a bone, particularly to the treatment of osteochondral defects in a cartilage and a bone adjacent to the cartilage in an individual by administering compositions to the individual comprising a biphasic biocompatible matrix in combination with platelet derived growth factor (PDGF) to at least one site of the osteochondral defect.	US 2013 0122095A1, 16 May 2013
35.	Candidates against infection [72]	The invention relates to the use of plasminogen/plas-min and its derivatives as agents for enhancing host defence against infection or other infectious diseases.	US 20160243204A1, 25 Aug 2016
36.	Antioxidant compositions and methods of use thereof [73]	Preparation of emulsion consists of highly polyunsaturated lipids from the natural ingredients and the various methods to prepare it.	USOO7118688B2, 10 Oct 2006
37.	Pyrimidine derivatives for the treatment of abnormal cell growth [74]	Use of pyrimidine derivatives for the management of abnormal cell growth like cancer in mammals.	USOO7208499B2, 24 April 2007
38.	Treatment of tissue with undifferentiated mesenchymal cells [75]	With this methods and constituents, defect of skin, bones and soft tissues will be treated.	US 2004O101959A1, 27 May 2004
39.	Molecular determinants of myeloma bone disease and uses thereof [76]	The validation and identification of molecular myeloma bone disease with the help of	USOO7642238B2, 05 Jan 2010

(*Continued*)

TABLE 13.10 (Continued)

Sr. No	Title of Patent	Remarks	Patent no.
		model of SCID rab mouse for primary myeloma.	
40.	Materials and methods for improved bone tendon bone transplantation [77]	For the efficient and easier surgery of reconstructing ligaments in the joints.	US 20030097179A1, 22 May 2003

13.8 SUDHA VARGA AS NUTRACEUTICALS AND FOOD SUPPLEMENTS

The term "nutraceutical" is used to describe these medicinally or nutritionally important functional foods.

Thousands of calcium supplements are available in the form of nutraceuticals.

1. They are used to cure calcium malabsorption by enhancing the diffusion constituent of absorption. They are commonly used as food supplement to prevent age-related osteoporosis. [78]
2. Calcium is used for chelating certain anions, mainly phosphate. It is used in chronic renal failure, where there is a reduction in phosphate absorption [79].
3. Symptomatic gastric acidity – calcium carbonate is used as an antacid between meals to neutralize gastric acidity in gastro-oesophageal acid reflux disease and peptic ulcer disease [79].

The formulations are mentioned in Table 13.11.

TABLE 13.11
Formulations of *Sudha Varga* considered as Food Supplement

S. No	Name	Indication	Dose
1.	*"Godanti bhasma"*	Rickets, Osteoporosis [80]	125–250 mg
2.	*"Kukkutandatwak bhasma"*	Rickets, supplement during pregnancy, lactation, dental eruption [80]	250–500 mg
3.	*"Ajasthi"*	Rickets, supplement during pregnancy, lactation, dental eruption [80]	250–500 mg
4.	*"Pravala pishti"*	Rickets with cough [80]	-
5.	*"Sringa bhasma"*	Strengthen bones and cartilages [80]	60–125 mg
6.	*"Shuktadi yoga"*	Calcium supplement [80]	125–250 mg
7.	*"Muktadi vati"*	Rickets. [80]	250–500 mg
8.	*"Balavati"*	Rickets. [80]	250–500 mg
9.	*"Balapanchabhadra churna"*	Rickets [80]	250–500 mg
10.	*"Sudhashataka yoga"*	Rickets. [80]	250–1000 mg
11.	*"Abha guggulu"*	Fracture healing [80]	250–500 mg
12.	*"Lakshadi guggulu"*	Fracture healing [80]	250–500mg

13.9 SUMMARY AND CONCLUSION

Bhasma (Nanomedicines) have been used and described in classical texts since ancient times. They are made using nanotechnology. Indian Government approved some departments for continuous research on nanomedicines. Calcium compounds used in *Ayurveda* are grouped under *sudha varga*. For preparation of *Bhasma*, various procedures are available, like *shodhana, marana* with the help of prescribed liquid media. They have gained therapeutic importance as calcium supplements in calcium deficiency to enhance normal growth and development. Apart from calcium supplements, they are also prescribed for conditions like *amlapitta, grahani, parinamashula, swasa, kasa, hridya roga* in *Ayurveda*. They are also used as food supplements and nutraceuticals. Finally, the chapter concludes with the idea that the use of *Sudha varg bhasmas (nanomedicines)* and other similar compounds, like pisti, is safe and eco-friendly if they are prepared according to the guidelines prescribed by the ministry of AYUSH, Government of India.

REFERENCES

1. National Institute of Health (2006). "National Institute of health roadmap for medical research: Nanomedicine", Nanomedicine. 2006. Accessed April 15, 2020Para 2.
2. European Science Foundation (2004). "Nanomedicine-An ESF-European Medical Research Councils forward look report", Strasbourg cedex, France ESF.
3. European Technology Platform on Nanomedicine (September, 2005). "*Nanotechnology for Health: Vision paper and basis for a strategic research agenda for nanomedicine*", EC Publication office.
4. Kumar A., Nair A. G., Reddy A. V. and Garg A. N. (2006). "Bhasmas: Unique ayurvedic metallic-herbal preparations, chemical characterization", *Biological Trace Element Research*, ED-109, pp. 231–254.
5. http://www.biospectrumindia.com/biospecindia/features/219860/nanotechnologyhealth-care/page/2#sthash.4b3hTYMv.dpuf (Last Accessed on 23-04-2020).
6. http://www.ibef.org/download/Healthcare-August-2015.pdf (Last Accessed on 21-04-2020).
7. Jain N. K. (2006). "Status of nanomedicine research in India", *Nanomedicine Nanotechnology Biology and Medicine*. ED-2, pp. 269–312.
8. Kumar A. and Desai P. N. (2013). "Overview of nanobiotechnology public R&D system in India", *ABDR*, ED-15, pp. 67–79.
9. Kumar A. (2014). "Nanotechnology development in India: an overview", *Research and Information System for Developing Countries*, ED-193, pp. 1–33.
10. Kumar A. and Desai P. N. (2014). "Mapping the Indian nanotechnology innovation system", *World Journal of Science, Technology and Sustainable Development*, ED-11, pp. 53–65.
11. Ali A. and Sinha K. (2014). "Emerging scenario of nanobiotechnology development in India", *EAR*, ED-II, pp. 1707–1727.
12. Ali A. and Sinha K. (2014). "Prospects of nanotechnology development in the health sector in India", *International Journal of Health Sciences and Research*, ED-2, pp. 109–125.
13. Ali A. and Sinha K. (2014). "Exploring the opportunities and challenges in nanotechnology innovation in India", *Journal of Social Science for Policy Implications*, ED-2, pp. 227–251.

14. Bhattacharya S. and Shilpa M. (2011). "Mapping nanotechnology research and innovation in India", *DESIDOC Journal of Library and Information Technology*. ED-31, pp. 349–358.
15. Anand M. (2014). "Nanoscience and nanotechnology", *Innovation in India: "Combining Economic Growth with Inclusive Development"* Ramani, S., Ed., Cambridge University Press: Cambridge, pp. 211–242.
16. Shefali, Gangwar R., Devi M., Chhabra P. and Prasad B. "Role of nano science in development of India", National Conference on 'Role of Science and Technology Towards Make in India' held on 5–7 March, 2016 at YMCA University of Science and Technology, Faridabad.
17. Sharm D. C. (2000). "India raises standards for traditional drugs", *Lancet*, ED-356, p. 231.
18. https://www.alibaba.com/product-detail/Quick-lime-Burnt-Lime-CalciumOxide_50039504166.html (Last Accessed on 22-04-2020).
19. https://www.kindpng.com/imgv/booiTh_sidewalk-chalkboard-white-transprent-chalk-clipart-black-and/ (Last Accessed on 20-04-2020).
20. https://www.indiamart.com/proddetail/loud-and-blowing-shankh-20866579933.html (Last Accessed on 23-04-2020).
21. https://sciencestruck.com/properties-uses-of-gypsum (Last Accessed on 20-04-2020).
22. https://www.kindpng.com/downpng/hJiiimR_stock-snail-shell-png-by-e-di-snail/ (Last Accessed on 23-04-2020).
23. https://webstockreview.net/pict/getfirst (Last Accessed on 23-04-2020).
24. https://www.kindpng.com/downpng/ihTxhxb_ring-top-cowrie-shells-ring-top-cowrie-hd/ (Last Accessed on 23-04-2020).
25. https://oman.desertcart.com/products/4479941-real-pond-turtle-shell (Last Accessed on 23-04-2020).
26. https://www.aliexpress.com/item/32870196928.html?aff_platform=promotion&sk=i6Ujaqn&aff_trace_key=750555b3406548eda26ba89481691dc5–1586796606752-06275-i6Ujaqn&terminal_id=e7511086bbb844de85923070bb67a9c2&aff_request_id=750555b3406548eda26ba89481691dc5–1586796606752-06275-i6Ujaqn (Last Accessed on 23-04-2020).
27. https://www.google.com/search?q=red+coral+shell+hd+picture&tbm=isch&ved=2ahUKEwi0nJKh8OXoAhXUNCsKHasPCBIQ2cCegQIABAA&oq=red+coral+shell+hd+picture&gs_lcp=CgNpbWcQA1CTwwNYvccDYIvMA2gAcAB4AIAB8wGIAdwFkgEFMC4zLjGYAQCgAQGqAQtnd3Mtd2l6LWltZw&sclient=img&ei=m5qUXvTiM9TprAGrn6CQAQ&bih=608&biw=1349&hl=en# imgrc=S5FIzE6-WeAVAM (Last Accessed on 23-04-2020).
28. https://www.amazon.in/HARSHALI-GEMS-Ratti-white-Gemstone/dp/B07CDQX212 (Last Accessed on 23-04-2020).
29. https://www.shutterstock.com/search/deer+antlers (Last Accessed on 23-04-2020).
30. https://www.freeimages.co.uk/galleries/festive/easter/slides/cracked_egg_shell.htm (Last Accessed on 23-04-2020).
31. https://www.turbosquid.com/3d-models/goat-skeleton-2–3ds/650792 (Last Accessed on 23-04-2020).
32. G. W. Ewing, (1985). "*Instrumental Method of Chemical Ananlysis*", McGraw-Hill, New York, vol. ED-5.
33. J. Kenkel (1992). "*Analytical Chemistry-Refresher Manual"*, Lewis Publication, Boca Raton.
34. Kapoor R. C., (2010). "Some observation on the metal-based preparations in the Indian System of Medicine", *Indian Journal of Traditional Knowledge*. 9 ED-3, pp. 562–575.

35. Bijjal A. G. (2008). "*Preparation and analysis of Tamra Bhasma by various procedures as per Rasa Tarangini*", M.D. dissertation. Bangalore, Karnataka: Rajiv Gandhi University of Health Sciences.
36. D. A. Skoog, F. J. Holler and T. A. Nieman (1998). "*Principle of Instrumental Analysis*", Thomson Learning, Crawfordsville, Vol. ED-5.
37. https://www.indiamart.com/proddetail/ayurvedic-patent-medicine-3363111133.html (Last Accessed on 23-04-2020).
38. https://patentimages.storage.googleapis.com/0e/39/37/70a361091cca6d/US8999278.pdf (Last Accessed on 23-04-2020).
39. https://patentimages.storage.googleapis.com/2f/fc/06/139beb4587cbe3/US6802980.pdf (Last Accessed on 23-04-2020).
40. https://patentimages.storage.googleapis.com/ce/09/3f/16bc7783394ae2/US7517401.pdf (Last Accessed on 23-04-2020).
41. https://patentimages.storage.googleapis.com/5e/f6/dd/1ad30030281b6b/US8865101.pdf (Last Accessed on 23-04-2020).
42. https://patentimages.storage.googleapis.com/c4/17/01/51048106ebb987/US9677144.pdf (Last Accessed on 23-04-2020).
43. https://patentimages.storage.googleapis.com/f8/6a/00/b8e030cbcb911e/US5223239.pdf (Last Accessed on 23-04-2020).
44. https://patentimages.storage.googleapis.com/ac/b9/2e/955d951290ef70/US6568842.pdf (Last Accessed on 23-04-2020).
45. https://patentimages.storage.googleapis.com/d2/ea/15/908fd9a2834307/US4871283.pdf (Last Accessed on 23-04-2020).
46. https://patentimages.storage.googleapis.com/b0/17/df/75d0e536ea7361/US4737356.pdf (Last Accessed on 23-04-2020).
47. https://patents.google.com/patent/US2564690A/en?q=lime&oq=lime&page=2 (Last Accessed on 23-04-2020).
48. https://patentimages.storage.googleapis.com/1e/88/56/701367a76f1422/US9295654.pdf (Last Accessed on 23-04-2020).
49. https://patentimages.storage.googleapis.com/5b/c0/e3/205b89683e60a4/US8323699.pdf (Last Accessed on 23-04-2020).
50. https://patentimages.storage.googleapis.com/e7/58/e0/53b47e70956948/US20150237904A1.pdf (Last Accessed on 23-04-2020).
51. https://patentimages.storage.googleapis.com/0c/4d/59/fed807f6da3610/US20190192603A1.pdf (Last Accessed on 23-04-2020).
52. https://patentimages.storage.googleapis.com/7b/78/3f/e411b63e7d75c2/US20050170009A1.pdf (Last Accessed on 23-04-2020).
53. https://patentimages.storage.googleapis.com/f3/cc/cf/2f477aa38fc9b1/US10342897.pdf (Last Accessed on 23-04-2020).
54. https://patentimages.storage.googleapis.com/73/76/26/cad2c197328873/US8349722.pdf (Last Accessed on 23-04-2020).
55. https://patentimages.storage.googleapis.com/f9/bf/6f/8a0856f156fe67/US6858072.pdf (Last Accessed on 23-04-2020).
56. https://patentimages.storage.googleapis.com/52/45/c6/267cf6bbae3bfe/US20050226830A1.pdf (Last Accessed on 23-04-2020).
57. https://patents.google.com/patent/US4208309A/en?q=pearl&oq=pearl&page=16 (Last Accessed on 23-04-2020).
58. https://patentimages.storage.googleapis.com/f6/9c/e3/5df1a7c71a079f/US8278096.pdf (Last Accessed on 20-04-2020).
59. https://patentimages.storage.googleapis.com/85/f0/4e/fdf214a5dd518e/US20120164269A1.pdf (Last Accessed on 23-04-2020).

60. https://patentimages.storage.googleapis.com/79/3e/3c/25e49a485b4cea/US20120090557A1.pdf (Last Accessed on 23-04-2020).
61. https://patentimages.storage.googleapis.com/8d/36/86/6eefad370748dc/US8067364.pdf (Last Accessed on 23-04-2020).
62. https://patentimages.storage.googleapis.com/1b/68/de/3d5cbb3cac6a51/US20140107806A1.pdf (Last Accessed on 23-04-2020).
63. https://patentimages.storage.googleapis.com/ac/c3/bb/444db9fd0066a9/US20140287088A1.pdf (Last Accessed on 23-04-2020).
64. https://patentimages.storage.googleapis.com/21/3a/09/87ae0ef9c451d9/US7339090.pdf (Last Accessed on 23-04-2020).
65. https://patentimages.storage.googleapis.com/a6/cf/ca/9eb7c38fceb4cb/US20100310552A1.pdf (Last Accessed on 23-04-2020).
66. https://patentimages.storage.googleapis.com/72/f3/61/f4fd97298c9f1e/US20130131804A1.pdf (Last Accessed on 23-04-2020).
67. https://patentimages.storage.googleapis.com/fe/8a/54/fba3ed0adfd1c7/US20180127475A1.pdf (Last Accessed on 23-04-2020).
68. https://patentimages.storage.googleapis.com/a5/99/67/c19e5e7b926326/US7780873.pdf (Last Accessed on 20-04-2020).
69. https://patentimages.storage.googleapis.com/06/05/6e/70c39c515287aa/US6432710.pdf (Last Accessed on 20-04-2020).
70. https://patentimages.storage.googleapis.com/ba/c5/df/b731baa91c4cbc/US8101184.pdf (Last Accessed on 20-04-2020).
71. https://patentimages.storage.googleapis.com/f7/ea/c1/3cdf1a4336b6b5/US20130122095A1.pdf (Last Accessed on 20-04-2020).
72. https://patentimages.storage.googleapis.com/4a/15/62/125cdccfd27879/US20160243204A1.pdf (Last Accessed on 20-04-2020).
73. https://patentimages.storage.googleapis.com/f8/5f/a8/ffa31e474568ed/US7118688.pdf (Last Accessed on 23-04-2020).
74. https://patentimages.storage.googleapis.com/a1/cf/78/50f8b0ace84b12/US7208499.pdf (Last Accessed on 23-04-2020).
75. https://patentimages.storage.googleapis.com/0a/b0/15/1cfb2d1f3fd715/US20040101959A1.pdf (Last Accessed on 23-04-2020).
76. https://patentimages.storage.googleapis.com/57/2b/7e/fd053e42c3b076/US7642238.pdf (Last Accessed on 23-04-2020).
77. https://patentimages.storage.googleapis.com/f6/28/c2/eabcca0969b7b6/US20030097179A1.pdf (Last Accessed on 23-04-2020).
78. Jack D. B. (1995). "Keep taking the tomatoes - the exciting world of nutraceuticals", *Molecular Medicine Today*, 1, pp. 118–121.
79. Shin C. and Kim K. (2015). "The risks and benefits of calcium supplementation", *Endocrinology and Metabolism (Seoul).* ED-30, pp. 27–34.
80. Li K., Wang X. F., Li D. Y., Chen Y. C., Zhao L. J., et al. (2018). "The good, the bad, and the ugly of calcium supplementation: A review of calcium intake on human health", *Clinical Interventions in Aging*, ED-13, pp. 2443–2452.

14 Biological and Clinical Perspectives of Nano Quantum Dots for Cancer Theranostics

Bakul Tikoo, Gagandeep Singh, Ashok Kumar Yadav, Rajiv Kumar, Gurpal Singh, and Ashish Suttee

14.1 INTRODUCTION TO CANCER THERANOSTICS

The organized consolidation of personalized *diagnostics* and *therapeutics* is termed as *theranostics*. This platform incorporates an imaging agent for investigation followed by providing the therapeutic agent for the treatment of the diagnosed ailment. This approach results in augmentation of the therapy effectiveness, reduced occurrence of adverse events, improved patient engagement, and reduction in patients' overall therapy expenditure.

More recently, there have been major developmental strides in the field of *Cancer Theranostics,* which combines the accurate diagnosis and concurrent therapy of cancer, aimed at early-stage diagnosis, accompanied by fastidious treatment with properly calculated doses at pre-defined time intervals and trailed by consistent monitoring of the progress of therapy.

Cancer comprises a set of many heterogeneous diseases delineated by uncontrolled cellular division occurring as a result of various genetic as well as epigenetic factors. Early diagnosis is an essential advancement required in this field of therapy so as to facilitate successful treatment of patients through surgery, radiotherapy, chemotherapy or immunotherapy.

Currently, chemotherapeutic drugs face numerous drawbacks such as severe adverse effects, development of resistance and suboptimal efficacy [1]. More interests have interest has been diverted towards engineering nano-sized formulations for cancer theranostics. This cutting-edge technology of biocompatible endogenous nano-formulations will build the way forward in the course of simultaneous delivery of cancer diagnostics and therapeutics [2].

14.2 EXISTING PLATFORMS

14.2.1 Nanoparticles

Nanoparticles are small in size with subcellular structures, making them favorable candidates for cancer theranostics due to their promising potential to readily accumulate at the site of the disease where they can be visualized with the help of imaging setups to better understand their tumor-targeting ability. Additional attributes, such as a leaky tumor physiology, allow nanoparticles to extravasate into tumor tissues, enhance permeability and retention (EPR) effect due to poor lymphatic drainage. The high drug-loading capacity due to their high surface area-to-volume ratios preclude nanoparticles from being readily cleared from the body, thereby extending their circulation time in the blood. Thus, nanoparticles form a highly versatile platform in the arena of cancer theranostics, as they can be loaded with therapeutics and diagnostics of varying natures and may also be surface-functionalized with targeting ligands (Figure 14.1).

Hence, since nanoparticles are advantageous in increasing the target-to-background contrast in imaging and localizing within the target tissue, thereby reducing toxic adverse effects, they prove to be conducive in cancer theranostics. Among the multitude of extensively studied nanoparticles, dendrimers, micelles, protein conjugates, linear and branched polymers have been employed in developmental evaluations in the field of theranostics by functionalizing with imaging agents. Nucleic acids, such as plasmids, antisense oligonucleotides, ribozymes, DNAzymes, aptamers, siRNA, have also existed as tools of traditional "gene therapy," where faulty copies of a gene are replaced with functional ones.

In recent times, enormous efforts have been made to establish methods for manufacturing adequate and reliable delivery vehicles, such as virus-based therapeutic delivery involving RNA and/or DNA, non-viral therapeutic delivery utilizing liposomes, cell-penetrating peptides, and some inorganic nanomaterials. These vehicles have been labeled with organic dyes, allowing the use of multiple

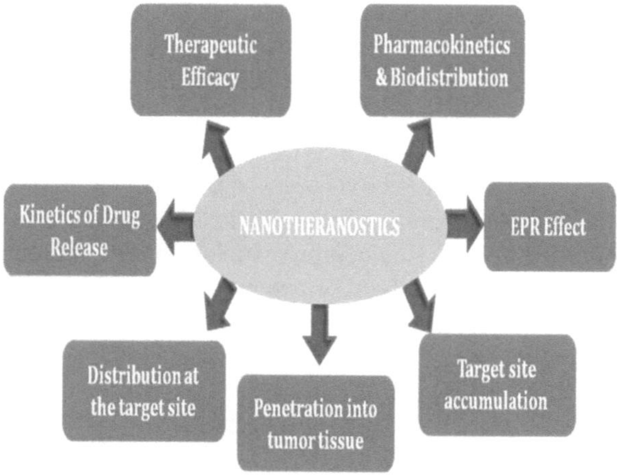

FIGURE 14.1 Schematic Diagram Emphasizing the Advantages of Nanotheranostic Platforms [1].

refined imaging tools, e.g. computed tomography (CT), positron emission tomography (PET), magnetic resonance imaging (MRI), single photon emission computed tomography (SPECT), and ultrasound (US), to fuel these approaches toward the development of theranostic systems. Despite these achievements, labeling polymeric vehicles with fluorescent dyes is restricted by certain limitations, such as fast fluorescent decay, high cost of gene guns and other equipment required, photobleaching, and non-uniform labeling of vehicles.

Protein-based nano-platforms have also generated great interest as theranostic agents due to their biodegradability, low toxicity, biocompatibility, ease of fabrication and ability to achieve targeted therapy.

The field of nano-oncology holds promise to develop new theranostic structures that will be able to perform diagnosis and targeted therapy efficiently. Therefore, the aforementioned nanoparticles exhibit exclusive (Figure 14.2) physical and chemical properties for active targeting and provide imaging as well as therapeutic actions against cancer and other life-threatening diseases.

14.2.1.1 Metallic and Non-Metallic Nanoparticles

Nanotheranostics exhibit electrical, biological, magnetic and optical properties, making them appropriate molecules for functionalization with imaging agents. They may be fabricated from two types of materials, i.e. organic and inorganic. Organic

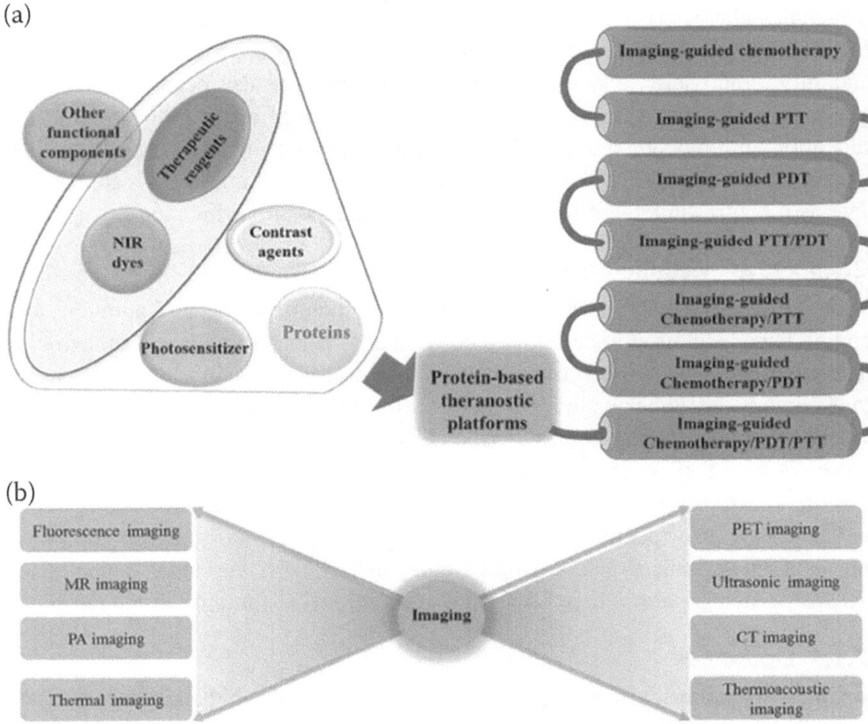

FIGURE 14.2 Molecular Imaging Techniques Employed in Nanotheranostics [3].

nanoparticles, involving distinct biopolymers such as lipoproteins, liposomes, and dendrimers, have more clinical significance. Nonmetallic nanoparticles, on the other hand, have biocompatibility, site-targeted operation, and often form covalent links with the imaging agent. Recently, metallic nanoparticles like quantum dots (QDs) and superparamagnetic iron oxide nanoparticles (SPIONs) have gained interest and are being efficiently used as contrasting materials. These nanoparticles can be rapidly transformed into nanotheranostics by loading them with therapeutic drugs [4,5].

14.2.1.2 Gold Nanoparticles

Because of their superior biocompatibility, their unique optical and photothermal properties and well-studied surface modification techniques, Gold nanoparticles are commonly used for multifaceted probes. Gold nanoparticles are applied in cancer therapy using techniques such as photothermal therapy (PTT), photodynamic therapy (PDT) and photo-triggered drug release. PTT is a therapy arbitrated through light in which gold nanoparticles absorb light, resulting in the generation of heat that burns the cancer-causing cells. The geometry of gold nanoparticles directly influences their absorption and scattering properties. This property can be exploited in selecting the required size range of the nanoparticles in clinical applications (Table 14.1) [7].

14.2.1.3 Iron Oxide Nanoparticles

IONPs have amassed great interest in the last decade converging on their biomedical application owing to their vital physicochemical nature observed in the nano-range. This includes characteristic tractable properties like size, superparamagnetism, high surface-to-volume ratio, high saturation magnetization, easy separation methodology, crystallinity, nontoxicity, and biocompatibility. These have also been referred to as magnetic nanoparticles. Like AuNPs, magnetic NPs also offer flexibility for surface modification with biocompatible molecules, which improve the targeting ability. The supermagnetic nature of IONPs additionally provides a biomedical application avenue as a contrasting agent for many magnetic diagnostic techniques [8].

14.2.1.4 Other Metallic Nanoparticles

A wide array of metals, such as Palladium, Platinum, Copper, Cadmium and Selenium, have been used in addition to conventional metals to prepare nanoparticles with theranostic applications. Given their simple process of synthesis, high photo-thermal conversion efficiency, low production costs and the ability to conduct repeated treatments without altering optical properties, copper NPs are gaining more importance. Due to their exceptional optical and catalytic properties, palladium nanoparticles have also been employed in theranostic applications. Palladium nanomaterials have been previously documented for use as prodrug activators, as photothermal agents, and in anticancer and/or antimicrobial therapy. On the other hand, nanoparticles employing cadmium and selenium are used less commonly in theranostics.

14.2.1.5 Liposomes

Liposomes are spherical lipid vesicles composed of a double-membrane structure consisting of amphiphilic lipid molecules. By encapsulating hydrophilic molecules inside the liposomal aqueous core domain or entrapping hydrophobic

TABLE 14.1
Various Metals Utilized Clinically at the Nano-platform [6]

Nanoparticles	Size (nm)	Surface functioning material	Diagnostic and contrast agent	Targeting agents	Therapeutic agents	Activators
Gold	<100	CTAB and poly(acrylic acid)	Fluorescein isothiocyanate (FITC)	A33 single chain antibody	Gold nanoparticles (Photothermal)	Light
Silver	~90	*Olax scandens* leaf extract	*Olax scandens* leaf extract	-	*Olax scandens* leaf extract conjugated silver nanoparticles	pH
Copper	10	Sn 2	Copper NPs	Alpha vs beta 3 integrin	Fumagilin prodrug	pH/enzyme
Palladium	~4.4	Reduced glutathione (GSH)	Pd nanoparticles	-	Doxorubicin	pH
Platinum	<120	Cyclic arginine glycine-aspartic acid (Crgd) tripeptide	Tetraphenysilole fluorore	Alpha vs beta 3 integrin	Pt(IV) prodrug	Enzyme
Cadmium and selenium	~100	Hydroxypropyl cellulose poly (acrylic acid) (HPCPAA)	HPC-PAA—CdSe hybrid nanogels	-	Temazolomide	pH
Polymer	~68	Polyglutamic acid (PGA)	-	Carbonicanhydrase IV (CA4)	Paclitaxel	Enzyme
Silica	~70	Polyethylene glycol and fe_3O_4	Rhodamine B isothiocyanate	-	Doxorubicin	-
Carbon	80-400	Gold and poly (4-vinylphenol)	Gold	-	Gold and carbon (Photothermal)	-

ones within the liposomal bilayer, they have been used effectively as nanocarriers for the delivery of many drugs and diagnostic agents. Like most nanoparticles, liposomes also offer easy surface modification with targeting molecules. Their enhanced permeability and retention (EPR) effect results in their selective accumulation within cancerous tissues not only passively, but also by targeting the angiogenic marker or cancer cells specifically. The imaging and surface modification multimodalities of liposomal theranostic agents render them quite useful for individualized visualization of their in vivo tumor-targeting and pharmacokinetic properties. Liposomal technology offers additional attributes such as prediction of the therapeutic efficacy combined with valuable information from each imaging technique [4–6,9–21].

14.2.1.6 Dendrimers

Dendrimers are large polymers. They are highly branched, radially symmetrical nano-sized macromolecules with a typical symmetric central core. Dendrimers offer a variety of biological properties such as self-assembly, polyvalency, electrostatic interactions, chemical stability, solubility, and low cytotoxicity, which makes them particularly useful in the biomedical area wherein these polymers can be applied for in vitro diagnosis, in gene therapy as vectors to transfer genes through the cell membrane, in regenerative medicine, as drug-delivery systems and as imaging agents in MRI when conjugated with other molecules [20].

14.2.1.7 Polymeric Nanoparticles

Also known as Polymeric Nanospheres, they serve as bioactive polymeric drugs, polymeric conjugates with therapeutic drug and/or contrasting agents, and as conjugates when combined with proteins. Chemotherapy has several adverse effects since drug molecules are unevenly distributed into the body. Polymer-drug conjugates may come into play in such instances by prolonging the circulation time of the drug, improving the target specificity, and enhancing the permeability and retention effect. The polymer backbone can be conjugated with targeting moieties like antibodies, peptides, and/or small molecules to further increase the target specificity. These approaches may augment the production of more of such polymeric NPs to provide a range of chemotherapeutic and diagnostic agents for numerous biomedical applications [4–6,9–19].

14.2.1.8 Carbon Nanotubes

Carbon nanotubes (CNTs) are carbon allotropes produced in the form of tiny tubes made of graphite (carbon) sheets rolled into nanoscale-diameter cylindrical tubes (Figure 14.3). Carbon nanotubes exhibit exceptional chemical, electrical, and mechanical properties with high elastic modulus. Chemical functionalization of CNTs has been shown to enhance solubility in many solvents, to improve their electronic properties, and to cause significant de-bundling. However, CNTs suffer from a disadvantage concerning their use in biochemistry and biomedical applications, i.e. they are highly hydrophobic and customarily form insoluble aggregates. Due to the low solubility of CNTs in many solvents, it is quite difficult to isolate one from the other [18].

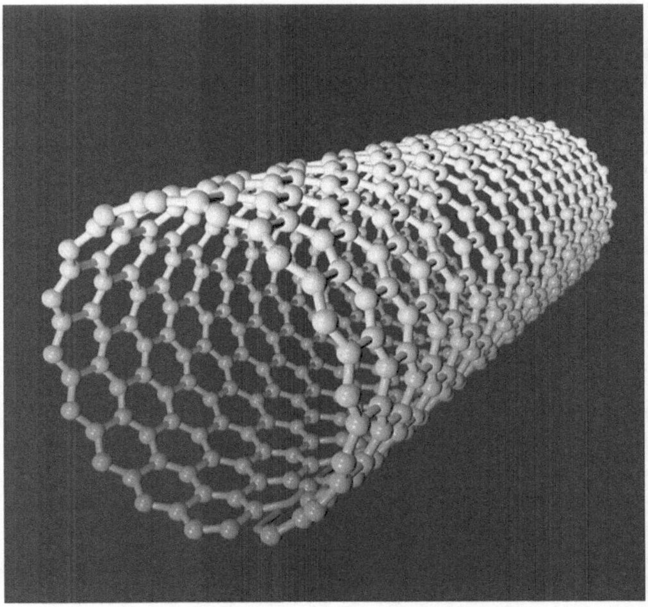

FIGURE 14.3 Basic Framework of Carbon Nanotubes [18].

14.2.1.9 Quantum Dots

Quantum dots (QDs) are colloidal crystals with sizes in the nanometric range and are composed of small semiconductor materials that exhibit quantum mechanical properties. These semiconductor particles are made small enough so that the quantum effects come into action, thus reducing the electron energies in the particles. Since energy influences wavelength, the optical properties of these particles can be finely tuned, depending on their size. Thus, particles can be fabricated to emit or absorb specific wavelengths (colors) of light, merely by controlling their size. Smaller QDs (2 nm) present blue fluorescence emission (380–440 nm), while larger particles (5 nm) have red fluorescence emission (605–630 nm). QDs are robust and stable light emitters and are not as susceptible to photobleaching as organic dye molecules. This photostability makes them very useful in observing cells for a long period of time. Different surface modifications of QDs can be achieved to visualize labeling of whole cells and tissue. QDs can be employed effectively in the field of theranostics, especially in the delivery and reporter systems of transfection therapies in vivo [2,3,22–28].

14.3 MOLECULAR IMAGING AND ITS IMPLICATION IN CANCER DIAGNOSIS

The diagnostic and therapeutic strategies for chemotherapy can be immensely boosted with the help of novel molecular imaging methods [27]. Emerging molecular enhancers for imaging modalities such as CT, US, PET and MRI will expedite faster and more authentic diagnoses, particularly for solid tumors, which is essential for effective surgical therapeutic intervention [5].

Nanotechnology breakthroughs have led to the production of different nanoparticles that are fabricated as diagnostic or molecular imaging tools for cancer detection. Due to their effectiveness in chemotherapy, various nano-range materials have been employed in drug formulation and have also been granted approval for clinical purposes [28]. Garnering contemporaneal diagnostic molecular imaging of biomarkers, therapeutic drug delivery, and continuous monitoring of therapeutic progress is of major significance in the field of nanotheranostics. Till now, several nanotheranostics have been revealed, but not many have been extrapolated clinically due to drawbacks such as low biodegradability, bioavailability, stability, and biocompatibility [4].

Customarily, improvement in drug treatment is viewed as the principal catalyst in the fight against cancer. However, in the case of tumors of solid tissues, early-stage detection must be taken into account equally, if not more critical for effective treatment, since it facilitates a surgical remedial approach. It is highly useful to have knowledge of biomarkers, which can help us envision the most effective therapies or estimate an early therapy response in the treatment course. Molecular diagnostic imaging has a important role to play in complementing and mitigating some of the shortcomings of conventional biomarkers by yielding the opportunity to achieve non-invasive, replicable assessments of the entire body [1]. Future research must be focused at interfacing the biochemical and genetic process leading to cancer development, instead of radiation-induced tumor degeneration, therapeutic drug treatment or surgical excision since the latter therapies are toxic to healthy tissues as well. A wide range of new biomarkers have been identified as a result of increasing and intensive curiosity aimed towards developing deeper insights about the pathogenesis of cancer. A majority of these biomarkers may be used for cancer diagnosis and treatment (Table 14.2). Such technologies, together with diagnostic imaging techniques, have the potential to revolutionize the treatment of cancer [6].

14.4 SIGNIFICANCE OF BIOMARKERS

Biomarkers, or "Biological Markers", refer to naturally occurring molecules or genes capable of defining a specific pathological or physiological mechanism or disease [15,16]. They are a measurable indicator of the biological state or condition that can be detected in blood, other body fluids, or tissue-examination responses. Evidence of successful implementation of biomarkers for diagnosis, screening and management of cancers, such as breast and prostate cancers, has led to earlier diagnoses, increased survival and lower morbidity rates, thus corroborating the clinical relevance of this concept. Moreover, delving into newer biomarkers such as PD-1 and CTLA4, and new classes such as microRNAs and exosomes, coupled with the prospect of closer ties between the realms of molecular biology and biotechnology confers the beginning of a new era of biomarker discovery for precision medicine in cancer. Hence, diagnostic markers can be utilised to direct therapeutic decisions in the field of cancer theranostics with the objective of individualising patient therapy [5,6,17].

TABLE 14.2
Few Oncogenes Which Are Predominantly Expressed on Some Tumors [6]

Oncogene	Chromosomal location	Tumor
Cyclin D1	11q 13	Breast, others
KRAS	12p 12.1	Pancreas, colon, lung
ERBB2/Nue	17q 11.2-17	Breast, ovary
N-RAS	1p 13.2	Thyroid, melanoma
C-myc	8q 24	Carcinomas, lyonphomas
N-myc	-	Neuroblatoona

14.4.1 Pharmacogenomics

Genetic polymorphisms have been increasingly utilised, especially with respect to drug-metabolizing enzymes that can predict treatment efficacy or complications due to anti-cancer drugs. Genomic variation can lead to differential drug responses in individual patients, affecting drug absorption, metabolism, pharmacodynamics and excretion [10]. The increased understanding of disease provided by pharmacogenetic research is now also being incorporated into the drug development process in order to optimize therapeutic benefits and minimize the risk of toxicity in the individual patient [13]. The identification of genetic alterations that increase the risk for developing cancer is useful for predisposition testing with mutational screening and counseling as part of the established subspecialty of cancer genetics [6].

14.4.2 Proteomic Biomarkers

Proteomics is a valuable technology used in the development of novel and more effective drugs following the identification and characterization of disease-causing proteins [11]. Protein biomarkers are often identified in basic science studies of cancer cells as overexpressed proteins. Given the proven ability to adapt a protein-based immunoassay on to a standard clinical platform, the translation of protein discoveries to a clinical test should be quite rapid and efficient. The difficulty in establishing a clinical test is often at the level of developing antibody pairs for sandwich immunoassays when multiple protein analytes must be assayed in a body fluid such as serum, plasma or urine. Novel proteomic biomarker discovery technologies are being developed using quantitative isotopic labelling and improved mass spectroscopy algorithms [12–14].

14.4.3 Metabolomic Biomarkers

Metabolomics is the systematic analysis of the small-molecule metabolites produced by normal or abnormal cellular processes [11]. In general, metabolomics is focused on chemical profiles using a variety of analytical technologies. Metabolomics is widely used to investigate numerous aspects of nutrition using a variety of samples ranging from plants and foods to human and animal tissues and biofluids. Metabolic patterns and biomarker classifiers for tumor staging and stratification have been developed for breast cancer, prostate, and renal cell carcinoma. Given the well-known changes in the glycolytic pathways, apoptosis, and phosphometabolic changes that occur upon carcinogenic progression, the changes in the metabolic profile of adenine nucleotide profiles provide a rich source for biomarker discovery. The integration of metabolomics with other omics-related technologies may provide more specific classifiers of alterations related to cancer stage, grade, response to therapy, and prognosis [13].

14.4.4 Early Detection of Cancer

In order to detect cancer at its earliest stages, when it is most curable, there is a need for biomarkers to detect individuals harboring occult cancers. One approach for accomplishing this objective is to detect molecular fingerprints of an organ in the process of developing a cancer and then to define biomarkers suitable as targets for treatment prior to a significant tumor burden [2]. Effective biomarker identification depends on multiple levels of study design, each of which must be optimized to ensure the utility of a biomarker or a panel of biomarkers for this specific clinical application – early detection [15]. The success of biomarkers for the early detection of cancer is measured by the fact they should not only detect disease early but also reduce the mortality of cancer [9].

14.5 QUANTUM DOTS: A NEW DEVELOPMENT IN CANCER DIAGNOSIS

The improvements in cancer diagnosis and imaging have greatly enhanced due to applications of various types of nano-molecular imaging agents, such as quantum dots (QDs), to correctly diagnose, manage, and treat malignant cancer. QDs are almost spherical NCs, which consist practically of semiconductor materials. These materials are created from elements, where s and p are valence electrons that include elements from groups IV, II–VI, III–V, or IV–VI in the periodic table [22]. The most striking property of semiconductor QDs is the massive modification of the optical properties according to the size, typically with diameters in the range of 2–8 nm consisting of ~100–1000 atoms [3]. Advantages of highly fluorescent QDs over luminescent dyes include their high extinction coefficients, robust control over optical properties, sharp emission bands, and decreased sensitivity to photobleaching (Figure 14.4) [25].

Strong and balanced fluorescence seemingly enables revelation of many cancer biomarkers in tissue biopsies, blood assays, and as molecular imaging agents for diagnosis.

14.5.1 Characteristics of Quantum Dots for in vivo Imaging and Cancer Research

Quantum dots usually consist of cadmium-selenium (Cd-Se) or cadmium-tellurium (Cd-Te) cores. As aforementioned, the electronic characteristics of QDs are determined by

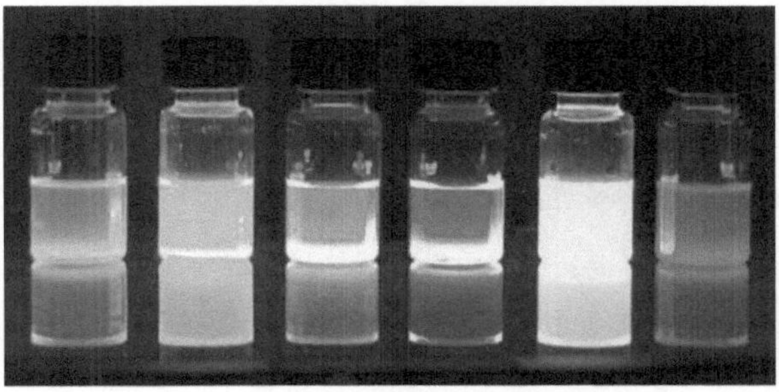

FIGURE 14.4 Vibrant Fluore scence of Quantum Dots Observed Under UV Light [26].

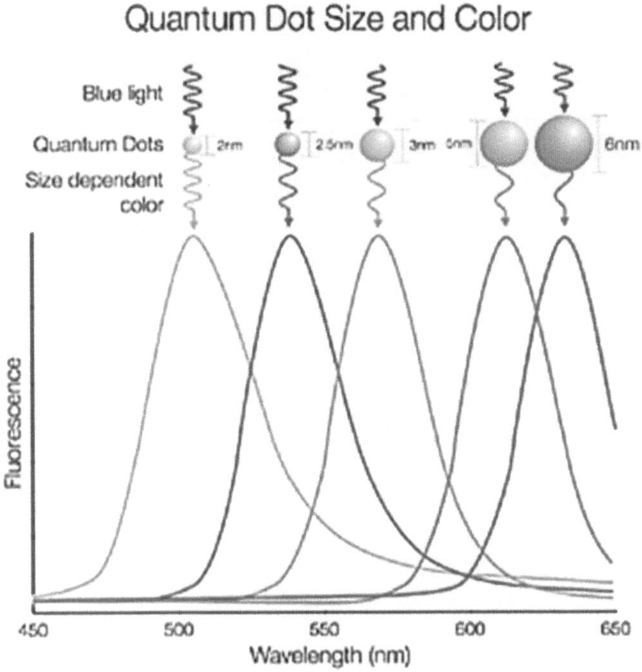

FIGURE 14.5 Fluorescence Spectra of Various Sizes of QDs [27].

their size and shape, which means their emission wavelengths can be controlled by tuning their size. Typically, smaller QDs (e.g. radius of 2~3 nm) emit shorter wavelengths, generating colors such as violet, blue or green, while bigger QDs (e.g. radius of 5~6 nm) emit longer wavelengths, generating colors like yellow, orange or red (Figure 14.5). Their highly tunable optical properties based on their size are fascinating, leading to a variety of research and commercial applications [26].

An intrinsic band gap is a known property of semiconducting materials, which is inversely proportional to the size of QDs. The electrons can be excited by absorbing incident light from the valence to the conduction band, leaving behind a hole. Thus, an *exciton* is formed by bond formation between the electron and the hole. Upon

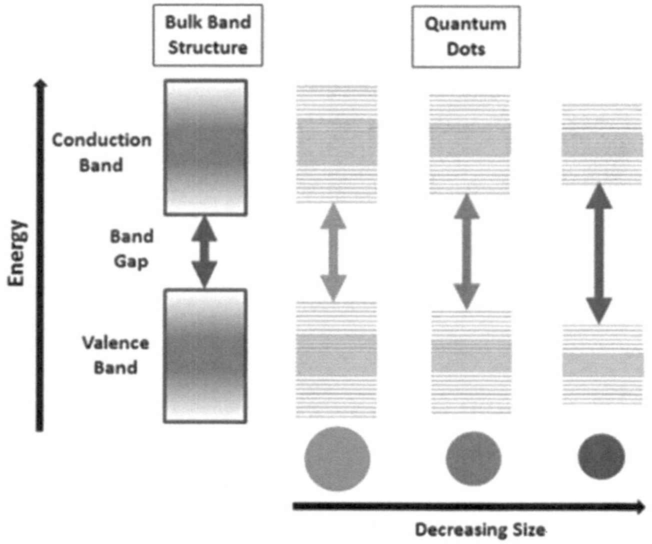

FIGURE 14.6 Effect of Size on the Electronic Structure of Quantum Dots [27].

recombination (i.e. the return of the excited electron to its ground state) of this *exciton,* a photon is emitted at a longer wavelength. This phenomenon is called fluorescence. When the synthesized QDs are too small in size to be compared with the wavelength of the electron, the Quantum Confinement Effect is observed (Figure 14.6). Once these confined *excitons* are excited by a light beam, they re-emit light (i.e. fluoresce) with a narrow and symmetrical emission spectrum that depends directly on the nanocrystal size [27]. The summarized advantages/ disadvantages are given in Table 14.3.

TABLE 14.3
Advantages and Disadvantages of Quantum Dots

Advantages	Disadvantages
Quite stable and can be handled more easily during manufacturing.	Due to their large physical size, it is difficult for them to cross biological membranes.
Highly efficient in converting shorter wavelengths to longer wavelengths.	Certain types of QDs may be toxic to cells.
Availability of numerous, simple and cost-effective methods of synthesis.	Their extended stability and lifetime may render them useless in cases where QDs are required to biodegrade immediately.

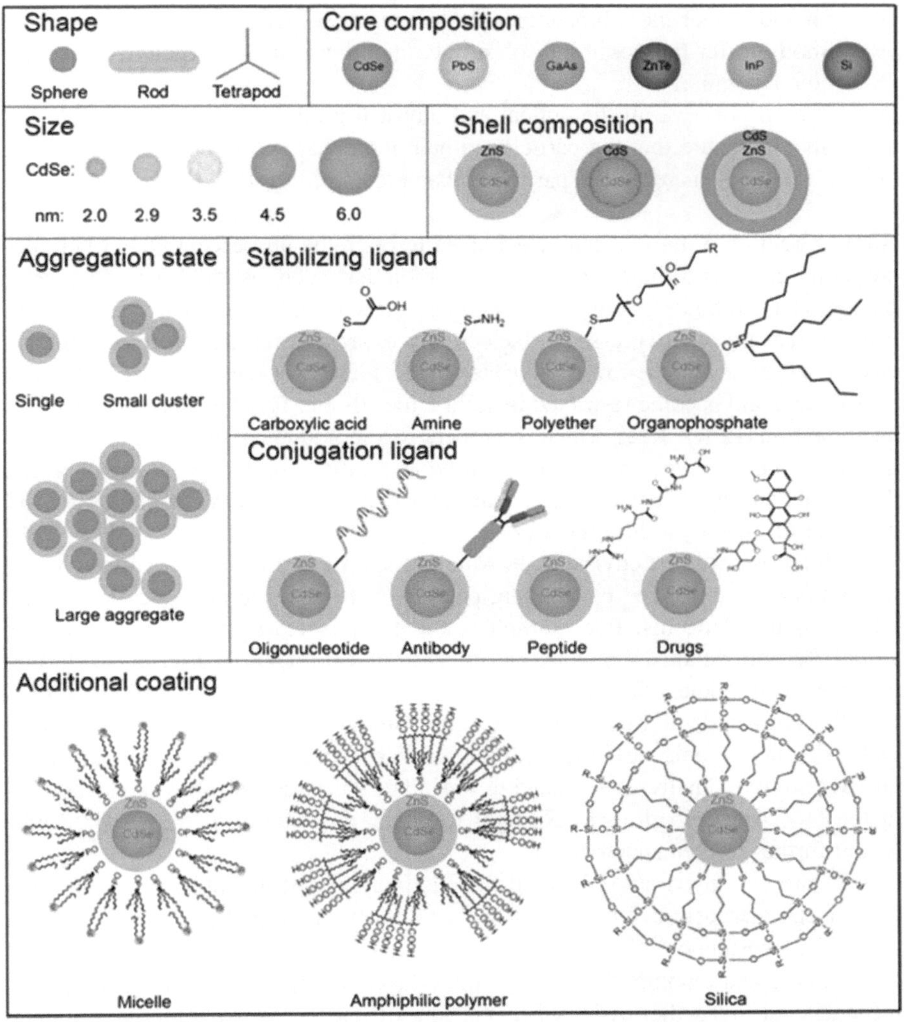

FIGURE 14.7 Various Ways of Fabrication of Quantum Dots to Improve Theranostic Properties [3].

14.5.2 Applications of Quantum Dots-based Biomedical Molecular Imaging

The high electronic density of QDs makes them excellent contrasting agents for molecular imaging. Having a wide imaging range from the level of the whole body (macro-scale) down to the nanometer resolution (Figure 14.7), QDs have the unique ability to visualize images at numerous length scales. Any modifications of the outer surface of QDs is required to meet the following criteria:

- Should render them biocompatible and water soluble;
- Should offer the possibility of surface modification with reactive groups for bioconjugation;
- Should preserve all the optical and physical properties;
- Should ensure that the particles remain monodispersed; and
- Should not increase the particles' diameter significantly [3].

Active targeting of tumors can be achieved through the fluorescent QDs when they are combined with binding ligands or moieties such as antibody fragments, monoclonal antibodies, folic acid, peptides, growth factors, carbohydrates, or receptors that are overexpressed or selectively expressed on cancer cells. Utilizing passive targeting and their restrictive size range, these QDs have a strong inclination to penetrate and become restricted in solid tumor tissue. The enhanced permeability and retention (EPR) effect, which is a repercussion of atypical biological features of the tumor microenvironment interpolating a faulty vasculature of tumor and a dearth of draining of waste material through lymphatic vessels, facilitates passive targeting of QDs to solid tumors [27].

A situation could be envisaged in which cancer detection and patient care could be significantly enhanced by imaging peptide-coated QDs at all scales, using various imaging platforms. For example, patients at increased risk for lung cancer would be intravenously injected with color-labeled QDs fabricated with bioengineered antibodies specialized for cancer-associated cell surface markers prior to bronchoscopy that will be capable of exciting and visualizing the emission from the QDs. This may enable earlier detection of cancer by providing molecular specificity and sensitivity. Finally, upon making the diagnosis, targeted QDs could be irradiated by X-rays or infrared (IR) light to induce heating-up of the tumor, which would further trigger apoptosis [4].

QDs are employed not only as diagnostic imaging agents but also as a platform to conceal therapeutic moieties as well as many hydrophilic and hydrophobic agents. Encapsulation of lipophilic drugs can be accomplished between the inorganic core and amphiphilic polymer outer layer, whereas lyophilic agents can be incapacitated over the hydrophilic portion of the outer amphiphilic polymer, through covalent or noncovalent bonds. The nanometric size and surface functionalization characteristics of these magical bullets prevent them from being readily eliminated through the kidneys, thereby extending circulation in the blood pool.

Not only are QDs a commendable alternative to magnetic and radioactive imaging, these engineered NCs serve as excellent carriers for delivering chemotherapeutic drugs and genes for altering tumor cells. QDs hold massive capabilities for the detection of many cancer markers simultaneously and hold tremendous promise for sorting out the complex gene expression profiles of cancers, thereby providing accurate clinical diagnosis. Recently, QDs have been widely used as a sensitive probe for screening cancer markers in fluids, specifically tissue biopsies and, most importantly, for tissue detection. No doubt, QDs have become an indispensible tool for targeting, imaging, and performing specific therapeutic functions [3,25,26].

14.6 CHALLENGES

The field of theranostics remains fairly new but is evolving at an extraordinarily rapid pace. Until now, theranostics have struggled to enter clinical trials and concerns about uncertainty and/or discrepancy between the optimal concentrations of therapeutic and imaging agents present a major challenge in their clinical extrapolation (Figure 14.8).

i Currently, the bulk of nanomedicines employed clinically depend on passive targeting, i.e. the EPR effect. More efforts need to be initiated to better understand the *in vivo* behavior of passively and actively targeted nanotheranostics, as well as of those that can be externally stimulated to discharge their contents at the target site.

ii The crux of personalized cancer therapy lies in the intelligent application of theranostic biomarkers, which can be identified in biological samples like serum, urine, tissue, or by molecular imaging but must be rigorously validated.

iii For many complicated nanotheranostic platforms with compound structures prepared in laboratories, it may be challenging to carry out replication in another lab and large-scale manufacturing.

iv There is a paucity of clear FDA guidelines to provide adequate information about the approval of nanotheranostics.

v It has been shown that various nanotheranostic particles induce cytotoxicity, genotoxicity, and immunotoxicity in relation to their nanometer size. The risk-to-benefit ratio needs to be evaluated before employing them clinically (Figure 14.8).

Emerging nanotheranostic formulations still have a long way to go to allow sensitive biomarker detection, molecular *in vivo* imaging of tumor targets, and target-specific delivery of therapeutic agents [23,24].

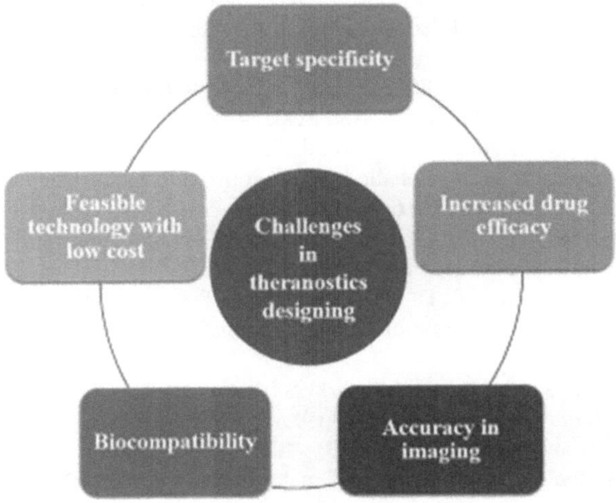

FIGURE 14.8 Schematic Diagram Showing the Challenges of Nanotheranos-tics [5].

14.7 FUTURE PROSPECTS

A wide variety of theranostic platforms that are based on distinct nanostructures show great potential as cancer theranostics. Cancer prevention will be enhanced with the help of tools based on molecular diagnostics and interventions, thus implementing preemptive medicine. Molecular diagnostic imaging techniques that truly represent and measure cancer characteristics will influence early-stage cancer detection and clinical management of patients. The combination of in vitro molecular diagnostics and entire-body molecular imaging readouts is expected to grow dramatically in the future and be incorporated into modern cancer therapies that will provide greater efficacy and cost savings. Of the myriad of nano-sized platforms utilized in the field of theranostics, QDs have generated massive interest among cancer researchers. These systems are immensely popular because of their well-known ability to act as specific markers for cellular and molecular structures and for surveillance of biochemical and physiological activities in live cells. While nanomaterials still have many challenges to overcome for their clinical development, the advancement of technology, the aggravation of clinical research, and the layout and fabrication of nanomaterials will aid significantly in the curation of safe and effective cancer theranostics. The field of cancer theranostics is set to revolutionize the future of healthcare delivery and aims to fulfill the current unmet needs leading to the ultimate eradication of cancer [23,24].

REFERENCES

1. Arranja A., Pathak V., Lammers T. and Shi Y. (2017). "Tumor-targeted nanomedicines for cancer theranostics", *Pharmacological Research*, 115, pp. 87–95.
2. Chen, X. and Wong, S. (2014). "Cancer Theranostics", *Cancer Theranostics*, pp. 3–8.
3. Bentolila, L. A. (2005). "Quantum Dots for Molecular Imaging and Cancer Medicine", *Discovery Medicine*, 5, pp. 213–218.
4. Enrico C. (2018). "Nanotheranostics and theranostic nanomedicine for diseases and cancer treatment", *Design of Nanostructures for Theranostics Applications*, pp. 41–68.
5. Siddhardha B. and Parasuraman P. (2019). "Theranostics application of nanomedicine in cancer detection and treatment", *Nanomaterials for Drug Delivery and Therapy*, pp. 59–89.
6. Hussain, T. and Nguyen, Q. T. (2014). "Molecular imaging for cancer diagnosis and surgery", *Advanced Drug Delivery Reviews*, 66, pp. 90–100.
7. Yeh, Y.-C., Creran, B. and Rotello, V. M. (2012). "Gold nanoparticles: preparation, properties, and applications in bionanotechnology". Nanoscale, 4(6), pp. 1871–1880.
8. Ali, A., Zafar, H., Zia, M., ul Haq, I., Phull, A. R., Ali, J. S. and Hussain, A. (2016). "Synthesis, characterization, applications, and challenges of iron oxide nanoparticles. Nanotechnology", *Science and Applications*, 2016(9), pp. 49–67.
9. Burgess, K., Rankin, N. and Weidtab, S. (2014). "Chapter 10 – Metabolomics", *Handbook of Pharmacogenomics and Stratified Medicine*, pp. 181–205.
10. Yu, L. R., Stewart, N. A. and Veenstra, T. D. (2010). "Chapter 8 - proteomics: the deciphering of the functional genome", *Essentials of Genomic and Personalized Medicine*, pp. 89–96.
11. Tainsky, M. A. (2009). "Genomic and proteomic biomarkers for cancer: A multitude of opportunities", *Biochimica et Biophysica Acta*, pp. 176–193.
12. Kovac, J. R., Pastuszak, A. W. and Lamb, D. J. (2013). "The use of genomics, proteomics and metabolomics in identifying biomarkers of male infertility", *Fertility and Sterility*, 99, pp. 998–1007.

13. Begg, K. and Tavassoli, M. (2017). "Biomarkers towards personalised therapy in cancer", *Drug Target Review*, 4(2), pp. 26–30.
14. Madamsetty, V. S., Mukherjee, A. and Mukherjee, S. (2019). "Recent trends of the bio-inspired nanoparticles in cancer theranostics", *Frontiers in Pharmacology*, 10, pp. 1264.
15. Ma, E. S. K. and Wong, C. L. P. (2010). "Cancer biomarker and molecular theranostics". *Journal of the Hong Kong College of Radiologists*, 13, pp. S42–S50.
16. Thakur, M. L. (2009). "Genomic biomarkers for molecular imaging: predicting the future". *Seminars in Nuclear Medicine*, 39(4), pp. 236–246.
17. Ulaner, G. A., Riedl, C. C., Dickler, M. N., Jhaveri, K., Pandit-Taskar, N. and Weber, W. (2016). "Molecular imaging of biomarkers in breast cancer," *Journal of Nuclear Medicine*, 57(Supplement_1), pp. 53S–59S.
18. Saifuddin, N., Raziah, A. Z. and Junizah, A. R. (2013). "Carbon nanotubes: a review on structure and their interaction with proteins," *Journal of Chemistry*, 2013, pp. 1–18.
19. Chan, J. M., Valencia, P. M., Zhang, L., Langer, R. and Farokhzad, O. C. (2010). "Polymeric nanoparticles for drug delivery", *Methods in Molecular Biology*, 624, pp. 163–175.
20. Abbasi, E., Aval, S. F., Akbarzadeh, A., Milani, M., Nasrabadi, H. T., Joo, S. W., Hanifehpour, Y., Koshki, K. N. and Pashaei-Asl, R. (2014). "Dendrimers: synthesis, applications, and properties", *Nanoscale Research Letters*, 9(1), p. 247.
21. Yue, X. and Dai, Z. (2018). "Liposomal nanotechnology for cancer theranostics", *Current Medicinal Chemistry*, 25(12), pp. 1397–1408.
22. Tripathi, S., Kaur, G., Khurana, R., Kapoor, S. and Singh, B. (2015). "Quantum dots and their potential role in cancer theranostics", *Critical Reviews in Therapeutic Drug Carrier Systems*, 32(6), pp. 461–502.
23. Yan, S., Zhao, P., Yu, T. and Gu, N. (2019). "Current applications and future prospects of nanotechnology in cancer immunotherapy", *Cancer Biology and Medicine*, 16(3), pp. 486–497.
24. Langbein T., Weber W. and Eiber M. (2019). "Future of theranostics: an outlook on precision oncology in nuclear medicine", *Journal of Nuclear Medicine*, 60(Supplement 2), pp. 13S–19S.
25. Bera, D., Qian, L., Tseng, T. K., & Holloway, P. H. (2010). Quantum dots and their multimodal applications: a review. Materials, 3(4), 2260–2345. https://doi.org/10.3390/ma3042260.
26. Medintz, I. L., Mattoussi, H., & Clapp, A. R. (2008). Potential clinical applications of quantum dots. International journal of nanomedicine, 3(2), 151–167. https://doi.org/10.2147/ijn.s614Chilton A., "The Properties and Applications of Quantum Dots" [Accessed from: https://www.azoquantum.com/Article.aspx?ArticleID=31].
27. Neha Bajwa, Neelesh K. Mehra, Keerti Jain & Narendra K. Jain (2016) Pharmaceutical and biomedical applications of quantum dots, Artificial Cells, Nanomedicine, and Biotechnology, 44(3), 758–768, DOI: 10.3109/21691401.2015.1052468.
28. Kelkar S. and Reineke T. (2011). "Theranostics: combining imaging and therapy", *Bioconjugate Chemistry*, 22(10), pp. 1879–1903.

15 Quantum Mechanics of Wound Healing: Nano-bio Interface of Wound Bed and Wound Dressing

Garima Shandilya, Kirtan Tarwadi, and Sachin Chavan

15.1 INTRODUCTION

There lies an interface between our body and this entire universe, which forms 16% of our physical body weight – Skin, the largest organ in our body. Skin is the foundation of the integumentary system, which includes our hairs, nails, specialized glands and nerves. It is made up of many layers of cells and lineages, including epidermis, dermis, hypodermis, keratinocytes, fibroblasts, and extracellular matrix. It also plays key roles in protecting, sensing, and regulating complex processes of physical sensation on pressure-sensitive skin components – merkel cells – conserving and releasing warmth from the body [1]. The skin effectively seals the internal organs and absorbs pressure, shocks and injury insults with flexible collagen, which makes up the dermis layer. It requires a lot of energy to maintain the healthy state of the skin functioning. It involves various mechanisms of maintaining co-ordination between the physical forces arising from mechanical forces and change in energy densities, resulting in chemical changes. These quantum changes regulate the organ's mechanics for performing essential biological tasks.

15.2 WHAT HAPPENS WHEN INJURY OCCURS?

Whenever minor cuts, deep lesions or traumatic gash occur on the skin, it ruptures the epidermis layer following invasion deep into hypodermis, leaking blood vessels, fragmented muscles and sometimes breaking bones (in traumatic cases). This results in changing energy alignment, chemical and physical arrangement and biofilm formation near and on the wound area [2]. These changes upshot cascade of signal transfers, ions movement, mechanical stress and stretch, overlapping cells and miscellaneous chemistry in multicellular organisms.

15.3 HOW DOES THE BODY REACT TO AN INJURY?

Multicellular organisms have a fundamental feature of self-repair of wounds through collective cellular movement attributed to cell crawling, '*purse-string*' contraction, stress signals and force patterns, in order to close the wound initially to prevent blood loss, invasion of micro-organisms and later, the body's immune system takes over to the wound site for remodeling the damaged tissues.

Wounds are compared with *'large biological building sites'*, where degraded dead tissues are replaced with a new cell assembly of extracellular matrix and collagen. Wound anabolism causes a series of biological events of harmonizing hormones for energy production, protein synthesis and breakdown, which begins with hemostasis and progressess through inflammatory response, formation of new connective tissue, epidermis and eventually remodeling [3]. The entire process is triggered by physical contraction, stress signals and adequate nutrients like vitamin C and proteins to aid healing.

The biology and cytology of cells attune the physiomechanics of cell build-up and tissue reconstruction. Wound repair within epithelial monolayers incorporates cell coordination for the congregation of branched and piled actin networks to synchronize cell movement through mechanical forces [6]. The transfiguration of cell-substrate abrasion and actin network criss-cross is determined by the rate at which reflexive muscle movement happens between cells, dermis and epidermal monolayers [4]. This quantum mechanism describes a robust physical representation explaining collective cell coordination through equilibrium and non-equilibrium comportment to dynamically modulate the cell-tissue mechanical output.

Various overlapping phases of cell derivation include mainly four stages-

1. Hemostasis
2. Inflammation
3. Proliferation
4. Tissue remodeling

15.3.1 *Hemostasis*

The first and foremost response to skin abuse comes from destruction of local blood vessels by the bruise. Immediate stoppage of local hemorrhage is achieved by platelet activation and assemblage, forming a temporary fibrin clot consisting of insoluble fibers.

Hemostasis is a spontaneous detainment or prevention of blood loss from injured or damaged vessels by physiological processes. It consists of three steps:

1. Vasoconstriction
2. Formation of temporary hemostatic plug
3. Defensive action

Cell crawling is coordinated by calibrating mechanical stresses taking place at cell interfaces between cell lineages, dermis, hypodermis, and extracellular matrix (ECM). The regulated continuance of this calibration determines the movement of epithelium along mucosa membranes and modulating renovation of epithelial wounds. Epithelial wound restoration is steered by the chip-in of differential relocation and coordination of spontaneous energy production and mechanical forces. This involves fabrication and contractility of unalike actin architectonics moving forward at different times.

At the early stages of wound repair, cells in proximity and distal to the wound migrate to pack the space. Migration inspired by 'cell-crawling' is driven by lamellipodial protrusions coupling focal adhesions, inducing contraction and ameboid motility of biological machines.

15.3.1.1 *Physiology of platelets*

In order to avert blood leakage, platelets and coagulation factors such as thrombin, pivotal factor V, VII, X, XII act in a coordinated manner to close the wound [5]. The platelets play an important role in sealing the wound and then a variety of coagulation factors add to form fibrin strands, which get stabilized as the clot grows.

The activation of coagulation factors can occur through two mechanisms: intrinsic and extrinsic. Extrinsic activation starts with exposed molecules of damaged vessel walls, such as tissue factor, which activates factor VII and which, in turn, triggers the formation of a factor X. The intrinsic pathway consists of various coagulation factors exciting each other in a chain reaction to activate factor X. This is a point where extrinsic and intrinsic pathways merge. Factor X plays an important role in coagulation cascade. Here Xa and Va combines and activates or catalyze thousands of thrombin. This new thrombin further activates platelets and intensify formation of fibrin. After this, fibrin forms a mesh, which stabilizes the platelet plug and arterial clot. This quantum physiology of platelets prevents blood loss, providing frontline protection from external environment [8].

15.3.2 *Inflammatory Response*

It is a non-specific defense and healing by the body to tissue damage or injury. It is initiated within minutes of infection or injury. This mechanics results in metabolic, physical and chemical activity, creating an environment conductive to healing and hostile to invading pathogens. Inflammation is characterized by redness, edema, pain and heat at the site of wound [6]. This channels four changes in the blood vessels.

> Redness and heat during inflammation is the result of increase in vascular diameter, which slows blood flow. Increase in vascular permeability. The

endothelial cells are generally packed together tightly with the blood vessels but during inflammation they have gaps between them. This results in a fluid exiting from the blood and getting accumulated in local tissues which outturns edema and pain. This fluid, which is called '*exudate*', consists of complement proteins and binding lectin, which fights invading pathogens and clears surface by keeping them out of site from the wound.

Endothelial cells activate cell-adhesion molecules that promote binding of circulating leukocytes, also called white blood cells. Clotting at the site of microinfection prevents pathogens from getting into circulation with blood.

15.3.2.1 *The Purpose of Inflammatory Response*

1. It allows to defend itself from invading microbes. The increased diameter and activated endothelial cells result in leukocytes being attached to the endothelium and then migrating into tissues to kill microbes. This process of leukocytes leaving the blood stream and entering tissues is called Extravasation.
2. It induces local blood clotting, which creates a physical barrier for infection to spread in the blood stream.
3. It promotes repair of damaged tissues [9].

15.3.2.2 *What Triggers the Inflammatory Response*?

A state of inflammation is set up when tissues are damaged or when pathogens or foreign invaders are recognized by other WBCs. Either of these liberates inflammatory mediators, which triggers an inflammatory response. Macrophage and neutrophils secrete prostaglandins, leukotrienes, platelet–activating factors, which are lipid mediators of inflammation. Macrophages secrete cytokines, which are substances released by cells of the immune system that affect other cells. One example of cytokines is chemokines, which produce chemotaxis, that is, the movement of cells or part of cells in a direction corresponding to the gradient of an increasing or decreasing concentration of the source of chemokines [10,11].

Two main inflammatory mediators are CVa and Tumor Necrosis Factor. CVa stimulates respiratory or oxidative burst and increases vascular permeability, which makes macrophage and neutrophils ready for battle with pathogens, and increases adhesion of certain molecules on the endothelium, which releases histamine and TNF from the mast cells.

TNF are produced rapidly by macrophages upon pathogen detection. It is a potent activator of endothelial cells. In succession, wound repair stages including lamellipodial protrusions concurring with multi-cellular bundles of actomyosin, also described as '*purse strings*', assemble at wound edges initiating contraction, pulling cells forward. The dynamics of closure and string movement depends upon flexure of wound and can arise in the presence or absence of underlying adhesion.

15.3.3 *Proliferation*

As an immediate temporary response to an injury, a clot or scab is formed as a protective barrier to restore the function of the skin. To attain permanent closure of the wound gap, 'proliferation, migration and contraction' activate a cell army to replenish lost and damaged tissues. This amalgamation of quantum movements within cells starts off within hours and the time required to heal varies and depends on age and health of tissues as well as on the size and location of the wound.

Re-epithelialization of damage is achieved by fusion of proliferation and migration of cells by keratinocytes in the vicinity of the wound. Kerationcytes alter cell-cell and cell-matrix adhesions, enabling their movement from fibrin strands and collagen. Migrating cells collect actin-rich lamellar protrusions for cell-crawling and upregulate the expression of proteolytic enzymes to bore a pathway at the interface between scab and viable tissue [12].

15.3.3.1 *Dermis Formation*

Fibroblasts in the neighborhood of a wound respond by making granulation tissues, which enable some connective tissue contraction. Circulating fibroblast and bone-marrow progenitor cells divide and migrate to the healthy dermis at the wound site to deposit new stroma, replacing the fibrin clot, which was temporary deposited earlier. Cooperatively, fibroblasts and myofibroblasts help in wound closure and contribute to the synthesis, bundling and alignment of collagen fibers into strands, which is the primary constituent of the scar [7].

15.3.4 *Resolution or Tissue Remodeling*

Wound resolution initiates many changes in the dermis.

1. Blood vessels within the scar are sifted and form a functional network when matured.
2. Earlier deposited extracellular matrix is remodeled.
3. This rebalance is done by a delicate balance of collagen synthesis, bundling and degradation.
4. Inflammatory response is resolved once the healing is completed, neutrophils are removed from wound site, and neutrophils and macrophages return to vasculature.

15.4 HEALING MECHANICS

Healing is a compounded biological process involving a well-ordered and prompt sequence of events and phases, which overlap and influence each other. The healing phases strictly followed by minor cuts and acute gashes progress through each stage towards successful tissue remodeling, maturation and wound closure [13]. The pathophysiological process is different for different types of wounds and varies according to the host factor.

When there is misbalance in any of the phases of the wound healing mechanism, it results in non-healing or chronic wounds. These wounds malfunction to heal in a physiologically ordered sequence of events, hindering morphological, clinical, biochemical, and microbiological differences, when compared to acute wounds. The misbalance results lodging in a particular wound stage, mostly inflammation and granulation phase, impeding progression toward wound healing.

15.5 MECHANICS OF BIOFILMS

Biofilms are 'complex biological systems,' which are structurally and dynamically a *'tridimensional microbial consortia,'* which closely pack microorganisms to the wound surface or to one another within the epopolysaccharide matrix (EPS). Biofilms can be envisioned as primitive multicellular organisms characterized by defense, adaptation, and pathogenesis. Chronic wounds or non-healing wounds are impacted in wound healing by biofilms, which delay inflammatory and maturation stages [14]. Upon research, it was found that polymicrobial biofilms weaken wound healing more significantly than monomicrobial biofilms, potentially due to synergistic interactions among bacteria expressing different virulence phenotypes. A hypothesis also suggested that biofilms might also help in maintaining wound homeostasis.

A biofilm allows bacteria and host to establish different social interactions, struggling or liaisoning together to form extracellular polymeric membranes. An increasing number of chronic incidences and biofilm infections need alternative therapeutic agents. Nanotechnology has revolutionized new ways in medicine by opening ways for antimicrobial coatings incorporating nanoparticles and their function as nanodrugs. Resistance to a large variety of infectious agents and foreign particles can be achieved by mere low concentrations of nanoparticles and nanostructured coatings. These coatings or dressings can contribute to the modulation of microbial colonies and biofilms formation in wounds. Biofilm formation occurs in five steps:

1. Wound contamination by fixing of microorganisms and settlement of host tissues.
2. Initially, microorganism adherence is reversible, which results in easy detachment of microbes by spontaneous physical or chemical methods and these are more susceptible to antibodies.
3. Maturation of biofilm is led by mucopolysaccharide matrix, which is composed of microbes and host molecules (polysaccharides, lipids, proteins and nucleic acid), which make biofilms tolerable to antibiotics and immune control.
4. Small organic compounds accomplish inter-bacterial communication via complex signaling networks, named quorum sensing.
5. Different bacteria species constitute different architectures of biofilm.

Delayed healing and microbial aggregation are consequences of biofilm establishment and depend on the host response to it through innate and adaptive immunity.

These biofilms are partially protected against the action of neutrophils, including phagocytosis, degranulation, and development of neutrophil extracellular traps [15]. Microbial virulence, microbial composition and diversity and composition of the extracellular matrix determine the efficiency of the immune defense. The physical and ecological stability of biofilms can contribute to the selection of more resistant or more virulent strains, which determine immune pressure to wound. Enzymes can also degrade collagen and other proteins as a result and cause harm to the host tissues and delay wound healing [16].

15.6 WHY ARE EXTERNAL AGENTS LIKE WOUND DRESSINGS AND COATINGS NECESSARY?

An effective wound-management strategy involves wound dressings as external agents aimed to prevent and treat infections, promote healing and prevent scarring. Wound-repair mechanics require an adequate balance between tissue damage and tissue repair, which should be maintained during inflammatory and remodeling phases. Various therapeutic options to treat this misbalance are available in this modern world [17]. Most infections can be intercepted by selecting correct high antibiotic pressure dressings and antimicrobial agents for highly resistant bacteria and pathogens. The risk of chronic and non-healing wounds is related to nosocomial infections and high antibiotic-resistant pathogens. Testing on the first line of treatment in minor and acute infections revealed that microbial tolerance and antibiotic therapy administered in non-toxic doses cannot eradicate biofilm infections and bactericidal concentrations. Also, systemic antibiotic therapy has lower availability at the site of infection and can increase the risk of microbial drug resistance. There is a fine line between the beneficial effects of antibiotic therapy like eradication of planktonic bacteria and biofilm disruption, its pathogenic effects, developing bacterial resistance and tolerance to antibiotics [18]. To move this border line towards an advantageous side, wound dressings play a very important role.

15.6.1 *Wound Dressings*

Wound dressings are engineered tools to facilitate rapid recovery of injuries. The dressings are mimicked to provide essentials vital for wound healing, exactly the same way the body's repair mechanism works. Wound dressing, when placed on the wound bed, forms a protective layer between the wound bed and the physical world. Then a number of processes work simultaneously, similar to the four stages of wound repair.

- **Initial step is to prevent blood loss**: This is done by wound dressing as it forms a layer and collagen wound dressing will form a cohesive gel sealing the space between wound bed and dressing.
- **Cleaning the wound**: The gel wound dressing has a property to pull out the

exudate residing within wound bed and simultaneously cleaning the area to eliminate microbial contamination.

- **Antimicrobial Nanoparticles**: To win the battle against microbes, bacteria, pathogens, nanoparticles behave as cytotoxic elements entering cell membrane and inducing DNA mutation for cell termination.
- **Healing agents transfer**: This is to provide wounds with proper nutrients and components that provide a sanitized positive healing environment and increase the rate of recovery. Aloe vera [20], glycerin, honey, *curcuma longa*, cinnamon, neem and other medicinal plants have been used in traditional medicine, serving multiple purposes as healers, nutrient donors, anti-microbial and anti-inflammatory elements [20].
- **Collagen dressings**: These provide the essential collagen fibers to the wound externally so that wound closure happens fast and is extra beneficial for chronic wound injuries. Collagen enhances movement of numerous types of cells, including chemotaxis, fibroblasts, keratinocytes, boosting tissue growth in wound bed.

Collagen derivatives, such as gelatin, gellen, chitosan, agarose, etc., are commonly used in biomedical engineering for tissue regeneration and scaffold engineering [21]. High abundance, low cost, biocompatibility, biodegradability, and low antigenicity of these wound-dressing materials make them ideal candidates in biomedicine. These materials can easily form a natural nanofiber structure, which is essential for skin regeneration. The structure, diameter and arrangement of these fibers recognize integrin receptors in the cells, which are crucial for cell adhesion [22].

15.6.2 *Drug-loaded dressings*

They provide essential drugs and antibiotics and play a key role of antibodies provided externally to favor wound repair. It is essential to provide drugs to wounds that are chronic and deep so as to protect them from infections and increase rapidity for healing.

15.6.3 *Easy Application and Removal of Dressings*

Hydrogels or collagen dressings [23] are easy to apply and wipe out from wounds as they adhere directly to the nanopores of the skin. Collagen wound dressings have gained attention due to their unique properties as they are eco-friendly, obtained from natural elements, less or not at all foul by-products, easily recyclable and no requisite for complex equipment to apply or remove [24].

15.6.4 *Advanced Wound Dressings and Coatings*

Wound dressing is aseptic pad or compressed coating applied to wound or injury to promote healing and epithelialization, further protecting the wound from distress. Wound dressings are a better option to cover the wound as they make direct contact with the damaged skin edges, unlike bandages. Modern dressings are self-adhesive and sometimes require bandages to hold dressings onto place. Numerous materials and engineering tools were developed in these recent years to create better wound dressings and exemplary coatings in wound dressing design [25]. The important characteristics that advanced dressing must possess are:

- Be able to create a moist, clean, and warm environment.
- Must hydrate dry and sloughy wound edges.
- Remove excess exudate from wound bed
- Prevent desiccation and be atraumatic.
- Easy exchange of gases and ions.
- Impermeable to microorganisms.
- Is free of toxic or irritant particles.
- Movement of healing agents from dressings to wound.
- Maintain pH of skin.
- Can contour to wound shape.
- Easy to apply and remove from the injured part reducing the pain; and
- No sophisticated instruments required for applying dressings.

15.7 NANOTECHNOLOGY FOR WOUND MANAGEMENT

Nanotechnology offers potential applications and cutting-edge solutions to design and engineer efficient biomedical approaches to solve medical complications. A number of nanomaterials have been developed and proved to have remarkable applications in wound care and healing. Nanostructures and varied shaped nanoparticles (rod shape, sphere, triangular, core-shell) are incredible components that aim to reinforce therapeutic delivery of growth factors, antimicrobial agents, gene therapy vectors and others to the wound. The most explored approaches for management of wounds invoke development of nano-devices for (i) inflammation control; (ii) cellular proliferation and re-epithelization; and (iii) tissue remodeling.

Nanoparticles, engineered nanosystems and modified dressings include a variety of nanomaterials, anti-microbial and anti-fungal nanoparticles (organic and inorganic), functionalized and modified nanoparticles, bioactive nanosystems (nanoscaffolds, nanogels), nanodetectors, nanosensors and nanoparticles embedded systems for effective wound management. Recent advancement in the development of nanostructured wound coatings and wound dressing incorporating nanoparticles is the main solution for treating non-healing and chronic wounds. Optimization of nanomaterials and nanodressings can circumvent microbial contamination of wound and disrupt biofilm formation at the wound site, which delays or reduces the chances of healing [26].

Nanotechnology has acquired a lot of consideration in the biomedical field due to its promising and favorable outcomes giving best solutions to drastic medical problems. Nanoparticles were studied, researched and proved as optimistic candidates for wound treatment. Metallic silver and gold nanoparticles are used as antimicrobial agents against pathogenic bacteria and microbes, exhibiting remarkable tolerance to multiple antibiotics. Many research works have shown that nanotechnology has accomplished remarkable results in the treatment of bacterial and microbial infections. Nanoparticles can be variegated as coatings on implantable devices or biomaterials having antibacterial properties, fighting bacterial infections, enhancing wound healing by antibiotic delivery systems and controlled drug delivery, microbial diagnosis through bacterial detection systems and vaccines. Several processes, including induction of oxidative stress, metal ion release, exudate suction and non-oxidative means which promote anti-microbial and anti-fungal actions of nanoparticles. Studies suggest that silver nanoparticles (AgNPs) effectively offset electric charge on the surface of bacterial membranes, disrupting their permeability following bacterial downfall. Electrostatic binding of nanoparticles with the cell wall of bacteria results in rupturing the bacterial membrane and entering the bacterial cell to destroy its nucleus, ensuring bacterial death [27].

Nanoparticles have shown to damage the robustness, resting potential, stimuli integration and depolarization of membrane, which results in loss of primary functions of cell such as ion and gas exchange, hindering internal electric charge, lysis, cellular respiration and energy conversion, which ultimately leads to cell death. High concentrations of ROS (reactive oxygen species) induced by nanoparticle interaction with cell membrane can damage DNA or RNA or persuade mutations of microbes, which ultimately leads to deactivating microbes. Production of ROS is effective in inducing cytotoxicity by nanoparticles, which can be obtained either indirectly or directly: indirect toxicity by perturbation in the cellular respiratory chain and direct toxicity by nanoparticle adhesion [28].

15.8 QUANTUM BEHAVIOR OF NANO-BIO INTERFACE

When wound dressings are applied to an open wound site, they form an interface connecting two different worlds working together for one motive as a wound-healing mechanism. Advanced wound dressings containing nanotechnology constitute the nanosphere, and the open wound with all the living mechanics of cells and biological events comprise the biosphere. This interaction configures the Nano-bio interface [29]. This conformational intramolecular interaction manifests incredible quantum mechanics to revive the usual biological affairs as before the injury. Figure 15.1: (Wound Healing mechanism and Nano-bio interface for wound management) perfectly shows nano-bio interface in wound dressings.

Collagen wound dressings contour the wound surface perfectly, as shown in Figure 15.1 (Wound Healing mechanism and Nano-bio interface for wound management). Epithelial monolayers are adhered to collagen-coated hydrogels or wound dressings creating small holes and initiating ablation process, which induce rapid outward retraction in surrounding cells. Wound-dressing curves onto the wound surface leaving no space for interaction of outer environment with the damaged site [30]. Collagen agents in dressings enhance cell syllable structure, actin dynamics and function-modulating pharmacotherapy by formation of lamellipodia or purse strings. Despite differences in monolayer viscoelasticity, wound closure mechanics is independent of substrate stiffness or mechanotransduction. Differential cytoskeletal tension and stiffness or reaction to collagen substrate leads to differences in cell–substrate adhesion and spreading, dramatically affecting cell

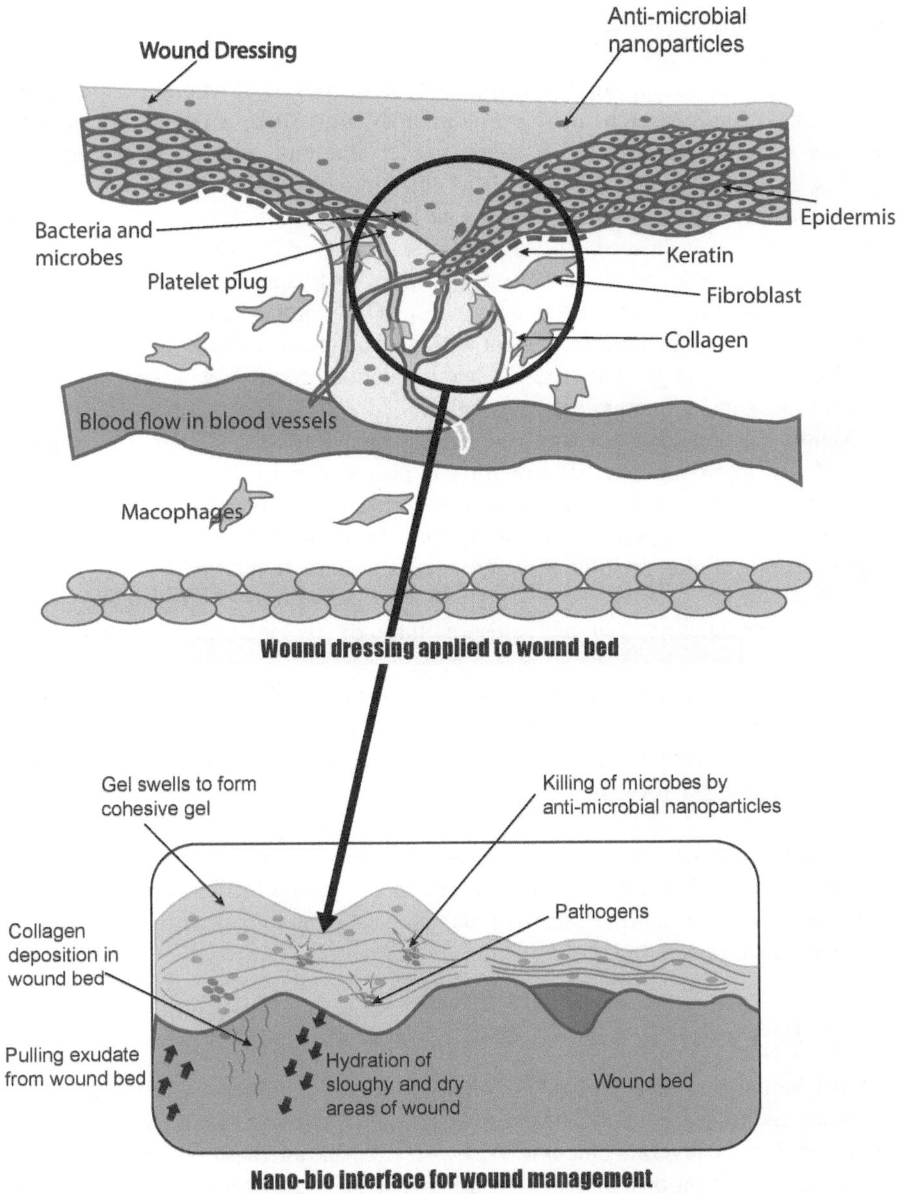

FIGURE 15.1 Wound Healing Mechanism and Nano-bio Interface for Wound Management.

migration and dictating friction between monolayer and dressing substrate. Tissues develop powerful action forces using actin-protein synthesis and attune these forces against external loading by dressings. Body immune resistance is referred to as 'tensional or energy homeostasis' with respect to maintaining a mechanical equilibrium in cell colonies, traction localized to colony boundaries and total elastic strain-stretch energy, which increases linearly as the size of colony gets localized to ruling edges of drifting cell monolayers [31].

In the wound-healing process, cell density is restrained to wound periphery and drive elastic strain-stretch energy to diminish with time, signaling to turn-off multiple on-going tasks such as shape-size oscillations, altering membrane mechanics, regulating clustering forces and cell biology. However, the strain energy drops rectilinearly with shrinking wound perimeter, suggesting leading edge tension during dynamics of closure. As velocity is inversely related to energy density, the architecture of cells and effective power does not change, compensating cell-migration and purse-string mechanism [32]. This compensation is regulated by substrate stiffness, actomyosin content and focal adhesion stability, which may also be applicable to a single cell. These relate regulation of cytoskeletal machineries to regulate mechanical energy at tissue-scales.

Quantitative scenario for mechanisms driving wound closure in an epithelial sheet shows that collective cell crawling is responsible for initial steps of wound closure but, at later stages of the process, involve cooperation between cell crawling and contraction of a supracellular actomyosin ring at the leading edges of the wound where a supracellular versatile structure serves at least two purposes.

1. It contributes to wound closure through its well-known purse-string mechanism.
2. It transmits part of its contractile force to the substrate through focal adhesions that are mainly tangential to the wound. These contractile forces induce a displacement of underlying gel towards wound area and thus tend to steer the monolayer forward.

Forces in single or collective cell systems are different from leading-edge dynamics and force patterns. Therefore, search for new mechanotransduction strategies as well as broader context of morphogenesis in wound closure and management is beneficial for future advancements [33].

15.8.1 *Role of pH in Wound Management*

The pH value of wound milieu indirectly or directly influences all biochemical reactions taking place in the healing process. However, it is so far a neglected parameter for the overall outcome. The pH value is an important parameter for therapeutic interventions in wound care and a key determinant for metabolism during wound healing. The body's inbred guarding system prevents bacteria from entering open sites by producing pus in the wound. This pus shifts the pH value towards acidic milieu. The correlation between skin pH and the bacterial contamination level decides whether the wound is progressing towards a positive environment for recovery or resulting in long-term inflammation [34].

In healing of critical wounds, body groupsall physiological acidosis on a temporary basis, resulting from several contributing factors working simultaneously to maintain pH of damaged site throughout the duration of healing. Organic acids, like lactic acid, are generated during the healing process, increasing the demand for O_2 with a sudden rise in local CO_2 due to tissue perfusion in the wound space. The production of lactic acid is linked with increase in glycolysis during the phase of increased collagen production as healing progressess, which reaches its physiological peak at later stages of wound healing.

Epithelial sheets covering the injury follow long-range coordination of motions, fluctuating forces, energy levels, grappling all chemicals to build-up tension in tissues, flesh to enhance cell crawling and accelerating wound assuage. Epithelial sheets display different shapes: finger-like lumps for epithelial edges and bulk sheets as spirals of motile cells. Multicellular organisms have a remarkable property to reform themselves even from severe damage to their original forms. Thus, wound healing is nature's pivotal process for regaining basic tissue and flesh structure and restoring their biological functions.

Quantum mechanics of wound healing shows that a very simple cut or interruption in skin can invoke an avalanche of cell signaling, with planar cell polarity directing interactions between polarization of neighboring cells, spreading of epithelial colonies, adjusting chemical balance and sustaining mechanical force patterns. Single cells coordinate their mobility forces and velocity in the direction where the damage occured to provide various nutrients and collagen to wound. Lamellipodia protrusive sheets filled with actin filaments hidden beneath neighboring cells generate motility forces to compel lamellipodium to exert force in the direction of the cell's velocity to quickly realign with the cell's direction and fill the gap formed. A biological perspective of this type of interaction can easily be imagined as a construction site where cell architects work together to set up the damaged wall [35].

15.8.2 *Nutrients in Wound Management*

Nutrition is mostly outlined in each wound healing phase and other vital processes in signal generation, migrating cells, macrophages, leukocyte, collagen to wound site, balancing chemical changes. Essential building units such as cells, enzymes need vitamins, amino acids, minerals, natural compounds, herbal extracts, target DNA-regulating transcription factors, cytokines, extracellular matrix proteins and glycosaminoglycan for proper functioning, maintaining and regulating basic life events and also plays an important role in the wound-healing process. Clinical evidence of dietary supplements administration supports that satisfactory nutritional status is crucial for promoting healing of wounds, synthesis of collagen, new blood vessels and exactly duplicating the genetic mechanism of action and cells by all biological machines to complete the task [36].

New technologies in which enzymes are added in wound dressings have made it possible to fabricate interactive dressings that detect pathogens with their fine-tuned properties, prevent wound infection, kill microbes and promote wound healing. Wound dressings with a synchronized degradation property, heals wound by maintaing adequate moisture to avert drying of wound edges, balancing optimal ion and nutrient movement, and regulating pH of wound. Giving importance to antimicrobial, anti-inflammatory, healing agents and drug loads to be incorporated in dressings is a needed milestone that can help develop controlled release of drugs and healing agents as and when required, thereby avoiding the difficulty and toxicity associated with topical administration of concentrated and heavy drug loads [37].

Further, despite the success of advanced dressings, some wound dressings exhibit poor mechanical properties, which require considerable research efforts for further improvement. This can be done by adding nanoparticles, growth factors or other agents as strengthening molecules into a hydrogel network or coats. These molecules, when applied to wounds externally, can invigorate granulation-tissue formation, progress wound healing and enhance epithelialization [38].

The limited therapeutic activity of growth factors and their high cost require dedicated research efforts to synthesize effective dressings for all at affordable costs. The healing agents called "*protective antigen*," which are present in wound-dressing nanopores, penetrate cell walls and change ion charge, thus reflecting a change in voltage across the cell membrane and encouraging ion flow through the pore. Healing agents also secrete other proteins called "*lethal factor*" and "*edema factor*," which get easily bonded to nanopores, opening flow of ions through the channel as the wound proceeds to progressive stages of healing [39].

The researchers are pursuing their work on several fronts to modify advance dressings and coats such as adding more colors, textures, cloth-like characteristics to the materials, real-time monitoring of wound progress and sustained release of drugs and healing complexes in wound dressings.

15.8.3 *Energy Conservation in Wounds*

Studying wound healing from the viewpoint of energy conservation incorporates basic diminutions and physics laws on wound healing, which provide different insights into wound repair. Calculating how much energy is taken to move cells, growth factors, blood, collagen, healing agents to wound cavity, removing dead cells, tissues, vessels and comparing this to the total energy required to run basic metabolism gives us an extra energy estimation required during the repair process [40]. Scientists have also considered a mathematical model of energy usage by all metabolic processes and concluded energy requirements into three parts:

> Energy required for the immune system to combat infection, energy required to maintain existing cell tissue and to grow new tissues, and energy requirement for growing new cells.

It was researched that the body requires approximately 20 kilo Joules per gram energy for every new tissue grown. This concludes that, in physical terms, wounds behave as a black hole for energy, trapping forces and directing them for repair.

However, the total energy expense available for doing all the tasks, including vital life function and maintenance cannot be exceeded; hence proper nutrients and healing agents are of utmost importance to conserve energy sources. Various predictions and other factors can be explained well by performing animal tests. Results on how much time a wound takes to heal, or the wound-closure rate, will open an amazing insight to understand the laws of physics that contribute to biological processess [41].

15.9 CONCLUSIONS

Understanding wound-healing science, factors involved in management and regeneration, role of external agents, pH, nutrients, energy conversation involving quantum physics, quantum chemistry, quantum biology, quantum mechanics in every stage of wound-healing helps us to seek and embrace nature's wisdom. Innovative biotechnology and nanotechnology approaches in development of next-generation wound-dressings including enzymes, nanoparticles, coatings, sensors, plant-derived herbs and natural compounds, controlled drug reservoirs, fighting mechanism to deal with infections and contaminations are proofs how science can lead to novel approaches and unprecedented opportunities for the betterment of humankind.

REFERENCES

1. Shaw, T. J. and Martin, P. (2009) "Wound repair at a glance", *Journal of Cell Science*, **122**, pp. 3209–3213.
2. Sonnemann, K. J. and Bement, W. M. (2011) "Wound repair: Toward understanding and integration of single-cell and multicellular wound responses", *Annual Review of Cell and Developmental Biology*, **27**, pp. 237–263.
3. Kuipers, D. et al. (2014) "Epithelial repair is a two-stage process driven first by dying cells and then by their neighbours", *Journal of Cell Science*, **127**, pp. 1229–1241.
4. Robson, M. C., Steed, D. L. and Franz, M. G. (2001) "Wound healing: Biologic features and approaches to maximize healing trajectories", *Current Problems in Surgery*, 38, pp. 72–140.
5. Arnout J., Hoylaerts M. F. and Lijnen H. R. (2006) "Haemostasis", *Handbook of Experimental Pharmacology*, 176 Pt 2, pp. 1–41. PMID:17001771, DOI: 10.1007/3-540-36028-x_1.
6. Shaw T.J. and Martin P. (2009) "Wound repair at a glance", *Journal of Cell Science*, 122, pp. 3209–3213. doi: 10.1242/jcs.031187.
7. Broughton, G., Janis, J. E. and Attinger, C. E. (2006) "The basic science of wound healing", *Plastic and Reconstructive Surgery*, 117(7 suppl), pp. 12S–34S.
8. Ghoshal K. and Bhattacharyya M. (2013) "Overview of platelet physiology its hemostatic and nonhemostatic role in disease pathogenesis", *The Scientific World Journal*, 2014, p. 781857. https://doi.org/10.1155/2014/781857.
9. Libby P. (2007) "Inflammatory mechanisms: The molecular basis of inflammation and disease", *Nutrition Reviews*, 2007(65), pp. S140–S146.
10 Jameson, J. M., Sharp, L. L., Witherden, D. A. and Havran, W. L. (2004) "Regulation of skin cell homeostasis by gamma delta T cells", *Frontiers in Bioscience*, 9, pp. 2640–2651.
11. Cumberbatch, M., Dearman, R. J., Griffiths, C. E. and Kimber, I. (2000) "Langerhans cell migration", *Clinical and Experimental Dermatology*, 25, pp. 413–418.
12. Cohen I. K. and McCoy B. J. (1983) "Wound healing", *Biochemistry and Physiology of the Skin*. Goldsmith, L. A. (ed.). Oxford University Press, London, pp. 462–470.
13. Lambert W.C., Cohen P.J., Klein K.M., and Lambert M.W. (1985) *Cellular and Molecular Mechanisms in Wound Healing: Selected Concepts. From the Departments of Pathology and Medicine and the Medical Class*, UMDNJ, New Jersey.

14. Phillips P. L., Wolcott R. D., Fletcher J. and Schultz G. S. (2010) "Biofilms made easy", *Wounds International*, 1(3).
15. Carver C. (2017) "How to identify biofilm in a wound", *Wound Source*. http://www.woundsource.com/blog/how-identify-biofilm-in-wound. Published August 18, 2015. Accessed December20.
16. Donlan R. M. (2002) "Biofilms: Microbial life on surfaces", *Emerging Infectious Diseases*, 8(9), pp. 881–890.
17. Rivera, A.E. and Spencer J.M. (2007) "Clinical aspects of full-thickness wound healing", *Clinical Dermatology*, 25, pp. 39–48.
18. Ayello E. A., Baranoski S., Kerstein M. D. and Cuddigan J. (2003) "Wound treatment options", Baranoski S. and Ayello E. A. (eds.). *Wound Care Essentials: Practice Principles*. Lippincott Williams & Wilkins, Philadelphia, PA, p. 138.
19. Atiba A., Ueno H., and Uzuka Y. (2011) "The effect of aloe vera oral administration on cutaneous wound healing in type 2 diabetic rats", *Journal of Veterinary Medical Science*, 73(5), pp. 583–589. https://doi.org/10.1292/jvms.10-0438.
20. Shedoeva A., Leavesley D., Upton Z. and Fan C. (2019) "Wound Healing and the Use of Medicinal Plants", *Hindawi Evidence-Based Complementary and Alternative Medicine Volume*, Article ID 2684108, 30 pages, https://doi.org/10.1155/2019/2684108.
21. Fleck C. A. and Chakravarthy D. (2007) "Understanding the mechanisms of collagen dressings", *Advances in Skin & Wound Care*, 20(5), pp. 256–259.
22. Schultz G. S. and Mast B. A. (1998) "Molecular analysis of the environment of healing and chronic wounds: Cytokines, proteases, and growth factors", Wounds, 10(6 Suppl F), pp. 1F–9F.
23. Zheng Y., Liang Y., Zhang D., Sun X., Liang L., Li J., and Liu Y.-N. (2018) "Gelatin-based hydrogels blended with gellan as an injectable wound dressing", *ACS Omega*, 3(5), pp. 4766–4775. DOI: 10.1021/acsomega.8b00308.
24. Grant M. E. and Prockop D. J. (1972) "The biosynthesis of collagen", *The New England Journal of Medicine*, 286(4), pp. 194–199.
25. Buhus G., Peptu C., Popa M. and Desbrieres J. (2009) "Controlled release of water-soluble antibiotics by carboxymethyl cellulose- and gelatin-based hydrogels crosslinked with epichlorohydrin", *Cellulose Chemistry and Technology*, 43, pp. 141–151.
26. Mihai, M. M., Dima, M. B., Dima, B. and Holban, A. M. (2019) "Nanomaterials for wound healing and infection control", *Materials (Basel, Switzerland)*, 12(13), p. 2176. https://doi.org/10.3390/ma12132176.
27. Pourjavadi A. and Soleyman R. (2011) "Silver nanoparticles with gelatin nanoshells: photochemical facile green synthesis and their antimicrobial activity", *Journal of Nanoparticle Research*, 13, pp. 4647–4658.
28. Alberti T., Coelho D. S., Voytena A., Pitz H., de Pra M., Mazzarino L., Kuhnen S., Ribeiro-do-Valle R. M., Maraschin M. and Veleirinho B. (2017) "Nanotechnology: A promising tool towards wound healing", *Current Pharmaceutical Design*, 23(24), pp. 3515–3528. doi: 10.2174/1381612823666170503152550.
29. Hamdan S., Pastar I., Drakulich S., Dikici E., Tomic-Canic M., Deo S. and Daunert S. (2017) "Nanotechnology-driven therapeutic interventions in wound healing: Potential uses and applications", *ACS Central Science*, 3(3), pp. 163–175. doi: 10.1021/acscentsci.6b00371.
30. Griffith L. G. (2002) "Emerging design principles in biomaterials and scaffolds for tissue engineering", *Annals of the New York Academy of Science*, 961, pp. 83–95.
31. Farooqui R. and Fenteany G. (2005) "Multiple rows of cells behind an epithelial wound edge extend cryptic lamellipodia to collectively drive cell-sheet movement", *Journal of Cell Science*, 118 (Pt 1), pp. 51–63.
32. Tambe D. T., et al. (2011) "Collective cell guidance by cooperative intercellular forces", *Nature Materials*, 10(6), pp. 469–475.

33. Serra-Picamal X., et al. (2012) "Mechanical waves during tissue expansion", *Nature Physics*, 8(8), pp. 628–634.
34. Schneider Lars, A., Korber, A., Grabbe, S. and Dissemond J. (2007) "Influence of pH on wound-healing: A new perspective for wound-therapy?", *Archives of Dermatological Research*, 298(9), pp. 413–420, DOI 10.1007/s00403-006-0713-x.
35. Hunt T. K., Twoney P., Zederfeldt B. and Dunphy J. E. (1967) "Respiratory gas tension and pH in healing wounds", *American Journal of Surgery*, 114(2), pp. 302–307.
36. Palmieri, B., Vadalà, M. and Laurino, C. (2019) "Nutrition in wound healing: Investigation of molecular mechanisms, a narrative review", *Journal of Wound Care*, 28(10), pp. 683–693.
37. Van Anholt R. D., Sobotka L., Meijer E. P., et al. (2010) "Specific nutritional support accelerates pressure ulcer healing and reduces wound care intensity in non-malnourished patients", *Nutrition*, 26(9), pp. 867–872. DOI: https://doi.org/10.1016/j.nut.2010.05.009.
38. Scholl D. and Langkamp-Henken B. (2001) "Nutrient recommendations for wound healing", *Journal of Intravenous Nursing*, 24(2), pp. 124–132.
39. Abe T., Abe Y. and Aida Y. (2001) "Extracellular matrix regulates induction of alkaline phosphatase expression by ascorbic acid in human fibroblasts", *Journal of Cellular Physiology*, 189(2), pp. 144–151. DOI: https://doi.org/10.1002/jcp.10011.
40. Basan M., Elgeti J., Hannezo E., Rappel W.-J. and Levine H. (2013) "Alignment of cellular motility forces with tissue flow as a mechanism for efficient would healing," *Proceedings of the National Academy of Sciences*, 110(7), pp. 2452-2459. DOI: 10.1073/pnas.1219937110
41. Apell, S. P., Neidrauer M., Papazoglou E.S. and Pizziconi V. (2012) "Physics of Wound Healing I: Energy Considerations", [physics.med-ph]-arXiv:1212.3778.

16 Ongoing Challenges with the Safety and Toxicity of Nanoparticles in the Field of Medicine

Kalvatala Sudhakar

16.1 INTRODUCTION

In nanotechnology, a particle is described as a small entity that acts as a whole in terms of transport and properties. Nanoparticles possess tremendous potential for therapeutics delivery [1]. The rapid development of nanotechnology means that each day, new nanostructures and new opportunities for their use are developed [2]. The area of nanomedicine is as broad, if not greater, as the world of small-molecule drugs. It may be unjustified to make broad assumptions about the possible toxicity of small-molecule drugs, since they are effective for a range of uses, from inactive drugs (e.g. sugar pill-glucose) to euthanasia drugs (pentobarbital:- ending a life in a painless manner) [3]. The nanoparticle (diameter < 100 nm) has a broad reactive surface, which can interfere positively with biological processes and contribute to toxic effects, particularly, in comparison with typical micro-scale substances (molecular diameter represented in microns) [4]. The adaptation of traditional nanoparticles legislation, the introduction of mandatory legislation for currently unregulated nanoparticles-containing products and the establishment by authorities of an electronic database for the efficient extraction of nanomedicinal knowledge is important for any distribution of nanoparticles in the body and is a prerequisite for any nanodrug delivery [5]. The standards for assessing nanospecific hazardous properties must be continually revised and tailored to the state-of-the-art of knowledge [6]. Numerous experiments have been carried out to better explain the effect of nanomaterials on human safety, and to help us create healthier and non-toxic materials [7]. Nanomaterial medicines that operate at the intersection of matter and life show great potential to enhance patient treatment [8]. The toxicity grade for a bulk material can be approximately determined by three factors (chemical composition, dose, and exposure route) [9]. Other nanoproperties include small size, form and reactivity, retaining period and dissemination in the body after breaching biological-barrier membranes, as well as sub-cellular and molecular interactions that play a qualitative role in assessing toxicity, i.e. the hazardous ability of the nanomaterial and the non-nanoscale comparable product that vary considerably [6]. Toxicity is a crucial aspect to be considered when assessing its potential for biomedical purposes, particularly in vivo activities [1]. The prons and cons of delivery cargo are important for any formulation scientist.

16.2 NANODRUG DELIVERY SYSTEM

16.2.1 Silver Nanoparticles

In recent times, silver nanoparticles (AgNPs) have become one of the most researched and investigated nanostructures emerging from nanotechnology, as nanosilver-oriented components have shown their use for a variety of therapeutic activities to be important, overwhelming and encouraging [10]. Although AgNPs have significant benefits that advocate them for novel and biomedical purposes, their toxicity (Figure 16.1) has only recently become an intense topic of research [10,11]. AgNPs do have a range of pitfalls and some limitations because of their nanotoxicity [11].

At present, however, there is very restricted and sometimes contradictory evidence on the toxicity of AgNPs, which has been largely derived from in vivo studies [12,13]. There has been minimal research to determine nanosilver toxicity. Using in-vitro assay, AgNP toxicity was shown to induce oxidative stress and impaired mitochondrial function in rodent mouse hepto-cells at low degrees of exposure. By interrupting mitochondrial activity and allowing the cell membrane

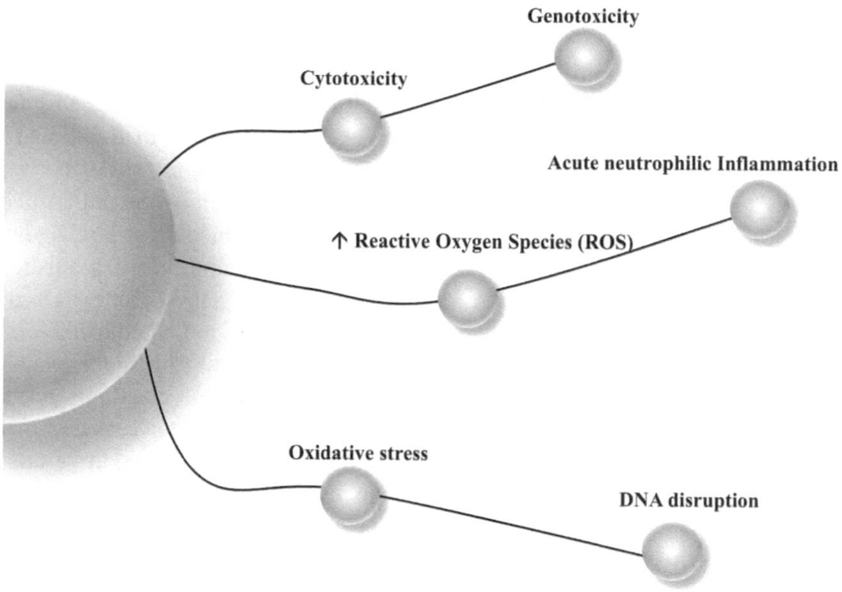

FIGURE 16.1 Toxicity of Silver Nanoparticles.

to leak, silver nanoparticles are poisonous to germline stem cells in in vitro mouse [11]. Ag-NPs have the ability to cause genotoxicity through oxidative stress in Sprague-Dawley rat bone-marrow cells [14]. In BEAS-2B cells, Ag-NPs exhibit genotoxic effects, and the oxidative stress caused by Ag-NPs may be a significant factor in their genotoxic effects [15]. Polyvinylpyrrolidone and citrate-AgNPs induce haemolysis and are acquired by erythrocytes. In fact, researchers have shown that AgNPs cause oxidative stress and eryptosis [16,17].

16.2.2 Carbon Nanotubes

CNTs for biomedical purposes, like those of drug-delivery systems as well as biomaterials, are under investigation [18]. Despite their many special physical and chemical properties, CNTs play a significant role in drug delivery as a cargo system [19]. Toxicity relies on various properties of CNTs, such as single wall or multiple wall, volume, aspect ratio, diameter, degree of aggregation, functional group attached to CNTs quality, composition, and dosage [18,19]. Carbon nanotubes are potential drug-delivery agents; nevertheless, their pulmonary toxicity can be a major drawback to their practical application [19]. It appears that the size of CNTs is important to their toxic capacity [20]. The physical properties of CNTs are liable for pulmonary toxicity in animals as inhalation of fine nanoparticles via the pulmonary networks is one of the most generally recorded types of CNT transmission as drug delivery [21]. Respiratory exposure to SWCNTs could induce acute pulmonary and cardiovascular responses. Respiratory exposure to SWCNTs containing different metal contents could induce acute pulmonary and cardiovascular responses. Inflammation biomarkers, oxidative stress, and cell disruption were substantially increased after 24 hour access to SWCNTs in bronchoalveolar fluid lavage. Elevated amounts of endothelin-1 in BALF and plasma and angiotensin I-converting (ACE-I) enzymes in plasma indicated endothelial impairment in pulmonary circulation and peripheral vascular thrombosis [22]. CNTs exhibit exceptional cell-transfection capabilities. CNTs also have the ability to enter cells, irrespective of specific groups, on the surface edge of CNTs, enabling the transport of intracellular drug molecules and genes, including protein. CNTs can either exit the body via urinary excretion or accumulate in secondary organs, staying indefinitely if the immune system fails to eliminate them [23–28]. The fate and toxicity of carbon nanotubes depend on different functional groups, length and surface area of CNTs. Hydroxylated single-wall carbon nanotubes are scattered rapidly across the whole body and accrue in the bone. Every coin has two sides; similarly, CNTs have some robust properties and some limitations, such as low dose loading. If the drug level is to be increased in the body, more CNTs need to be used to maintain the concentration of the drug in the body. But increasing the CNTs' concentration in cells may increase cell toxicity. In order to overcome these problems, CNTs can linked or be incorporated into nanovesicles liposomes, which act as drug carriers in the nanotrain drug-delivery system.

Zhu et al. studied the nanotrain drug delivery of DOX–SWCNTs–liposome. It was formulated to have the double effect of CNTs and liposomes to target and increase the DOX content in the tumor site for a long time. Long MWCNTs produced the most harm to DNA and enhanced the total amount of cells in the abdominal lavage fluid. MWCNTs of varying lengths are responsible for various degrees of granuloma development. The shorter size of MWCNTs, which show high crystallinity in nature demonstrate cytotoxicity in vitro and eventual in vivo inflammation and mesotheliomagenicity [22]. CNTs can exercise an oxidative response, which activates inflammatory, genotoxic and cytotoxic effects [20]. CNTs infiltrate the cell membranes, which are lipid bilayers in nature, leading to oxidative stress that can contribute to inflammation and cytotoxicity. Since CNTs behave as a foreign body to cell, foreign body response is elicited and chemicals are released to eliminate CNTs from the cell [21]. Fiber-like CNTs have properties reminiscent of asbestos and cause some of the same disease outcomes when they are inhaled into the lungs of laboratory mice [29]. CNTs are strong pulmonary fibrogen inductors, characterized by the over-deposition of collagen fibers and the scaring of affected tissues, which induce interstitial, bronchial, myofibroglyphic, lung and pleural fibrosis [30]. Because of the multiple applications and significance of CNTs, their thresholds of toxicity and impacts on the human body pose a global concern [21]. Generally, simply dispersed CNTs are more toxic than the covalently modified ones, but the toxicity of simply dispersed CNTs is still very low, even with long-term observation [31].

It has been observed that pristine MWCNTs with a large aspect ratio, surface hydrophobicity and metallic impurities were found to inflict serious hepatotoxicity and oxidative damage in rodents; however, the effect was repaired after 28 days of therapy. Conversely, carboxylic acid oxidized CNTs with shorter lengths, water-soluble surfaces and high aqueous dispersibility have been found to be less harmful and more biocompatible than their pristine equivalents [32]. Lacerda et al. indicated that serum-dispersed pristine MWCNTs were far more deleterious than amino-MWCNTs [33]. Amino and polyethylene glycol (PEG) groups and Pluronic F108 can reduce CNT cytotoxicity; while albumin coating can specifically reduce SWCNT toxicity, Pluronic F108 decreases the MWCNTs toxicity in lungs [34–38].

16.2.3 Dendrimers

The usage of polymeric nanoparticles such as dendrimers in the transport of therapeutic molecules and genes, has given rise to a significant area in the biomedical field [39]. The toxic effects of dendrimers are typically identified by haemolytic toxicity, cytotoxicity and haematological toxicity in the biological process [40] (Figure 16.2). The cytotoxicity of dendrimers relies strongly on the amount and type of specific surface-groupings. Cationic dendrimers are mostly extremely toxic, while anionic and neutral dendrimers have mild to no adverse effects [40,41]. The generation-dependent toxicity of higher-generational dendrimers polyamidoamine (PAMAM) G4, G5 and G6 has been documented to create nanoscale holes in the lipid bilayer, resulting in greater toxicity [39]. Recent research has shown that functionalized amine-terminated cationic polyamidoamine dendrimers lead to a toxic effect, which when given intravenously to mice and zebrafish show blood-clot

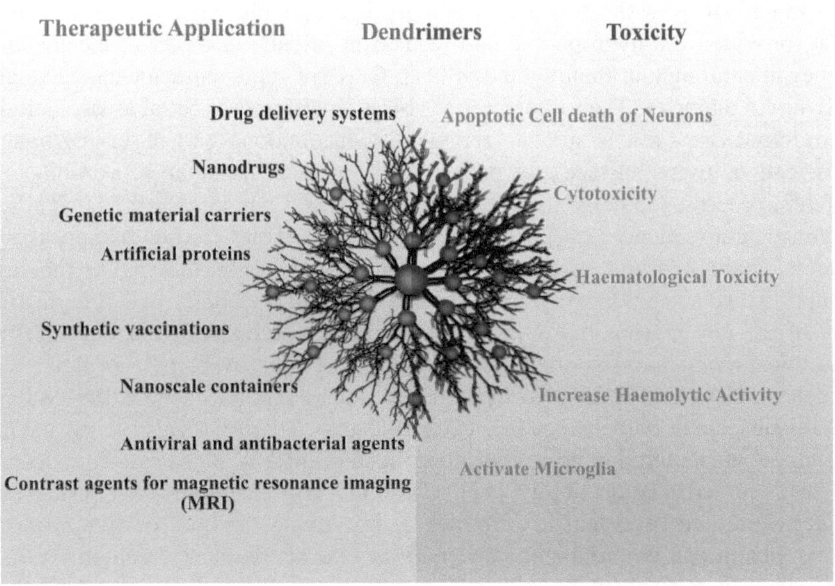

FIGURE 16.2 Balance of Therapeutic Potential Along with Toxicity Profile of Dendrimers.

formation and activate platelets, which lead to fatal complications, whereas neutral and anionic dendrimers of the same type revealed no detectable vascular complications [39]. Dendrimers G4 of cationic PAMAM are harmful for the larvae of Zebrafish and rely on the dosage and length of exposure [39]. The level class of PAMAM toxicity is hydroxyl-terminated$<$carboxyl-terminated$<$amine-terminated dendrimers [39,42–44]. The severity and nature of toxicity responses rely, therefore, on the generation and dosage of dendrimers [43]. The higher generation of cationic dendrimers shows a toxicity profile in zebrafish embryos when compared to anionic dendrimers. The strongest predictor of dendrimer toxic effects is perhaps the surface charge. Dendrimer category and generations are other possible sources of the toxic effects of dendrimers [39]. Cationic PAMAM dendrimers have shown skin-irritant properties while being used as a topical formulation in a rat model [44]. Several dendrimers are toxic, owing to their positively charged surfaces [45]. The charge of the end groups of the cationic dendrimers appeared to be the major reason for the in-vitro toxicity [44]. A higher dose of uncoated Poly(propyleneimine) dendrimers triggered toxicity, but surface alteration almost absolutely eliminated this toxic impact [45].

16.2.4 Quantum Dots

Quantum dots (QDs) form another category of NPs with a strong therapeutic use potential. The knowledge of the physical-chemical properties and toxicity of manufactured nanoparticles is important for environmental and safety risk assessment [46]. Fresh QDs are essentially hydrophobic but not clinically beneficial, provided the hydrophobic cap formed in organic solvents in the metalloid framework throughout their synthesis [47]. QDs are semiconductor nanocrystals 2 to 10 nm in diameter. Their fluorescence ability in different spectral areas, including the infrared one [48], is suitable for identifying, marking and observing/imaging cells, cell or tissue surfaces, or pathogenic biological substances, as well as for different processes in cells, tissues, and the body as a whole, which has significant diagnostic consequences [49]. The determination variables for QD toxicity are QD volume, charge, dosage, external cover bioactivity (thin film material or functional groups), as well as oxidative, photolytic and mechanical stability [47] (Figure 16.3). One of the key reasons that QDs are not extended to clinical imaging and pharmaceutical application to humans is the uncertainty over their negative consequences [50,51]. The in vivo ovarian function is influenced by CdSe/ZnS QDs and its subsequent influence on in vitro fertilization. The results also show that QDs disrupt oocyte maturation, lower hormone receptor mRNA expression, and decrease the in vitro fertilization ability [52]. Cadmium and selenium are considered to trigger acute and persistent toxic effects in vertebrates and are of significance to human health and environment, especially as two of the most commonly utilized component metals in key QD complexes [47].

16.2.5 Other Nanoparticles

Gold nanorods are appropriate for therapeutic application in the field of medicine and cancer therapy and are normally injected directly into systemic circulation. Gold nanorods are detrimental to the vascular endothelium, which contributes to diminished aortic ring relaxation [53]. Silica-based nanoparticles have pioneered in the field of targeted and controlled release of drug-delivery systems. However, toxicity is

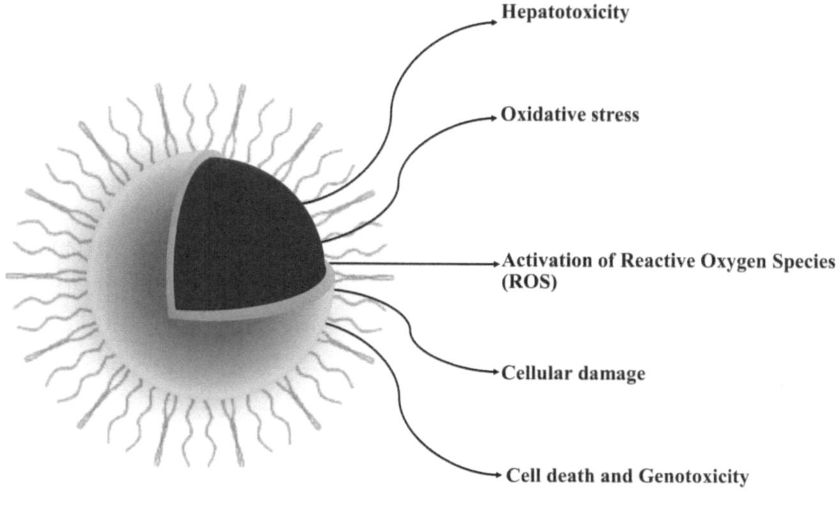

FIGURE 16.3 Imaging Agent to Drug Delivery Path with Toxicity Profile of QDs.

TABLE 16.1
List of Some Nanoparticles Showing Toxicity Profile

Nanoparticles	Mechanism	Toxicity	References
ZnO nanoparticles	Functional compression of mitochondrial in cells and increased oxidative stress,	Mitochondrial damage, cell cycle arrest at G2/M, apoptosis, genotoxicity	[58]
Gold Nanoparticle	Prompt ROS development after reaching the cells and then contribute to additional oxidative stress-related cytotoxicity (in vitro study:- high concentration of AuNPs)	DNA damage, cell death (apoptosis and necrosis) and cell cycle arrest, nitric oxide NO is catalyzed by metal ions Gold Nanoparticle and peroxynitrite is developed by NO reacting with O_2, which can disrupt DNA, proteins	[59]
MWCNT	Inflammation is mediated by surface area dose and length of CNT	Carcinogenicity and considerable loss of cell viability	[60]
Gold nanorods with CTAB	Presence of the stabilizer CTAB, it causes many serious effects on cell	Cytotoxicity	[53]
Silica nanoparticles	Increased levels of ROS and decreased levels of glutathione suggesting ↑ oxidative stress.	Cell membrane damage	[55]
Cadmium telluride quantum dots	Prompt of lipid peroxidation in cells and activation of reactive oxygen species (ROS)	Cellular damage. Damage to plasma membranes, mitochondria and nucleus.	[61]
AgNPs	Oxidative stress, DNA disruption and manipulation of cytokine expression and ROS ↑	Cell death by either apoptosis or necrosis, Genotoxicity	[62]
Citrate-coated Ag NPs	Inflammation, ↑ROS, eryptosis, ↑ cytosolic Ca2+	Acute neutrophilic inflammation in the lungs	[62]

associated to silica nanoparticles. The response to Silica-based nanoparticles in vitro resulted in increased rates of reactive oxygen species (ROS) and decreased rates of glutathione, suggesting elevated oxidative stress [54]. At large concentrations, silica nanoparticles have been shown to be toxic by decreasing cell viability or cell proliferation, and by releasing lactic acid dehydrogenase from cells, showing disruption to the membranes [1,55]. The cytotoxicity of silica to human cells relies extensively on its metabolic activity, but could be greatly decreased by augmenting or coating silica with chitosan polymers [55]. Supramagnetic metal oxides, such as iron oxide, can be used as magnetically guided nanoparticles for drug delivery. Iron Oxide Nanoparticles show a toxicity profile at high doses, such as inhibition of acetylcholinesterase enzyme in red blood cells (RBCs) and brain cells, coupled with induction of aspartate and alanine aminotransferase enzyme in the hepatic cell and serum, which may trigger detrimental effects in the biochemical profile [56].

16.2.6 Cellular Mechanisms of Nanoparticle Toxicity

Nanoparticle penetration, if exposed to the body through different routes, via skin, the lung or the intestinal tract, can contribute to a broad range of toxicological effects when nanoproducts are generated, used and disposed of [14] (Table 16.1). Engineered nanomaterials have the potential to connect with biological structures, producing as probable pathways of toxicity, reactive oxygen species (ROS) [13,14]. Cell cycle arrest often varies because of the form of nanoparticle. Many pathways can include toxicity caused by nanoparticle exposure. Altered signaling pathways disrupt cellular homeostasis, which results in cellular injury. Nanotoxicity may result in proliferation suppression (by the arrest of cell cycle). The cells are doomed to death (apoptosis or necrosis) if they cannot resolve the tension and repair the damage [7]. Toxicological tests have found that smaller nanoparticles (100 nm) have more detrimental respiratory and inflammatory effects than larger particles produced from the same substance. Metallic nanoparticles smaller than 30 nm in size travel rapidly through the blood-circulation environment, whereas non-metallic nanoparticles (4–200 nm) travel very slowly or are stagnant [57]. NPs raise the apoptotic amount due to mechanical tension on the cell surface induced by particle-cell interactions [7,57].

16.3 CONCLUSION

Nanoparticles, nanotechnology, their use in the field of medicine, their applications and, most notably, their health concerns are still ignored. The usage of nanoparticles as drug-delivery systems should be looked at from both sides of the coin, with respect to their beneficial properties and toxicity profile. The unique physical and chemical properties of nanoparticles have given rise to health issues, which could not be forecast simply by taking the safety risks of the preceding bulk substance. The medical profession has recently begun to react to the scarcity of knowledge by engaging in the area of nanoparticle toxicology. However, FDA has approved many nanoparticle drug-delivery systems, but a clear picture on safety and toxicity is required.

REFERENCES

1. Hossain, S., Chowdhury, E. H. and Akaike, T. (2011). "Nanoparticles and toxicity in therapeutic delivery: The ongoing debate", *Therapeutic Delivery*, 2(2), pp. 125–132. DOI: 10.4155/tde.10.109.
2. Krajewska, A., Kwiecien-Obara, E., Kolodziej, M. and Szponar, J. (2013). "Nanopaticles cardiotoxity–review of the literature", *Przegl Lek*, 70(8), pp. 628–632. https://www.ncbi.nlm.nih.gov/pubmed/24466707.

3. Wolfram, J., Zhu, M., Yang, Y., Shen, J., Gentile, E., Paolino, D., Fresta, M., Nie, G., Chen, C., Shen, H., Ferrari, M. and Zhao, Y. (2015). "Safety of nanoparticles in medicine", *Current Drug Targets*, 16(14), pp. 1671–1681. DOI: 10.2174/1389450115666140804124808.
4. Hydzik, P. (2012). "Nanoparticles toxicity–selective examples", *Przegl Lek*, 69(8), pp. 486–489. https://www.ncbi.nlm.nih.gov/pubmed/23243914.
5. Hock, S. C., Ying, Y. M. and Wah, C. L. (2011). "A review of the current scientific and regulatory status of nanomedicines and the challenges ahead", *PDA Journal of Pharmaceutical Science and Technology*, 65(2), pp. 177–195. https://www.ncbi.nlm.nih.gov/pubmed/21502077.
6. Becker, H., Herzberg, F., Schulte, A. and Kolossa-Gehring, M. (2011). "The carcinogenic potential of nanomaterials, their release from products and options for regulating them", *International Journal of Hygiene and Environmental Health*, 214(3), pp. 231–238. DOI: 10.1016/j.ijheh.2010.11.004.
7. Huang, Y. W., Cambre, M. and Lee, H. J. (2017). "The toxicity of nanoparticles depends on multiple molecular and physicochemical mechanisms", *International Journal of Molecular Science*, 18(12), 2702. DOI: 10.3390/ijms18122702.
8. Alidori, S., Thorek, D.L.J., Beattie, B. J., Ulmert, D., Almeida, B. A., Monette, S., Scheinberg, D. A. and McDevitt, M. R. (2017). "Carbon nanotubes exhibit fibrillar pharmacology in primates", *PLoS One*, 12 (8), p. e0183902. DOI: 10.1371/journal.pone.0183902.
9. Yan, L., Zhao, F., Li, S., Hu, Z. and Zhao, Y. (2011). "Low-toxic and safe nanomaterials by surface-chemical design, carbon nanotubes, fullerenes, metallofullerenes, and graphenes", *Nanoscale*, 3(2), pp. 362–382. DOI: 10.1039/c0nr00647e.
10. Burdusel, A. C., Gherasim, O., Grumezescu, A. M., Mogoanta, L., Ficai, A. and Andronescu, E. (2018). "Biomedical applications of silver nanoparticles: An up-to-date overview", *Nanomaterials (Basel)*, 8(9). DOI: 10.3390/nano8090681.
11. Mathur, P., Jha, S., Ramteke, S. and Jain, N. K. (2018). "Pharmaceutical aspects of silver nanoparticles", *Artificial Cells, Nanomedicine, and Biotechnology*, 46(sup1), pp. 115–126. DOI: 10.1080/21691401.2017.1414825.
12. Wen, H., Dan, M., Yang, Y., Lyu, J., Shao, A., Cheng, X., Chen, L. and Xu, L. (2017). "Acute toxicity and genotoxicity of silver nanoparticle in rats", *PLoS One*, 12(9), p. e0185554. DOI: 10.1371/journal.pone.0185554.
13. Patlolla, A. K., Hackett, D. and Tchounwou, P. B. (2015). "Silver nanoparticle-induced oxidative stress-dependent toxicity in Sprague-Dawley rats", *Molecular and Cellular Biochemistry*, 399(1–2), pp. 257–268. DOI: 10.1007/s11010-014-2252-7.
14. Patlolla, A. K., Hackett, D. and Tchounwou, P. B. (2015). "Genotoxicity study of silver nanoparticles in bone marrow cells of Sprague-Dawley rats", *Food and Chemical Toxicology*, 85, pp. 52–60. DOI: 10.1016/j.fct.2015.05.005.
15. Kim, H. R., Kim, M. J., Lee, S. Y., Oh, S. M. and Chung, K. H. (2011). "Genotoxic effects of silver nanoparticles stimulated by oxidative stress in human normal bronchial epithelial (BEAS-2B) cells", *Mutation Research*, 726(2), pp. 129–135. DOI: 10.1016/j.mrgentox.2011.08.008.
16. Ferdous, Z., Beegam, S., Tariq, S., Ali, B. H. and Nemmar, A. (2018). "The in vitro effect of polyvinylpyrrolidone and citrate coated silver nanoparticles on erythrocytic oxidative damage and eryptosis", *Cell Physiology and Biochemistry*, 49(4), pp. 1577–1588. DOI: 10.1159/000493460.
17. Bae, E.-J., Park, H.-J., Park, J.-S., Yoon, J.-Y., Kim, Y.-H., Choi, K.-H. and Yi, J.-H. (2011). "Effect of chemical stabilizers in silver nanoparticle suspensions on nanotoxicity", *Bulletin of the Korean Chemical Society*, 32(2), pp. 613–619. DOI: 10.5012/bkcs.2011.32.2.613.
18. Francis, A. P. and Devasena, T. (2018). "Toxicity of carbon nanotubes: A review", *Toxicology and Industrial Health*, 34(3), pp. 200–210. DOI: 10.1177/0748233717747472.

19. Kayat, J., Gajbhiye, V., Tekade, R. K. and Jain, N. K. (2011). "Pulmonary toxicity of carbon nanotubes: A systematic report", *Nanomedicine*, 7(1), pp. 40–49. DOI: 10.1016/j.nano.2010.06.008.
20. Johnston, H. J., Hutchison, G. R., Christensen, F. M., Peters, S., Hankin, S., Aschberger, K. and Stone, V. (2010). "A critical review of the biological mechanisms underlying the in vivo and in vitro toxicity of carbon nanotubes: The contribution of physico-chemical characteristics", *Nanotoxicology*, 4(2), pp. 207–246. DOI: 10.3109/17435390903569639.
21. Mohanta, D., Patnaik, S., Sood, S. and Das, N. (2019). "Carbon nanotubes: Evaluation of toxicity at biointerfaces", *Journal of Pharmaceutial Analysis*, 9(5), pp. 293–300. DOI: 10.1016/j.jpha.2019.04.003.
22. Liu, Y., Zhao, Y., Sun, B. and Chen, C. (2013). "Understanding the toxicity of carbon nanotubes" *Accounts of Chemical Research*, 46(3), pp. 702–713. DOI: 10.1021/ar300028m.
23. Ali-Boucetta, H., Al-Jamal, K. T., Muller, K. H., Li, S., Porter, A. E., Eddaoudi, A., Prato, M., Bianco, A. and Kostarelos, K. (2011). "Cellular uptake and cytotoxic impact of chemically functionalized and polymer-coated carbon nanotubes", *Small*, 7(22), 3230–3238. DOI: 10.1002/smll.201101004.
24. Kostarelos, K., Lacerda, L., Pastorin, G., Wu, W., Wieckowski, S., Luangsivilay, J., Godefroy, S., Pantarotto, D., Briand, J. P., Muller, S., Prato, M. and Bianco, A. (2007). "Cellular uptake of functionalized carbon nanotubes is independent of functional group and cell type", *Nature Nanotechnology*, 2(2), pp. 108–113. DOI: 10.1038/nnano.2006.209.
25. Georgin, D., Czarny, B., Botquin, M., Mayne-L'hermite, M., Pinault, M., Bouchet-Fabre, B., Carriere, M., Poncy, J. L., Chau, Q., Maximilien, R., Dive, V. and Taran, F. (2009). "Preparation of (14)C-labeled multiwalled carbon nanotubes for biodistribution investigations", *Journal of the American Chemical Society*, 131(41), pp. 14658–14659. DOI: 10.1021/ja906319z.
26. Antonelli, A., Serafini, S., Menotta, M., Sfara, C., Pierige, F., Giorgi, L., Ambrosi, G., Rossi, L. and Magnani, M. (2010). "Improved cellular uptake of functionalized single-walled carbon nanotubes", *Nanotechnology*, 21(42), p. 425101. DOI: 10.1088/0957-4484/21/42/425101.
27. Shi Kam, N. W., Jessop, T. C., Wender, P. A. and Dai, H. (2004). "Nanotube molecular transporters: Internalization of carbon nanotube-protein conjugates into Mammalian cells", *Journal of the American Chemical Society*, 126(22), pp. 6850–6851. DOI: 10.1021/ja0486059.
28. Simon, J., Flahaut, E. and Golzio, M. (2019). "Overview of carbon nanotubes for biomedical applications", *Materials (Basel)*, 12(4), p. 624. DOI: 10.3390/ma12040624.
29. Duke, K. S. and Bonner, J. C. (2018). "Mechanisms of carbon nanotube-induced pulmonary fibrosis: A physicochemical characteristic perspective", *Wiley Interdisciplinary Reviews - Nanomedicine and Nanobiotechnology*, 10(3), p. e1498. DOI: 10.1002/wnan.1498.
30. Dong, J. and Ma, Q. (2016). "Myofibroblasts and lung fibrosis induced by carbon nanotube exposure", *Particle and Fibre Toxicology*, 13(1), p. 60. DOI: 10.1186/s12989-016-0172-2.
31. Yang, S. T., Luo, J., Zhou, Q. and Wang, H. (2012). "Pharmacokinetics, metabolism and toxicity of carbon nanotubes for biomedical purposes", *Theranostics*, 2(3), pp. 271–282. DOI: 10.7150/thno.3618.
32. Jain, S., Thakare, V. S., Das, M., Godugu, C., Jain, A. K., Mathur, R., Chuttani, K. and Mishra, A. K. (2011). "Toxicity of multiwalled carbon nanotubes with end defects critically depends on their functionalization density", *Chemical Research in Toxicology*, 24(11), pp. 2028–2039. DOI: 10.1021/tx2003728.
33. Lacerda, L., Ali-Boucetta, H., Herrero, M. A., Pastorin, G., Bianco, A., Prato, M. and Kostarelos, K. (2008). "Tissue histology and physiology following intravenous administration of different types of functionalized multiwalled carbon nanotubes", *Nanomedicine (Lond)*, 3(2), pp. 149–161. DOI: 10.2217/17435889.3.2.149.

34. Chen, W., Xiong, Q., Ren, Q., Guo, Y. and Li, G. (2014). "Can amino-functionalized carbon nanotubes carry functional nerve growth factor?", *Neural Regeneration Research*, 9(3), pp. 285–292. DOI: 10.4103/1673-5374.128225.
35. Wang, X., Xia, T., Duch, M. C., Ji, Z., Zhang, H., Li, R., Sun, B., Lin, S., Meng, H., Liao, Y. P., Wang, M., Song, T. B., Yang, Y., Hersam, M. C. and Nel, A. E. (2012). "Pluronic F108 coating decreases the lung fibrosis potential of multiwall carbon nanotubes by reducing lysosomal injury", *Nano Letters*, 12(6), pp. 3050–3061. DOI: 10.1021/nl300895y.
36. Liu, Y., Ren, L., Yan, D. and Zhong, W. (2014). "Mechanistic study on the reduction of SWCNT-induced cytotoxicity by albumin coating", *Particle & Particle Systems Characterization*, 31(12), pp. 1244–1251. DOI: 10.1002/ppsc.201400145.
37. Perkins, B. L. and Naderi, N. (2016). "Carbon Nanostructures in Bone Tissue Engineering", *The Open Orthopaedics Journal*, 10, pp. 877–899. DOI: 10.2174/1874325001610010877.
38. Patlolla, A., Knighten, B. and Tchounwou, P. (2010). "Multi-walled carbon nanotubes induce cytotoxicity, genotoxicity and apoptosis in normal human dermal fibroblast cells", *Ethnicity & Disease*, 20(1 Suppl 1), pp. S1-65–S-72. https://www.ncbi.nlm.nih.gov/pubmed/20521388.
39. Pryor, J. B., Harper, B. J. and Harper, S. L. (2014). "Comparative toxicological assessment of PAMAM and thiophosphoryl dendrimers using embryonic zebrafish", *International Journal of Nanomedicine*, 9, pp. 1947–1956. DOI: 10.2147/IJN.S60220.
40. Jain, K., Kesharwani, P., Gupta, U. and Jain, N. K. (2010). "Dendrimer toxicity: Let's meet the challenge", *International Journal of Pharmaceutics*, 394(1–2), pp. 122–142. DOI: 10.1016/j.ijpharm.2010.04.027.
41. Janaszewska, A., Lazniewska, J., Trzepinski, P., Marcinkowska, M. and Klajnert-Maculewicz, B. (2019). "Cytotoxicity of dendrimers", *Biomolecules*, 9(8). DOI: 10.3390/biom9080330.
42. Svenson, S. and Tomalia, D. A. (2005). "Dendrimers in biomedical applications–reflections on the field", *Advanced Drug Delivery Reviews*, 57(15), pp. 2106–2129. DOI: 10.1016/j.addr.2005.09.018.
43. Mukherjee, S. P. and Byrne, H. J. (2013). "Polyamidoamine dendrimer nanoparticle cytotoxicity, oxidative stress, caspase activation and inflammatory response: Experimental observation and numerical simulation", *Nanomedicine*, 9(2), pp. 202–211. DOI: 10.1016/j.nano.2012.05.002.
44. Winnicka, K., Wroblewska, M., Sosnowska, K., Car, H. and Kasacka, I. (2015). "Evaluation of cationic polyamidoamine dendrimers' dermal toxicity in the rat skin model", *Drug Design, Development and Therapy*, 9, pp. 1367–1377. DOI: 10.2147/DDDT.S78336.
45. Ziemba, B., Janaszewska, A., Ciepluch, K., Krotewicz, M., Fogel, W. A., Appelhans, D., Voit, B., Bryszewska, M. and Klajnert, B. (2011). "In vivo toxicity of poly(propyleneimine) dendrimers", *Journal of Biomedical Materials Research Part A*, 99(2), pp. 261–268. DOI: 10.1002/jbm.a.33196.
46. Oh, E., Liu, R., Nel, A., Gemill, K. B., Bilal, M., Cohen, Y. and Medintz, I. L. (2016). "Meta-analysis of cellular toxicity for cadmium-containing quantum dots", *Nature Nanotechnology*, 11(5), pp. 479–486. DOI: 10.1038/nnano.2015.338.
47. Hardman, R. (2006). "A toxicologic review of quantum dots: Toxicity depends on physicochemical and environmental factors", *Environmental Health Perspectives*, 114(2), pp. 165–172. DOI: 10.1289/ehp.8284.
48. Altinoglu, E. I. and Adair, J. H. (2010). "Near-infrared imaging with nanoparticles", *Wiley Interdisciplinary Reviews - Nanomedicine and Nanobiotechnology*, 2(5), pp. 461–477. DOI: 10.1002/wnan.77.
49. Medintz, I. L., Uyeda, H. T., Goldman, E. R. and Mattoussi, H. (2005). "Quantum dot bioconjugates for imaging, labelling and sensing", *Nature Materials*, 4(6), pp. 435–446. DOI: 10.1038/nmat1390.

50. Ren, H. and Huang, X. (2010). "Polyacrylate nanoparticles: Toxicity or new nanomedicine?" *European Respiratory Journal*, 36(1), pp. 218–221. DOI: 10.1183/09031936.00022410.
51. Wegner, K. D. and Hildebrandt, N. (2015). "Quantum dots: Bright and versatile in vitro and in vivo fluorescence imaging biosensors", *Chemical Society Reviews*, 44(14), pp. 4792–4834. DOI: 10.1039/c4cs00532e.
52. Xu, G., Lin, G., Lin, S., Wu, N., Deng, Y., Feng, G., Chen, Q., Qu, J., Chen, D., Chen, S., Niu, H., Mei, S., Yong, K. T. and Wang, X. (2016). "The reproductive toxicity of CDSE/ZNS quantum dots on the in vivo ovarian function and in vitro fertilization", *Scientific Reports*, 6, p. 37677. DOI: 10.1038/srep37677.
53. Alkilany, A. M., Shatanawi, A., Kurtz, T., Caldwell, R. B. and Caldwell, R. W. (2012). "Toxicity and cellular uptake of gold nanorods in vascular endothelium and smooth muscles of isolated rat blood vessel: Importance of surface modification", *Small*, 8(8), pp. 1270–1278. DOI: 10.1002/smll.201101948.
54. Lin, W., Huang, Y. W., Zhou, X. D. and Ma, Y. (2006). "In vitro toxicity of silica nanoparticles in human lung cancer cells", *Toxicology and Applied Pharmacology*, 217(3), pp. 252–259. DOI: 10.1016/j.taap.2006.10.004.
55. Chang, J. S., Chang, K. L., Hwang, D. F. and Kong, Z. L. (2007). "In vitro cytotoxicitiy of silica nanoparticles at high concentrations strongly depends on the metabolic activity type of the cell line", *Environmental Science & Technology*, 41(6), pp. 2064–2068. DOI: 10.1021/es062347t.
56. Araujo, F., Shrestha, N., Granja, P. L., Hirvonen, J., Santos, H. A. and Sarmento, B. (2015). "Safety and toxicity concerns of orally delivered nanoparticles as drug carriers", *Expert Opinion on Drug Metabolism & Toxicology*, 11(3), pp. 381–393. DOI: 10.1517/17425255.2015.992781.
57. Crisponi, G., Nurchi, V. M., Lachowicz, J. I., Peana, M., Medici, S., Zoroddu, M. A. (2017). "Toxicity of nanoparticles: Etiology and mechanisms", pp. 511–546. DOI: 10.1016/b978-0-323-52733-0.00018-5.
58. Gao, F., Ma, N., Zhou, H., Wang, Q., Zhang, H., Wang, P., Hou, H., Wen, H. and Li, L. (2016). "Zinc oxide nanoparticles-induced epigenetic change and G2/M arrest are associated with apoptosis in human epidermal keratinocytes", *International Journal of Nanomedicine*, 11, pp. 3859–3874. DOI: 10.2147/IJN.S107021.
59. Khlebtsov, N. and Dykman, L. (2011). "Biodistribution and toxicity of engineered gold nanoparticles: A review of in vitro and in vivo studies", *Chemical Society Reviews*, 40(3), pp. 1647–1671. DOI: 10.1039/c0cs00018c.
60. De Jong, W. H. and Borm, P. J. (2008). "Drug delivery and nanoparticles: Applications and hazards", *International Journal of Nanomedicine*, 3(2), pp. 133–149. DOI: 10.2147/ijn.s596.
61. Lovric, J., Cho, S. J., Winnik, F. M. and Maysinger, D. (2005). "Unmodified cadmium telluride quantum dots induce reactive oxygen species formation leading to multiple organelle damage and cell death", *Chemistry & Biology*, 12(11), pp. 1227–1234. DOI: 10.1016/j.chembiol.2005.09.008.
62. AshaRani, P. V., Low Kah Mun, G., Hande, M. P. and Valiyaveettil, S. (2009). "Cytotoxicity and genotoxicity of silver nanoparticles in human cells", *ACS Nano*, 3(2), pp. 279–290. DOI: 10.1021/nn800596w.

17 Impacts of Nanotechnology on Pharmaceutical Sciences

Mohit Vij and Pankaj Wadhwa

17.1 INTRODUCTION

Nanotechnology is an emerging nanoscale technology that has real-world applications. This technology involves structures that measure between 1 nm and 100 nm in one or more dimensions [1]. One of the most significant contributions of nanotechnology is its ability to mold the structure of original materials into new nano-range materials that demonstrate an incredible difference in properties from those of original materials [2]. There are a few terms related to nanotechnology, such as nanomaterial, nanoparticles and nanostructures, which are often used interchangeably, but have different meanings. Nanomaterials are defined as pieces of matter with one or more external dimensions on nanoscale. If a certain matter has two or three external dimensions, it is called a nanoparticle. Nano-structured materials have nano-scale internal features, but they may be larger than 100 nm [3]. The employment of nanotechnology in health and pharmaceutical sciences is referred to as nanomedicine, which has opened new and exciting avenues for the prevention, therapeutics, and diagnosis of numerous diseases. Nanomedicine is made possible by exploiting improved and novel physicochemical properties of drug molecules at the nanoscale. In nanomedicine, the size limit of drug molecules extends up to 1000 nm. Nanotechnology endows drug molecules with properties such as site-specific drug-targeting, potential to cross physiological barriers, improved bioavailability, and tailored drug release. After this brief introduction, we will next discuss the applications of nanotechnology in the pharmaceutical sector.

17.2 APPLICATIONS OF NANOTECHNOLOGY IN PHARMACEUTICAL SCIENCES

Nanotechnology has a huge number of applications in the pharmaceutical sector. We have categorized this part into different subsections, highlighting the role of nanotechnology in fields such as drug delivery, imaging technology and many more [4].

17.2.1 Drug-Delivery Systems

Nanoparticle-based drug-delivery systems are more advantageous as compared to conventional systems, in terms of controlled release, with more drug-loading capacity, increased stability as well as specificity, a vast number of drug-administration routes for both hydrophilic and lipophilic molecules. In this drug-delivery system, drugs can be enclosed spherically or over the surface. After reaching the nanoparticles at the targeted site, the drug may be released via either degradation, diffusion or swelling. Apart from these, other factors, such as light or magnetic field, can also affect drug release by enforcing the impact of external energy. These delivery systems, such as carbon nanotubes, dendrimers, fullerenes, liposomes, nanoparticles, nanosuspensions etc., have drug carriers with a size of less than 1 μm or 200 nm as part of their structural component [5–7]. Lipid nanoparticles (liposomes) are a capable substitute to existing carriers for delivering insoluble drugs, and they can reach specific sites, protecting them from degradation. Apart from this, various nanoparticles and nano-scale structures can also act as pharmaceutically active compounds for cell-sorting procedures and cancer treatments.

Magnetic nanoparticles that have attached antibodies are commonly used to isolate adult stem cells for curing blood disorders. Upon injecting them into blood or bone marrow, they can bind to the target cells and can be easily recovered by using a magnet. Iron-oxide nanoparticles act similarly in tumor cells, where they increase the temperature above 40 °C and demolish the tumor cells. In line with this, many three-dimensional tree-like branched polymeric nano-scale molecules have been developed for the treatment of HIV and as a vaginal microbicide in pharma industry. Fullerenes, which are composed of carbon atoms and are mainly present in a hollow spherical form, have the ability to inactivate radicals via binding and are one of the leading approaches for Alzheimer's, Parkinson's, and cardiovascular diseases.

17.2.2 Nanotechnology in Imaging

Disease conditions can be easily identified in early phases by using imaging procedures. Molecular imaging is a technique used for investigating the various biological processes in organisms, such as cellular trafficking, gene expression, signal transduction and many more. Nanotechnology has played a significant role in transformation of existing imaging techniques where substances are injected, swallowed, or inhaled. The substances travel through the area being examined and release gamma rays in the form of energy. Examples of such methods include single photon emission computed tomography (SPECT), positron emission tomography (PET), etc. These imaging techniques can manipulate the different properties of nanoparticles to make them proficient in marking diseases at the cellular or even organelle level. It was also reported that alterations in liposomes can be made by placing a magnetic element through magnetic resonance imaging (MRI) to produce special views [8,9].

17.2.3 Biomaterials

Degradation of human organs and joints due to degenerative diseases has emerged as a major issue in the last few years. The use of biomaterials/implants is a good approach to address this issue. The biocompatibility, lifespan and performance of implant material can be improved using nanotechnology. Nanotechnology plays a significant role in the fields of antibiotic development, bone replacement materials, dental restoratives, as well as hard and soft tissue implants. In recent years, it was also found that nano-structured materials play a key role in the development of various types of electronic active implants, viz. pacemakers, bladder stimulators, implantable electronic drug delivery devices, etc.

17.2.4 Cosmetics

Before pharmaceutical products, nanotechnology has been used in the cosmetic industry for various innovative products. This can be substantiated by the fact that the first liposome-based anti-aging lotion was launched before the first liposomal drug. So, it can be said that nanotechnology plays a vital role in cosmetic industries by providing various innovative products. In the development of cosmetic products, the major concern is the transportation of vitamins or various plant-based substances into the deeper layers of the skin. So, in that case, nanotechnology-based nanosized delivery systems are usually preferable. In the next section, we will discuss briefly about the drivers of and challenges related to the development of nanotechnology.

17.3 DRIVERS FOR NANOTECHNOLOGY DEVELOPMENT [7]

There are lots of diseases that are associated with proteins, DNA and RNA, respectively. The diagnosis and treatment of such diseases is always a tough task with conventional technologies. In recent times, researchers have gained sufficient knowledge about designing and development of nano-scale material. Fusion of this knowledge with complete understanding of cell function and disease progression at molecular level leads to nano-medicine emergence. Other applications of nanomaterials are for effective targeting of cancerous tissues, efficient drug carriers like nanosponges and liposomes and as imaging agents for diagnostic purposes [9]. Nanomaterials are versatile and unique in nature, as their scale relates with the biomolecule scale. Hence, nanotechnology has great potential for pharmaceutical and medical applications [10].

In the pharmaceutical field, there are lots of issues we need to be addressed for effective disease treatment. Many drugs show adverse side effects, some drugs are unable to cross biological barriers, especially the blood-brain barrier, few diseases cannot be diagnosed at the early stages for effective treatment and limited lifespan of implants. To meet all these needs, novel nanomaterials could be a possible route. Some budding drivers for nanotechnology are listed below:

- Most anti-cancerous drugs have adverse side effects, which worsens patients' condition. But with the help of nanotechnology-based drug-delivery systems, only the required amount of drug can be delivered to cancerous tissues and this ultimately helps mitigate the other adverse effects associated with the drugs.

- Many therapeutically effective drugs have issues with their solubility and bioavailability, respectively. Currently, the pharmaceutical industry is successfully working on nanotechnology-based approaches like cyclodextrin-based nanosponges and liposome drug carriers to solve the issue of low drug solubility.
- Current therapies for cancer are expensive and have a lot of side effects. The pharmaceutical industry making progress in the development of cost-effective nanotechnology-based drugs and therapies that have limited or no side effects.
- To diagnose and treat diseases at the molecular or cellular level, nanotechnology-based contrast agents are being developed with the help of nanoscale carriers; however, this is still in the development phase.
- There are lots of in vitro diagnostic tests that can currently only be run in sophisticated laboratories. Here nanotechnology contributes toward the development of novel sensor systems that are highly specific and sensitive with ultimate miniaturization and which can help perform these tests at doctor's office or even at home.
- In the field of medical implants, there are certain issues like limited lifespan and biocompatibility. To meet these challenges, researchers are developing nanomaterial-based implants having a long lifespan with better biocompatibility.

17.4 CHALLENGES TO COMMERCIALIZATION OF PHARMACEUTICAL NANOTECHNOLOGY

With a development history of many years, nanotechnology has reached a matured stage. As per field experts, there are no scientific hurdles to the commercialization of nanomedicines. But there are some external factors, like non availability of capital, lack of technology transfer, intellectual property rights and regulatory-related concerns, which pose big challenges to the potential realization of pharmaceutical nanotechnology. Worldwide, a very small percentage of venture capital is spent on nanotechnology-based pharmaceuticals as compared to conventional pharmaceuticals. This restricted funding is responsible for slow commercialization of nanomedicines. Further lack of or very cautious investment by big pharmaceutical players on the clinical trial of novel nanomedicine is responsible for this. They are not courageous enough to come out from their regular investments and look forward to exploring the full potential of nanotechnology [11].

Material scientists have played a very big and important role in the field of nanotechnology and nanomaterials. These scientists have excellent knowledge about the fundamentals of nanotechnology but not about their applications related to the biological and pharmaceutical industry. This knowledge gap is a block in the commercialization of nanomedicines. By proper technology transfer and knowledge sharing between scientists and entrepreneurs of different fields, it will be beneficial to study the effects of these novel synthetic materials on cells and tissues for therapeutic benefits as well as to acquire regulatory approval for commercialization of nanomedicines.

For commercial success and sustainability of any pharmaceutical product, patent plays a very crucial role. The field of nanomaterials is very complex and multidisciplinary in nature. So, it's always a challenge to categorize it in specific field like physics, chemistry or biology [12]. Therefore, before investing in the field of nanomedicine, every industry or investor will carefully look into the patent potential of a specific nanomaterial. This apprehension and risk in the field of nanotechnology also act as a hurdle for its fast commercialization.

17.5 IMPACT OF NANOTECHNOLOGY ON PHARMACEUTICALS AND HEALTH CARE COSTS

In the past few years, pharmaceutical and health care innovations were primarily assessed with high quality, safety and efficacy, whereas cost effectiveness was a secondary consideration. But due to demographic changes, most of countries are now leading towards an aging society. Eventually, the cost of pharmaceutical innovations has become a key factor as nations' health care expenditure is expected to increase significantly. To overcome these challenges, we must look for pharmaceutical innovations that would be of high quality, efficient, safe and cost effective.

It has been identified by researchers that cancer treatment, cardiac related health issues, and neurodegenerative diseases require a lot of expense and are going to affect a huge population in near future. Taking this into consideration, nanotechnology-based medicines could be a solution to minimize treatments costs if researchers aim at nanotechnology-based innovations for the treatment of these major cost-involving diseases rather than diseases with minor costs involved. Secondly, nanomedicine has the potential to reduce personnel costs, by shortening the hospital stay as well.

17.6 RISKS ASSOCIATED WITH NANOTECHNOLOGY (NANOTOXICITY)

In this chapter, we have seen a broad range of applications of nanotechnology in the pharmaceutical and health fields. Likewise, it is self-evident that there could be many potential risks associated with nanotechnology like business, environmental, human health, safety and risks related to the protection of intellectual property [13]. Out of these, human health and safety related risk is of first and foremost importance here [14]. The toxicity of nanomaterials depends on their nature, particle size, surface charge and physiochemical properties. Nanoparticles can show greater toxicity and reactivity as compared to their equivalent bulk materials as they are small, have a large surface area and insolubility characteristics. Such characteristics will facilitate their entry into human body rapidly and may induce inflammation and suppress the immune system. Careful studies are required to check the threshold number of nanoparticles present inside the human body, which could be toxic to humans or animals. But unfortunately, there are no such studies or data available to prove the harmful effect of nanoparticles on human health. Moreover, researchers have suggested one promising way to prevent the potential health hazards: to make biodegradable nanomaterials. These nanomaterials will be degraded by water or enzymes inside the body to reduce the health risks and make them biocompatible. Accordingly, more research and information should be needed to compile an efficient database and proofs regarding the risks of nanomaterials to human health and safety. Further, we need to establish certain regulations that encourage prudent investment in nanotechnology-based innovations and social acceptance of final products.

17.7 CONCLUSION

Nanotechnology has come up as a new area of interest in the field of health and pharmaceuticals. It is considered as a collection of tools and ideas that can be applied in pharmaceutical meadow to tackle major pharmaceutical problems. It has great potential to overcome the limitations of conventional techniques through the use of nanoengineering tools. In spite of a large range of applications of nanotechnology, there are only few nano-based pharmaceutical products launched or available in the market. Although, worldwide, it is presently considered as one of the hottest topics in academic research as well as publication.

It has been observed that socio-economic and ethical challenges and issues like patenting, technology transfer and regulatory approval of nanomaterials restrict the large pharmaceutical and health care industries to invest open-heartedly in nanotechnology-based innovations. Therefore, it is widely acknowledged that we promptly need to address these hurdles to accelerate the transformation of nanotechnology-based laboratory research into industrial-scale pharmaceutical products of high efficacy and lower adverse effects.

REFERENCES

1. Kaehler, T. (1994). "Nanotechnology: Basic concepts and definitions", *Clinical Chemistry*, 40(9), pp. 1797–1799.
2. Bhattacharyya, D., Singh, S., Satnalika, N., Khandelwal, A. and Jeon, S.-H. (2009). "Nanotechnology, big things from a tiny world: a review, "*International Journal of u- and e- Service, Science and Technology*, 2(3), pp. 29–38.
3. K. Kulinowski and B. Lippy (2011). "Training workers on risks of nanotechnologies".
4. Wagner, V., Husing, B., Gaisser, S., and Bock, A.-K. (2006). "Nanomedicine: drivers for development and possible impacts", *European Commission Joint Research Centre*, Institute for Prospective Technological Studies, pp. 45–53.
5. Allen, T. and Cullis, P. R. (2004). "Drug delivery systems: entering the mainstream", *Science*, 303, pp. 1818–1822.
6. Duncan, R. (2004). "Nanomedicines in action", *The Pharmaceutical Journal*, 273, pp. 485–488.
7. Wagner, V. and Wechsler, D. (2004). Nanobiotechnologie II: Anwendungen in der Medizin und Pharmazie, VDI Technologiezentrum GmbH, Düsseldorf.
8. Ahmad, M. U., Ali, S. M. and Ahmad, I. (2012). "Applications of nanotechnology in pharmaceutical development", *Lipids in Nanotechnology*, AOCS Press, pp. 171–190.
9. Wickline, S. A. and Lanza, G. (2003). "Nanotechnology for molecular imaging and targeted therapy", *Circulation*, 107, pp. 1092–1095.
10. Ferrari, M. (2005). "Cancer nanotechnology: Opportunities and challenges", *Nature Reviews Cancer*, 5(3), pp. 161–171.
11. Allianz and OECD (2005). *Opportunities and Risks of Nanotechnologies*, Lauterwasser, C. (ed.), Allianz and OECD, München, Paris.
12. Nano werk (2006). Nanotechnology and intellectual property issues.
13. Kargozar, S. and Mozafari, M. (2018). "Nanotechnology and nanomedicine: start small, think big", *Materials Today: Proceedings*, 5, pp. 15492–15500.
14. Nasrollahzadeh, M., and Sajadi, S. M. (2019). "Risks of nanotechnology to human life", An *Introduction to Green Nanotechnology*, Academic Press, pp. 323–336.

18 Nanomaterials and Their Synthesis

Pawan Kumar, Vinod Kumar, Rajnish Kumar, Ravinder Kumar, and Dipen Kumar Rajak

18.1 INTRODUCTION AND BACKGROUND: NANOMATERIALS

Nanotechnology involves tailoring of materials at the atomic level to achieve unique properties at the nanoscale [1]. Nanotechnology produces materials smaller than 100 nm in at least one dimension [2]. Due to their inherent size, the physical, chemical and biological properties of nanomaterials differ from larger particles [3]. Nanomaterials can pass through skin and blood-brain barriers and exhibit both positive and negative impacts on the host body [4]. Hybrid nanomaterials are receiving popularity these days because they provide the ability to tune the properties of nanohybrids [5]. These hybrid or engineered nanoparticles have a wide range of applications in energy production [6], drug delivery [7], diagnostics [8], environmental remediation [9], and tissue engineering applications [10,11]. The global market has a high demand for nanomaterials, and it is expected that this demand will reach $98 billion by 2025 [12]. The characteristic of nanomaterials is that the ratio of surface area to volume is large, so the surface can be covered with many molecules [13]. Figure 18.1 demonstrates the relative size of numerous types of materials ranging from nano- to macro-scale [14]. Nanoparticles are not simple molecules; they are complex in nature and are mainly composed of three layers: (a) the surface layer, (b) the shell layer, and (c) the core (see Figure 18.2). Based on the dimensions of nanoscale (<100 nm), nanoparticles are zero-, one-, two- and three- dimensional [15], while based on morphology, they exhibit spherical, triangular, cubic, hexagonal, oval, prism, rod, and helical shapes [16]. Different forms of nanomaterials, including nanoparticles, nanofilms, nanoflakes, nanotubes, nanofibers, and nanocomposites, have been used to improve the mechanical, electrical, thermal and biological properties products [17].

In recent decades, a large number of nanomaterials have been synthesized using old-fashioned ceramic approaches, which comprise mixing and grinding powders of constituent oxides, carbonates, and other compounds, and heating them to high temperatures with transition milling when needed [18]. The choice of the synthesis technique can be a key factor in determining the effectiveness of a nanomaterial [19]. Several techniques have been used to manufacture various types of nanomaterials, such as electrospinning, hydrothermal, co-precipitation, micro-emulsion, ion-exchange, microwave, sol-gel, etc.

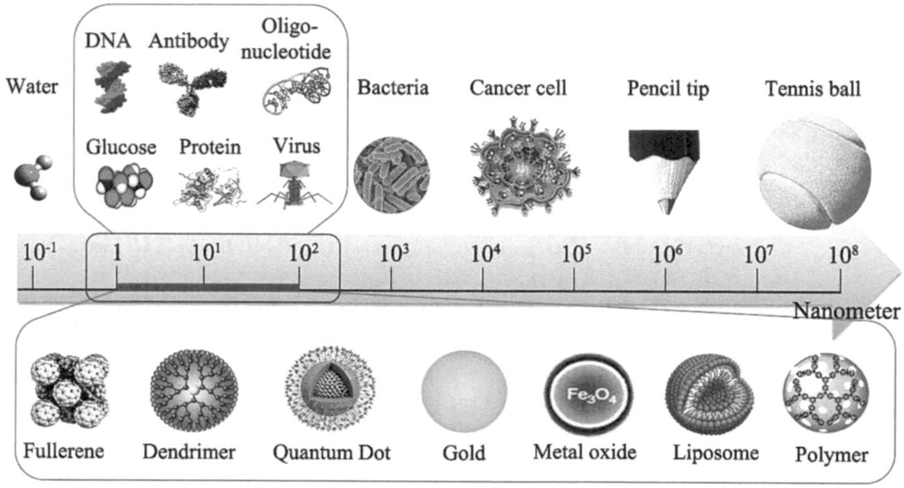

FIGURE 18.1 Nanoscale Integration of Materials

18.2 ROUTE OF SYNTHESIS OF NANOMATERIALS

There are various processes and materials involved in the synthesis of nanomaterials, which are described in this section.

18.2.1 Sol-gel

The sol-gel process is a wet-chemical technique, also known as chemical solution deposition, widely used for the preparation of glassy materials [20]. It consists of preparing a sol, followed by gelation and solvent removal [21]. Subsequently, a drying process is performed on the obtained gel, and the product produced according to the drying mode is easily converted into Xerogel or Aerogel [22]. This method has potential control over the textural and surface properties of the materials [23]. Various shape-controlled nanostructures, including nanofibers, nanospheres,nanoribbons,nanoflakes,nanorods,nanospheres, and nanotubes, can be successfully synthesized using the sol-gel technology [24]. Nanoparticles, including

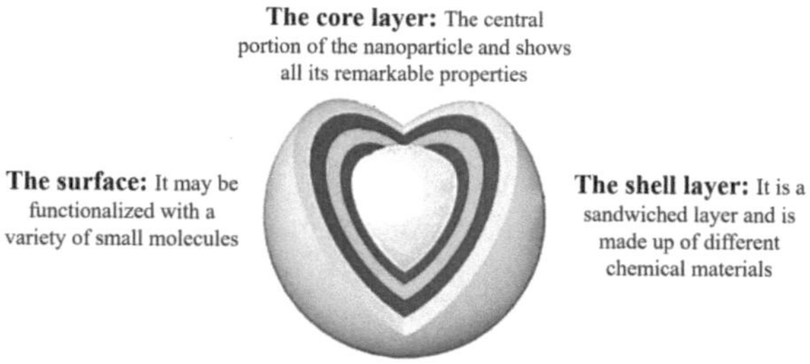

FIGURE 18.2 Composition of Nanoparticles

silver [25], TiO_2 (titania) [26], bioactive glasses [27–29], ZnO [30], ZrO_2 [31], nano-silica [32], SnO_2 [33], ZrB_2 [34], CuO [35], and many composites [36], have been successfully prepared using the sol-gel method.

18.2.2 *Hydrothermal*

Hydrothermal synthesis is a reaction-based approach for the preparation of different, highly crystalline nanoparticles [37]. The crystallinity of materials depends on the solubility of minerals in hot water under high pressure [38]. The formation of a single crystal can take place at a high vapor pressure level and a wide temperature range, above 100°C [39]. In the artificial hydrothermal synthesis process, a hydrothermal reactor 'Autoclave', containing a Teflon-lined container, is filled with a solution [40]. In this process, an aqueous mixture is heated in the autoclave above atmospheric pressure and above the boiling point of water [41]. The solvent properties, like polarity, dipole moment, polarizability and hydrogen bonding, of many compounds change dramatically under supercritical conditions [42]. During the hydrothermal reaction, the size of the particles is controlled by nucleation and grain growth processes [43]. Hydrothermal synthesis offers many advantages over conventional and non-conventional ceramic synthetic methods [44]. Highly crystalline ZnO [45], Cu-ZnO [46], Co-ZnO [47], TiO_2 [48], Fe_3O_4 [49], SnO_2 [50], NiO [51], MnO_2 [52], ZrO_2 [53], TiO_2/carbon [54] and many other types of nanomaterials have been synthesized by hydrothermal reaction.

18.2.3 *Electrospinning*

Electrospinning is an electrostatic ultra-fine or nanoscale fiber fabrication method performed under a strong electric field on a polymer solution or melt [55]. It has received more interest and attention in recent years due to its high efficiency, and flexibility for potential applications in different fields [56]. It is a convenient approach for the production of functional nanofibrous biomaterials for tissue-engineering applications [57]. The quality and performance of the nanofibrous membrane can be enhanced by modifying/combining with active molecules in different ways [58]. There are two ways, needle-less and needle-based, through which nanofibers can be produced using the electrospinning method [59]. The electrospinning process has several variants like bubble electrospinning, vibration electrospinning, siro-electrospinning, and magneto-electrospinning [60].

18.2.4 *Microwave Irradiation*

The microwave irradiation method is a novel technique used to synthesize nanoparticles with exact parameter control. Starting materials are heated to high temperatures in a short time using a high-frequency wave generated in the instrument [61]. The synthesis of nanostructured materials, whose growth is highly sensitive to reaction conditions, can be easily processed through microwave irradiation [62]. It is used in the synthesis of one-pot inorganic nanomaterials, including mono- and bimetallic nanomaterials, such as Au [63], Cu [64], ZnO [65], grapheme [66], Ag [67] nanoparticles and quantum dots, including CdSe [68], Na_2TeO_3 [69], CdTe/TGA [70].

18.2.5 *Green Synthesis*

Green synthesis is an emerging approach for the formation of stable, cost-effective, and non-toxic nanomaterials. It is a fast, affordable, and reproducible technique that involves involving microbes and plant extract as reducing agents. Green technology is eco-friendly and more beneficial as compared to physical and chemical approaches because it poses numerous stresses on the environment due to their toxic metabolites [71]. Different metal and metal oxides, including Au [72], Ag [73], CuO [74], UO_2 [75], Fe_2O_3 [76], TiO_2 [77]and ZnO [78] nanoparticles, can be easily produced through green approaches using various natural extracts.

18.3 SUMMARY

Nanotechnology improves daily life by improving the performance and efficiency of everyday objects. The methods used for fabrication of nanoparticles include physical, chemical, and biological processes that have been improved with time. Nanostructured materials, with different shapes and sizes, possess unique properties that make them applicable in different fields of science and technology. The use of green technology minimizes the use of chemicals and solvents for the synthesis of nanomaterials. In recent years, their amazing properties have made nanoparticles important in many fields such as health care, agriculture, energy and environment.

REFERENCES

1. Capek, I. (2006) "Chapter 1 Nanotechnology and nanomaterials", *Nanocomposite Structures and Dispersions*, Elsevier, Netherlands, (Vol. 23), pp. 1–69. https://doi.org/10.1016/S1383-7303(06)80002-5.
2. Cheng, X. (2014) "10 - Nanostructures: Fabrication and applications", In Feldman, M. (ed.), *Nanolithography: The Art of Fabricating Nanoelectronic and Nanophotonic Devices and Systems*, Woodhead Publishing, pp. 348–375. https://doi.org/10.1533/9780857098757.348.
3. Mourdikoudis, S., Pallares, R.M. and Thanh, N.T.K. (2018) "Characterization techniques for nanoparticles: Comparison and complementarity upon studying nanoparticle properties", *Nanoscale*, 10(27), pp. 12871–12934. https://doi.org/10.1039/C8NR02278J.
4. Sudak, N.L. and Harvie, J. (2018) "Chapter 108 - Integrative strategies for planetary health", In Rakel, D. (ed.), *Integrative Medicine (Fourth Edition)*, Elsevier, Netherlands, pp. 1016–1026. https://doi.org/10.1016/B978-0-323-35868-2.00108-0.
5. García, M.C. and Uberman, P.M. (2019) "Chapter 2 - Nanohybrid filler-based drug-delivery system", In Mohapatra, S.S., Ranjan, S., Dasgupta, N., Mishra, R. K., and Thomas, S. (eds.), *Micro and Nano Technologies*, Elsevier, Netherlands, pp. 43–79. https://doi.org/10.1016/B978-0-12-814033-8.00002-3.
6. Wang, H., Liang, X., Wang, J., Jiao, S. and Xue, D. (2020) "Multifunctional Inorganic Nanomaterials for Energy Applications", *Nanoscale*, 12(1), pp. 14–42. https://doi.org/10.1039/C9NR07008G.

7. Ghitman, J., Biru, E. I., Stan, R. and Iovu, H. (2020) "Review of hybrid PLGA nanoparticles: Future of smart drug delivery and theranostics medicine", *Materials & Design*, 193, pp. 108805. https://doi.org/10.1016/j.matdes.2020.108805.
8. Nguyen, K. T. and Zhao, Y. (2015) "Engineered hybrid nanoparticles for on-demand diagnostics and therapeutics", *Accounts of Chemical Research*, 48(12), pp. 3016–3025. https://doi.org/10.1021/acs.accounts.5b00316.
9. Giese, B., Klaessig, F., Park, B., Kaegi, R., Steinfeldt, M., Wigger, H., ... Gottschalk, F. (2018) "Risks, release and concentrations of engineered nanomaterial in the environment", *Scientific Reports*, 8(1), p. 1565. https://doi.org/10.1038/s41598-018-19275-4.
10. Kumar, P., Dehiya, B.S. and Sindhu, A. (2018) "Bioceramics for hard tissue engineering applications: A review", *International Journal of Applied Engineering Research*, 13(5), pp. 2744–2752. https://doi.org/10.3844/ajbbsp.2006.49.56.
11. Kumar, P. and Sindhu, A. (2018) "Materials for tissue engineering", In *Advances in Animal Biotechnology and its Applications*, Springer, Singapore, pp. 357–370.
12. Jeyaraj, M., Gurunathan, S., Qasim, M., Kang, M.-H. and Kim, J.-H. (2019) "A comprehensive review on the synthesis, characterization, and biomedical application of platinum nanoparticles", *Nanomaterials*, 9(12), p. 1719. https://doi.org/10.3390/nano9121719.
13. Navya, P.N. and Daima, H.K. (2016) "Rational engineering of physicochemical properties of nanomaterials for biomedical applications with nanotoxicological perspectives", *Nano Convergence*, *3*(1), pp. 1. https://doi.org/10.1186/s40580-016-0064-z.
14. Saallah, S. and Lenggoro, I.W. (2018) "Nanoparticles carrying biological molecules: Recent advances and applications." *KONA Powder and Particle Journal*, 35, pp. 89–111. https://doi.org/10.14356/kona.2018015.
15. Kolahalam, L.A., Kasi Viswanath, I.V., Diwakar, B.S., Govindh, B., Reddy, V. and Murthy, Y.L.N. (2019) "Review on nanomaterials: Synthesis and applications", *Materials Today: Proceedings*, 18, pp. 2182–2190. https://doi.org/10.1016/j.matpr.2019.07.371.
16. Gatoo, M., Naseem, S., Arfat, M., Dar, A., Qasim, K. and Zubair, S. (2014) "Physicochemical properties of nanomaterials: Implication in associated toxic manifestations", *BioMed Research International*, 2014, p. 498420. https://doi.org/10.1155/2014/498420.
17. Asmatulu, R., Nguyen, P. and Asmatulu, E. (2013) "Chapter 5 - Nanotechnology safety in the automotive industry", In Asmatulu, R. (ed.), *Nanotechnology Safety*, Elsevier, Amsterdam, pp. 57–72. https://doi.org/10.1016/B978-0-444-59438-9.00005-9.
18. Ganachari, D.S., Banapurmath, N., Salimath, B., Yaradoddi, J., Shettar, A.S., Hunashyal, A.M., ... Hiremath, G. (2019) "Synthesis techniques for preparation of nanomaterials", In *Handbook of Ecomaterials*, Springer, Cham, pp. 83–103. https://doi.org/10.1007/978-3-319-68255-6_149.
19. Khan, I., Saeed, K. and Khan, I. (2019) "Nanoparticles: Properties, applications and toxicities", *Arabian Journal of Chemistry*, 12(7), pp. 908–931. https://doi.org/https://doi.org/10.1016/j.arabjc.2017.05.011.
20. Sakka, S. (2016) "History of the sol–gel chemistry and technology BT", Handbook of Sol-Gel Science and Technology. Klein, L., Aparicio, M. and Jitianu, A., (eds.), Springer, Cham. https://doi.org/10.1007/978-3-319-19454-7_87-1.
21. Danks, A., Hall, S. and Schnepp, Z. (2015) "The evolution of "sol-gel" chemistry as a technique for materials synthesis", *Materials Horizons*, 3, pp. 91-112. https://doi.org/10.1039/C5MH00260E.
22. Bisson, A., Rigacci, A., Lecomte, D., Rodier, E. and Achard, P. (2003) "Drying of silica gels to obtain aerogels: Phenomenology and basic techniques", *Drying Technology*, 21(4), pp. 593–628. https://doi.org/10.1081/DRT-120019055.

23. Montes, D., Henao, J., Taborda, E.A., Gallego, J., Cortés, F.B. and Franco, C.A. (2020) "Effect of textural properties and surface chemical nature of silica nanoparticles from different silicon sources on the viscosity reduction of heavy crude oil", *ACS Omega*, 5(10), pp. 5085–5097. https://doi.org/10.1021/acsomega.9b04041.
24. Thiagarajan, S. Sanmugam, A. and Vikram, D. (2017) *Facile Methodology of Sol-Gel Synthesis for Metal Oxide Nanostructures*, In Chandra U. (ed.), IntechOpen, London. https://doi.org/10.5772/intechopen.68708.
25. Ahlawat, D., Kumari, R., Ahlawat, R. and Yadav, I. (2014) "Synthesis and Characterization of Sol–Gel Prepared Silver Nanoparticles", *International Journal of Nanoscience*, 13, p. 1450004. https://doi.org/10.1142/S0219581X14500045.
26. Hema, M., Arasi, A. Y., Selvi, T. and Anbarasan, R. (2012) "Titania Nanoparticles Synthesized by Sol-Gel Technique", *Chemical Science Transactions*, 2, pp. 239–245. https://doi.org/10.7598/cst2013.344.
27. Kumar, P., Dehiya, B. S. and Sindhu, A. (2019) "Ibuprofen-loaded CTS/nHA/nBG scaffolds for the applications of hard tissue engineering", *Iranian Biomedical Journal*, 23(3), pp. 190–199. https://doi.org/10.29252/.23.3.190.
28. Kumar, P., Dehiya, B. S. and Sindhu, A. (2019) "Synthesis and characterization of nHA-PEG and nBG-PEG scaffolds for hard tissue engineering applications", *Ceramics International*, 45(7), pp. 8370–8379. https://doi.org/10.1016/j.ceramint.2019.01.145.
29. Kumar, P., Saini, M., Dehiya, B. S., Umar, A., Sindhu, A., Mohammed, H., ... Guo, Z. (2020) "Fabrication and in-vitro biocompatibility of freeze-dried CTS-nHA and CTS-nBG scaffolds for bone regeneration applications", *International Journal of Biological Macromolecules*, 149, pp. 1–10. https://doi.org/10.1016/j.ijbiomac.2020.01.035.
30. Khan, M. F., Ansari, A. H., Hameedullah, M., Ahmad, E., Husain, F. M., Zia, Q., ... Aliev, G. (2016) "Sol-gel synthesis of thorn-like ZnO nanoparticles endorsing mechanical stirring effect and their antimicrobial activities: Potential role as nano-antibiotics", *Scientific Reports*, 6, p. 27689. https://doi.org/10.1038/srep27689.
31. Tyagi, B., Sidhpuria, K., Shaik, B. and Jasra, R.V. (2006) "Synthesis of nanocrystalline zirconia using sol–gel and precipitation techniques", *Industrial & Engineering Chemistry Research*, 45(25), pp. 8643–8650. https://doi.org/10.1021/ie060519p.
32. Dixit, C.K., Bhakta, S., Kumar, A., Suib, S.L. and Rusling, J.F. (2016) "Fast nucleation for silica nanoparticle synthesis using a sol–gel method", *Nanoscale*, 8(47), pp. 19662–19667. https://doi.org/10.1039/C6NR07568A.
33. Gu, F., Wang, S.F., Lü, M.K., Zhou, G. J., Xu, D. and Yuan, D.R. (2004) "Photoluminescence Properties of SnO_2 Nanoparticles Synthesized by Sol–Gel Method", *The Journal of Physical Chemistry B*, 108(24), pp. 8119–8123. https://doi.org/10.1021/jp036741e.
34. Zhang, Y., Li, R., Jiang, Y., Zhao, B., Duan, H., Li, J. and Feng, Z. (2011) "Morphology evolution of ZrB2 nanoparticles synthesized by sol–gel method", *Journal of Solid State Chemistry*, 184(8), pp. 2047–2052. https://doi.org/10.1016/j.jssc.2011.05.040.
35. Chand, P., Gaur, A. and Kumar, A. (2011) "Study of CuO nanoparticles synthesized by sol-gel method", *AIP Conference Proceedings*, 1393(1), pp. 211–212. https://doi.org/10.1063/1.3653684.
36. Guglielmi, M. and Martucci, A. (2016) *Sol–Gel Nanocomposites BT - Handbook of Sol-Gel Science and Technology*. Klein, L., Aparicio M., and Jitianu A., (eds.). Springer-Verlag, New York. https://doi.org/10.1007/978-3-319-19454-7_100-1.
37. Gan, Y. X., Jayatissa, A. H., Yu, Z., Chen, X. and Li, M. (2020) "Hydrothermal Synthesis of Nanomaterials", *Journal of Nanomaterials*, 2020, pp. 8917013. https://doi.org/10.1155/2020/8917013.
38. Tan, C., Liu, Z., Yonezawa, Y., Sukenaga, S., Ando, M., Shibata, H., ... Wakihara, T. (2020) "Unique crystallization behavior in zeolite synthesis under external high

pressures", *Chemical Communications*, 56(18), pp. 2811–2814. https://doi.org/10.1039/C9CC09966B.

39. Shimura, F. (2017) *Single-Crystal Silicon: Growth and Properties BT - Springer Handbook of Electronic and Photonic Materials*. S. Kasap and P. Capper, (eds.), Springer, Cham. https://doi.org/10.1007/978-3-319-48933-9_13.
40. Ledoux, G., Joubert, M. F. and Mishra, S. (2016) "3 - Upconversion phenomena in nanofluorides", Photonic and Electronic Properties of Fluoride Materials. Tressaud, A. and Poeppelmeier, K.R., (eds.). Elsevier, Amsterdam. https://doi.org/10.1016/B978-0-12-801639-8.00003-9.
41. Huang, G., Lu, C.-H. and Yang, H.-H. (2019) "Chapter 3 - Magnetic Nanomaterials For Magnetic Bioanalysis", *Environmental and Energy Applications, Micro and Nano Technologies*. Wang, X. and Chen, B. (eds.), Elsevier, Netherlands, pp. 89–109. https://doi.org/10.1016/B978-0-12-814497-8.00003-5.
42. Hayashi, H. and Hakuta, Y. (2010) "Hydrothermal Synthesis of Metal Oxide Nanoparticles in Supercritical Water", *Materials (Basel, Switzerland)*, 3(7), pp. 3794–3817. https://doi.org/10.3390/ma3073794
43. Denkbaş, E. B., Çelik, E., Erdal, E., Kavaz, D., Akbal, Ö., Kara, G. and Bayram, C. (2016) "*Chapter 9 - Magnetically based nanocarriers in drug delivery*", Grumezescu, A.M. (ed.). Elsevier, Netherlands, pp. 285-331. https://doi.org/10.1016/B978-0-323-42866-8.00009-5.
44. Shandilya, M., Rai, R. and Singh, J. (2016) "Review: hydrothermal technology for smart materials", *Advances in Applied Ceramics*, 115(6), pp. 354–376. https://doi.org/10.1080/17436753.2016.1157131.
45. Baruwati, B., Kumar, D. K. and Manorama, S. V. (2006) "Hydrothermal synthesis of highly crystalline ZnO nanoparticles: A competitive sensor for LPG and EtOH", *Sensors and Actuators B: Chemical*, 119(2), pp. 676–682. https://doi.org/10.1016/j.snb.2006.01.028.
46. Nair, M. G., Nirmala, M., Rekha, K. and Anukaliani, A. (2011) "Structural, optical, photo catalytic and antibacterial activity of ZnO and Co doped ZnO nanoparticles", *Materials Letters*, 65(12), pp. 1797–1800. https://doi.org/10.1016/j.matlet.2011.03.079.
47. Arshad, M., Azam, A., Ahmed, A. S., Mollah, S. and Naqvi, A. H. (2011) "Effect of Co substitution on the structural and optical properties of ZnO nanoparticles synthesized by sol–gel route", *Journal of Alloys and Compounds*, 509(33), pp. 8378–8381. https://doi.org/10.1016/j.jallcom.2011.05.047.
48. Ezema, C. G., Nwanya, A. C., Ezema, B. E., Maaza, M., Ukoha, P. O. and Ezema, F. I. (2017) "Hydrothermal synthesis of brookite TiO_2 nanoparticles for dye-sensitized solar cell", *Journal of Solid State Electrochemistry*, 21(9), pp. 2655–2663. https://doi.org/10.1007/s10008-017-3652-x.
49. Ge, S., Shi, X., Sun, K., Li, C., Uher, C., Baker, J. R., … Orr, B. G. (2009) "Facile hydrothermal synthesis of iron oxide nanoparticles with tunable magnetic properties", *The Journal of Physical Chemistry C*, 113(31), pp. 13593–13599. https://doi.org/10.1021/jp902953t.
50. Suthakaran, S., Dhanapandian, S., Krishnakumar, N. and Ponpandian, N. (2019) "Hydrothermal synthesis of SnO2 nanoparticles and its photocatalytic degradation of methyl violet and electrochemical performance", *Materials Research Express*, 6(8), p. 0850i3. https://doi.org/10.1088/2053-1591/ab29c2.
51. Cao, S., Peng, L., Han, T., Liu, B., Zhu, D., Zhao, C., … He, S. (2020) "Hydrothermal synthesis of nanoparticles-assembled NiO microspheres and their sensing properties", *Physica E: Low-Dimensional Systems and Nanostructures*, 118, p. 113655. https://doi.org/10.1016/j.physe.2019.113655.

52. Qiu, G., Huang, H., Dharmarathna, S., Benbow, E., Stafford, L. and Suib, S. L. (2011) “Hydrothermal synthesis of manganese oxide nanomaterials and their catalytic and electrochemical properties”, *Chemistry of Materials*, 23(17), pp. 3892–3901. https://doi.org/10.1021/cm2011692.
53. Behbahani, A., Rowshanzamir, S. and Esmaeilifar, A. (2012) “Hydrothermal synthesis of zirconia nanoparticles from commercial zirconia”, *Procedia Engineering*, 42, pp. 908–917. https://doi.org/10.1016/j.proeng.2012.07.483.
54. Maletić, M., Vukčević, M., Kalijadis, A., Janković-Častvan, I., Dapčević, A., Laušević, Z. and Laušević, M. (2019) “Hydrothermal synthesis of TiO_2/carbon composites and their application for removal of organic pollutants”, *Arabian Journal of Chemistry*, 12(8), pp. 4388–4397. https://doi.org/10.1016/j.arabjc.2016.06.020.
55. Zhong, W. (2016) “3 - Nanofibres for medical textiles", *Advances in Smart Medical Textiles: Treatments and Health Monitoring*. van Langenhove, L. (ed.), Elsevier, Netherlands, pp. 57–70. https://doi.org/10.1016/B978-1-78242-379-9.00003-7.
56. Bhardwaj, N. and Kundu, S. C. (2010) “Electrospinning: A fascinating fiber fabrication technique”, *Biotechnology Advances*, 28(3), pp. 325–347. https://doi.org/10.1016/j.biotechadv.2010.01.004.
57. Liang, D., Hsiao, B. S. and Chu, B. (2007) “Functional electrospun nanofibrous scaffolds for biomedical applications”, *Advanced Drug Delivery Reviews*, 59(14), pp. 1392–1412. https://doi.org/10.1016/j.addr.2007.04.021.
58. Selatile, M. K., Ray, S. S., Ojijo, V. and Sadiku, R. (2018) “Recent developments in polymeric electrospun nanofibrous membranes for seawater desalination”, *RSC Advances*, 8(66), pp. 37915–37938. https://doi.org/10.1039/C8RA07489E.
59. Zhou, F., Gong, R. and Porat, I. (2010) “Needle and needleless electrospinning for nanofibers”, *Journal of Applied Polymer Science*, 115, pp. 2591–2598. https://doi.org/10.1002/app.31282.
60. Zabar, N. and Al-Hazeem, A. (2018) *Nanofibers and Electrospinning Method*, IntechOpen, London. https://doi.org/10.5772/intechopen.72060.
61. Seekaew, Y., Arayawut, O., Timsorn, K. and Wongchoosuk, C. (2019) “Chapter Nine - Synthesis, characterization, and applications of graphene and derivatives”, *Carbon-Based Nanofillers and Their Rubber Nanocomposites*. Yaragalla, S., Mishra, R., Thomas, S., and Kalarikkal, N.(eds.), Elsevier, Netherlands, pp. 259-283. https://doi.org/10.1016/B978-0-12-813248-7.00009-2.
62. Bilecka, I. and Niederberger, M. (2010) “Microwave chemistry for inorganic nanomaterials synthesis”, *Nanoscale*, 2(8), pp. 1358–1374. https://doi.org/10.1039/B9NR00377K
63. Sunkari, S., Gangapuram, B. R., Dadigala, R., Bandi, R., Alle, M. and Guttena, V. (2017) “Microwave-irradiated green synthesis of gold nanoparticles for catalytic and anti-bacterial activity”, *Journal of Analytical Science and Technology*, 8(1), p. 13. https://doi.org/10.1186/s40543-017-0121-1.
64. Sreeju, N., Rufus, A. and Philip, D. (2016) “Microwave-assisted rapid synthesis of copper nanoparticles with exceptional stability and their multifaceted applications”, *Journal of Molecular Liquids*, 221, pp. 1008–1021. https://doi.org/10.1016/j.molliq.2016.06.080.
65. Hasanpoor, M., Aliofkhazraei, M. and Delavari, H. (2015) “Microwave-assisted synthesis of zinc oxide nanoparticles”, *Procedia Materials Science*, 11, pp. 320–325. https://doi.org/10.1016/j.mspro.2015.11.101.
66. Hassan, H., Abdelsayed, V., Khder, A. el R., Abouzeid, K., Terner, J., El-Shall, M. S., … El-Azhary, A. (2009) “Microwave Synthesis of graphene sheets supporting metal nanocrystals in aqueous and organic media”, *Journal of Materials Chemistry*, 19, pp. 3832-3837. https://doi.org/10.1039/b906253j.

67. Seku, K., Gangapuram, B. R., Pejjai, B., Kadimpati, K. K. and Golla, N. (2018) "Microwave-assisted synthesis of silver nanoparticles and their application in catalytic, antibacterial and antioxidant activities", *Journal of Nanostructure in Chemistry*, 8(2), pp. 179–188. https://doi.org/10.1007/s40097-018-0264-7.
68. Ung, T. D. T., Tran, T. K. C., Pham, T. N., Nguyen, D. N., Dinh, D. K. and Nguyen, Q. L. (2012) "CdTe and CdSe quantum dots: synthesis, characterizations and applications in agriculture", *Advances in Natural Sciences: Nanoscience and Nanotechnology*, 3(4), p. 43001. https://doi.org/10.1088/2043-6262/3/4/043001.
69. Melichar, L., Jarosova, M., Kopel, P., Adam, V. and Kizek, R. (2013) "Synthesis of quantum dots by microwave irradiation." In *NANOCON 2013 - Conference Proceedings, 5th International Conference*.
70. Ding, L., Peng, Z., Shen, W., Liu, T., Cheng, Z., Gauthier, M. and Liang, F. (2016) "Microwave synthesis of CdTe/TGA quantum dots and their thermodynamic interaction with bovine serum albumin", *Journal of Wuhan University of Technology-Mater. Sci. Ed.*, 31(6), pp. 1408–1414. https://doi.org/10.1007/s11595-016-1546-x.
71. Gour, A. and Jain, N. K. (2019) "Advances in green synthesis of nanoparticles", *Artificial Cells, Nanomedicine and Biotechnology*, 47(1), pp. 844–851. https://doi.org/10.1080/21691401.2019.1577878.
72. Vijaya Kumar, P., Mary Jelastin Kala, S. and Prakash, K.S. (2019) "Green synthesis of gold nanoparticles using Croton Caudatus Geisel leaf extract and their biological studies", *Materials Letters*, 236, pp. 19–22. https://doi.org/10.1016/j.matlet.2018.10.025.
73. Ahmed, S., Saifullah, Ahmad, M., Swami, B. L. and Ikram, S. (2016) "Green synthesis of silver nanoparticles using Azadirachta indica aqueous leaf extract", *Journal of Radiation Research and Applied Sciences*, 9(1), pp. 1–7. https://doi.org/10.1016/j.jrras.2015.06.006.
74. Naika, H. R., Lingaraju, K., Manjunath, K., Kumar, D., Nagaraju, G., Suresh, D. and Nagabhushana, H. (2015) "Green synthesis of CuO nanoparticles using Gloriosa superba L. extract and their antibacterial activity", *Journal of Taibah University for Science*, 9(1), pp. 7–12. https://doi.org/10.1016/j.jtusci.2014.04.006.
75. Hasan, S. and Ghosh, T. (2011) "Synthesis of uranium oxide nanoparticles in aqueous solutions", *Nuclear Technology*, 173, pp. 310–317. https://doi.org/10.13182/NT11-A11664.
76. Bibi, I., Nazar, N., Ata, S., Sultan, M., Ali, A., Abbas, A., … Iqbal, M. (2019) "Green synthesis of iron oxide nanoparticles using pomegranate seeds extract and photocatalytic activity evaluation for the degradation of textile dye", *Journal of Materials Research and Technology*, 8(6), pp. 6115–6124. https://doi.org/10.1016/j.jmrt.2019.10.006.
77. Thakur, B. K., Kumar, A. and Kumar, D. (2019) "Green synthesis of titanium dioxide nanoparticles using Azadirachta indica leaf extract and evaluation of their antibacterial activity", *South African Journal of Botany*, 124, pp. 223–227. https://doi.org/10.1016/j.sajb.2019.05.024.
78. Agarwal, H., Venkat Kumar, S. and Rajeshkumar, S. (2017) "A review on green synthesis of zinc oxide nanoparticles – An eco-friendly approach", *Resource-Efficient Technologies*, 3(4), pp. 406–413. https://doi.org/10.1016/j.reffit.2017.03.002.

Index